HIV and Gay Men

"There have been books on HIV histories and clinical virology; on pathophysiology of HIV disease; on gay men, too, but here, in one volume, key aspects of HIV and gay men: clinical, social and psychological perspectives are brought together, under one cover. Jaspal and Bayley have produced a truly contemporary text. This is a 'must' for contemporary practitioners; those of us old enough to remember the early days, to see how they have improved, and those young enough to know little about it. I will certainly commend this text to my students".

—Professor David Evans, OBE, NTF, *Professor in Sexualities and Genders: Health & Well-Being, University of Greenwich*

"It's 2020 and a new virus is sweeping round the globe for which there is no cure and no vaccine. Go back forty years and the world was grappling with another virus, a virus for which there is still no outright cure and no vaccine. However, this virus, HIV and the illness it causes, AIDS, can be successfully managed and are no longer life-threatening. We might even reach a time, in about ten years, when the virus is eradicated. Despite great advances in understanding how the virus works and how people deal with it, this can only happen if we no longer separate clinical research and social psychological work. This book does just that. Written by a social psychologist and a clinician, it explores in detail, and using examples from lived experience, how one particularly affected group of people, gay men, cope with and negotiate living with HIV/AIDS in sometimes very different contexts. This book is essential reading for clinical practitioners trying to gain insights into what makes people think, feel and behave in certain ways—a precondition for the success of any medical innovation and intervention—, for people living with HIV/AIDS trying to live as normal a life as possible, and, of course, for anybody interested in the social psychological study of health and illness".

—Professor Brigitte Nerlich, *Emeritus Professor of Language, Science and Society, University of Nottingham*

"Could HIV be eliminated by 2030? This cannot be done by medication alone, as this book shows clearly. Beliefs, behaviours and feelings need to change, and this book shows why, and how such changes might be made. This important collaboration between medicine and social psychology is needed to save lives from this mystifying and terrifying infection".

—Professor Kate Loewenthal, *Emeritus Professor of Clinical Psychology, Royal Holloway, University of London*

"The field of HIV and AIDS has seen enormous changes in the past few years, in virology and pharmacology, in treatment and prevention options and in terms of the meaning of the issues in the lives of the people most closely involved. This volume deserves to become a classic in the field, offering a contemporary glimpse into the lives of those who have been touched by HIV. Moreover it offers a thoroughgoing overview of clinical and psychosocial aspects of HIV medicine, so has something to offer the student, the academic, the clinician and the curious layperson."

—Professor Brian Brown, *Professor of Health Communication,
De Montfort University, Leicester, UK*

"The goal of ending HIV transmission in the UK by 2030 is a challenging one, but well within our reach. *HIV and Gay Men* sets out the clinical, social and psychological context and addresses the challenges in achieving this in a way that should inform researchers, policymakers, clinicians and activists alike."

—Dr Michael Brady, *National Advisor for LGBT Health, NHS England; Consultant
Physician in Sexual Health and HIV, Kings College Hospital, London;
Medical Director, Terrence Higgins Trust*

"This book—a collaboration by two leading experts on the impact of HIV amongst gay men—is an important contribution to understanding the history, evolution and current position of the HIV epidemic amongst gay men in the UK.
It takes you on a journey—from the early days of the epidemic in the UK and the death of Terry Higgins to a robust and thoughtful insight into HIV prevention, diagnosis, management and prognosis. The journey continues by highlighting the significant mental health impact of HIV amongst gay men and how important it is to ensure that services are accessible to meet these needs.
The journey ends but raising the tantalising prospect of the elimination of new HIV transmissions in the UK by 2030, highlighting some key actions that need to be taken to achieve this ambitious goal.
As a gay man living with HIV I want to thank Rusi and Jake for the care that they have taken in writing this important book—it's a must read."

—Ian Green, *Chief Executive, Terrence Higgins Trust*

"This book is invaluable for everyone working with gay men either with an HIV diagnosis or who might be at risk of one. Its multidisciplinary focus and consideration of the history and context of HIV is its strength, and several important perspectives are incorporated emphatically into one volume. Reading this book will enable the practitioner to understand HIV in depth from a variety of necessary contexts and—crucially—it highlights essential issues to consider in clinical practice."

—Dr Claire Bloxsom, *UKCP Registered Integrative Psychotherapist. Senior Lecturer in
Psychology, Counselling, and Psychological Therapies, Nottingham Trent University*

"This book can serve scholars and professionals being introduced to both clinical and social psychological dimensions of HIV, its history and its future. This reference book is very original and unique in its kind: it reviews the evidence and proposes recommendations. The clinical cases presented throughout this volume are provided for the benefit of people working with HIV in gay men".

—Dr Ismaël Maatouk, *Clemenceau Medical Center affiliated with Johns Hopkins
International, Beirut, Lebanon*

Rusi Jaspal • Jake Bayley

HIV and Gay Men

Clinical, Social and Psychological Aspects

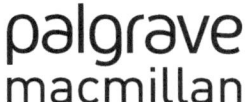

Rusi Jaspal
School of Social Sciences
Nottingham Trent University
Nottingham, UK

Jake Bayley
Barts Health NHS Trust
London, UK

ISBN 978-981-15-7225-8 ISBN 978-981-15-7226-5 (eBook)
https://doi.org/10.1007/978-981-15-7226-5

Cover illustration: © Joe Cummins / @JOE.DRAWS.THINGS

This Palgrave Macmillan imprint is published by the registered company Springer Nature Singapore Pte Ltd.
The registered company address is: 152 Beach Road, #21-01/04 Gateway East, Singapore 189721, Singapore

This book is dedicated to Dr Mags Portman, 1974–2019

Acknowledgements

It has felt very rewarding to write this book. Jake and I did so because we believed that academic psychology and clinical medicine needed to be brought together in order to effect positive change in clinical practice, to show how academic psychology could make a 'real-world' difference and, most importantly, to create a resource that might ultimately be used to enhance the lives of patients. I wish to express my gratitude to my many students over the years for encouraging me to write this book. In our classes, meetings and supervisions, they often lamented the absence of a comprehensive text on the clinical and social psychological aspects of HIV among gay men. I believe that this book provides just that. I am especially grateful to my PhD students for our intellectually stimulating conversations about the psychological aspects of HIV. Last but by no means least, I thank my beloved family—Ramesh, Asha, Jaya and Babak—for their support during the writing of this and other books.

RJ

I have very much enjoyed writing this book—especially the history of HIV, with a lot of help from Rusi. Our distinct specialties are a great combination as many patients I see in clinic can have psychological issues that the clinician needs to be aware of. This is especially important at a time when treatment options have allowed most patients to become undetectable with very few side effects. This book is dedicated to all of the patients I have had the good fortune to meet in my career. I continue to learn and grow from your stories and tales of bravery on a daily basis. I would also like to mention Dr Mags Portman, who sadly died well before her time and was a dear colleague and friend. She did more for the advancement of pre-exposure prophylaxis (PrEP) in the gay community in her short time than most people could hope to achieve in a life time. She is, and always will be, sadly missed. I would also like to say a special thank you to Joe Cummings (@joe.draws.things) for providing the art on the cover of the book—your generosity, like your art, is always first rate. I would also like to thank my family—Sid, Sue, John, Chas and Dan— for their unwavering support and ability to make me see the bright side in all occasions.

JB

Contents

List of Figures

1

Understanding the Clinical and Social Psychological Aspects of HIV

Introduction

Where there is life, there are viruses. Viruses have probably existed since the beginning of humankind. Many have come and gone and returned—influenza, smallpox and COVID-19 are just three of many millions of viruses on the planet. Human immunodeficiency virus (HIV) is undoubtedly one of the most unique, complex and deadly viruses that humankind has known. In the relatively short period in which it has existed, HIV has infected 74.9 million and killed 32 million people around the world. Moreover, HIV has brought about the stigma, isolation and ostracisation of those it has infected and affected. The short history of HIV has been characterised by hope and despair, as the condition has transformed from being life-limiting to life-changing. It has forced society and political institutions to confront pressing polemical issues, such as sexuality, morality and human rights, in novel ways. It is a condition that generates fear in some and indifference in others. HIV is changing both medically and socially—as more effective treatments emerge, societal perceptions of the condition are shifting. In the era of ever-improving

© The Author(s) 2020
R. Jaspal, J. Bayley, *HIV and Gay Men*, https://doi.org/10.1007/978-981-15-7226-5_1

antiretroviral therapy (ART), the ways in which individuals think about, and behave in relation to, HIV are similarly in flux.

Though a *human* immunodeficiency virus, some groups in society have been disproportionately affected by HIV. Acquired Immune Deficiency Syndrome (AIDS), which is late-stage HIV, was first observed in gay men who remain one of the most affected groups in Western, industrialised countries. Epidemics were later observed in intravenous drug users, heterosexual Haitians and sex workers, and HIV affects up to 25% of (mainly heterosexual) adult populations in some African countries. Yet, the association of HIV with gay men, in particular, is entrenched in societal thinking. HIV affects so many groups in society and, on both clinical and psychosocial levels, it affects these groups differently.

Today many people continue to die of AIDS when the communities in which they are embedded refuse to acknowledge HIV, stigmatise it and prohibit any discussion about the condition. In these communities, there is often very limited access to social or clinical support. The burden of HIV falls most heavily on the most marginalised groups in society, highlighting the usual fault lines of socioeconomic inequality. It is imperative to support those who are most affected, as many in these often marginalised communities feel stigmatised, disempowered and isolated. In this book, we highlight some of the remaining barriers to ensuring that all of those affected obtain access to effective clinical and psychological support.

This book focuses on the clinical and social psychological aspects of HIV among gay men. Gay men in Britain constitute a heterogeneous community—in terms of ethnicity, religion, social class and many other factors—with a rich history. Gay men have been around for a long time indeed, even though their presence has not always been explicitly acknowledged. They have faced, and continue to face, social, political and psychological ups and downs. Before delving into some of these challenges, it is advantageous to provide some definitions at the outset. After all, HIV, gay men, social psychology and clinical medicine have all been written about from distinct disciplinary, theoretical and epistemological perspectives. We must ensure a common understanding of these issues, which are discussed in the rest of this volume.

Some Definitions

HIV Risk or HIV Outcomes?

In this book, we focus both on HIV risk and on the experience of living with HIV, including clinical outcomes among those living with the condition. The principal aim is to understand the factors that can increase gay men's risk of HIV so that suitable interventions may be developed in order to mitigate these risk factors, that is, to *reduce* the incidence of HIV in this key population. Moreover, a key objective of this volume is to discuss the feasibility of Britain's target to achieve zero HIV infections by 2030.

Yet, we acknowledge that much existing research, theory and practice have focused on the prevention of HIV and sometimes neglected the identities, lives and wellbeing of people living with diagnosed HIV. It is important to examine the lives of people living with HIV in order to develop effective strategies and interventions for safeguarding their physical and psychological wellbeing. HIV medicine has advanced significantly to facilitate a good clinical prognosis for most people who are diagnosed early. We describe the ways in which the benefits of HIV medicine can be fully exploited.

It must also be acknowledged that the success of our HIV prevention efforts is dependent partly on the wellbeing of people living with HIV. After all, people living with HIV must first be tested and diagnosed in order for them to initiate ART. They must subsequently engage with HIV clinical care in order to acquire ART. And they must adhere to ART in order for treatment as prevention (TasP) to be a viable HIV prevention strategy (Maatouk & Jaspal, 2020a). Often, the reasons to test, be treated, and to adhere to ART are social psychological in origin.

The Focus on Gay Men

In this volume, we focus on gay men because this heterogeneous group remains disproportionately affected by HIV in Britain and other Western societies (see Chap. 2). This is not to say that other groups in society, such as bisexual men and women, trans women, cisgender women and heterosexual men, should not constitute the focus of HIV research. These too are important research foci. It is hoped that research into these communities will continue. However, these communities are not the focus of the present volume.

What exactly do we mean by 'gay men'? To address this question, it is important to note that there is a difference between sexual orientation and sexual identity. Sexual orientation can be thought of 'as a trait that predisposes an individual to experience sexual attraction to people of the same sex (gay), to people of the opposite sex (heterosexual), or to people of both sexes (bisexual)' (Jaspal, 2019, p. 19), while sexual identity refers to 'the individual's subjective perception, appraisal and categorisation of their sexual orientation' (p. 39). The two categories—sexual orientation and identity—are often aligned in that individuals tend to identify in a way that is consistent with their behaviour, but this is of course not always the case. For instance, a man may have sex exclusively with other men but regard himself as bisexual or even as heterosexual (e.g. Maatouk & Jaspal, 2020b).

A diverse range of categories have been used to describe sexual orientation and sexual identity, such as homosexual, gay, bisexual, heterosexual, straight and others. Many more categories have come into existence, and, undoubtedly, many more will be created to capture the nuances of one's sexual identity. In clinical research, the term 'men who have sex with men' (MSM) tends to be used to focus not on sexual orientation or identity but rather on sexual behaviour. It is accepted that some men who define themselves as heterosexual are mostly heterosexual but occasionally have sex with other men. It is understood that the use of sexual identity categories (e.g. gay, bisexual) with which patients do not identify could lead to disengagement from healthcare services. Therefore, a focus on behaviour, rather than identity, obviates some of the challenging tensions between sexual orientation and identity.

The reality is that a separate volume could be written about the HIV epidemic among each sexual orientation/identity group. The risk factors and care outcomes of heterosexual men are quite different from those of gay men, and those of bisexual men are different still. The lived experiences of men who identify with each of these categories appear to differ.

The level of stigma reported by bisexual men tends to be higher than that reported by gay men, for instance (Shilo & Savaya, 2012). In this volume, we focus principally on gay men, that is, same-sex attracted men who define themselves as gay. In Britain and other Western societies—the geographical focus of this volume—the vast majority of same-sex attracted men do self-identify as gay, have some level of involvement in what can loosely be described as 'the gay community' and exhibit some elements of shared experience. Most of the observations made in this volume are applicable principally to gay-identified men but may also be transferable to other groups of same-sex attracted men who do not identify as gay. When we discuss research into other groups of same-sex attracted men, such as bisexuals and other men who have sex with men, we make this clear.

Clinical and Social Psychological Aspects

In the title of this volume, we refer to clinical and social psychological perspectives. This is rather unusual—most volumes remain cautiously within the confines of one discipline. However, we believe that the clinical and social psychological dimensions of HIV go hand in hand. There will be only limited success in clinical care if we fail to understand the social and psychological worlds of patients, and the full potential of social psychological research into HIV cannot be fully exploited unless applied to real-world clinical contexts. This book aims to bridge these disciplinary perspectives, examining their convergences, divergences and the creative solutions that they can generate when used in conjunction.

Clinically, HIV is now a long-term manageable chronic disease. Exceptionally high levels of mortality and morbidity were the norm before the advent of effective ART, devastating many communities globally. There was an especially profound impact on gay communities in major cities. From a clinical perspective, the development of effective ART has been nothing short of life-saving for those living with HIV. Moreover, evidence showing that virally suppressed patients cannot pass HIV onto their sexual partners has been life-changing for patients (Tan, Lim, & Chan, 2020). The majority of those living with HIV in the

UK are now on effective ART and are at low risk of potentially fatal opportunistic infections and of infecting others.

We must look at the wider picture which involves identifying and resolving a range of psychological sequelae from HIV. This not only includes mood disorders and anxiety (which are disproportionately high in this group), substance use (which is particularly important in the context of 'chemsex' for gay men) including smoking and alcohol, but also the debilitating stigma that can impede access to clinical care and indeed to ART. Therefore, the clinical perspective espoused in this volume focuses on elucidating the social and psychological issues that can inhibit or undermine clinical health, including physical, psychological and social outcomes.

HIV affects people at multiple levels—individually, socially, politically, institutionally and so on. It is both an individual and public health concern. Social psychology is essentially the study of how the individual interacts with the social world—how the individual thinks, feels and behaves is understood to be shaped by society (Jaspal & Breakwell, 2014). Social psychology could be thought of in terms of the meeting-point between sociology (the study of societal structure) and psychology (the study of individual cognition and behaviour). Theories from social psychology enable us to understand, and sometimes to predict, individual thinking, social influence processes, interpersonal relationships and aspects of group behaviour.

As demonstrated repeatedly throughout this volume, these are important foci for the researcher interested in HIV. Social psychologists have a long-standing interest in addressing societal challenges which involve individual cognition. The HIV epidemic is undoubtedly one such challenge, and the ambitious zero-infections target is one that requires a multi-level response. A variety of methods are used in social psychology research to understand the ways in which people think and behave and, crucially, to predict how they will think and behave in particular contexts. Evidently, the ability to understand and to predict HIV risk awareness and behaviour is an important tool in HIV prevention, while the capacity to understand and predict engagement with care and adherence to ART will be vital for enhancing HIV care.

Case Studies

It is useful to begin our discussion of HIV among gay men by describing case studies that exemplify some of the social, psychological and clinical challenges confronted by gay men in the twenty-first century. It is similarly useful to consider how these challenges are in turn associated with HIV, that is, how they might increase one's risk of infection or one's risk of poor HIV outcomes. These case studies are intended to illustrate our rationale for focusing on the clinical and social psychological aspects of HIV among gay men, in particular. The cases are real but the individuals' names have been changed to prevent identification.

Case Study 1: Rob, an HIV-Negative White British Gay Man

Rob is a 23-year-old White British gay man from Sunderland in North-East England. As a child, Rob struggled with his weight and physical appearance and, even though he is clinically underweight, continues to view himself as overweight. He has a diagnosed eating disorder and often eats in secret. Rob has also struggled with anxiety and depression, which improved somewhat when he came out as gay. He no longer felt the need to hide his 'true identity' which provided some psychological relief. His family and most of his friends were accepting of his sexual identity and provided support. Last year, Rob decided to move to London which he thought would be more gay-friendly, but he has found the gay scene overwhelming. He has made some friends and often goes to gay bars and nightclubs but, contrary to expectations, finds it impersonal and devoid of a 'gay community'. In fact, he does not perceive any sense of community at all. His mental health issues have been resurfacing—he is feeling increasingly depressed and anxious, and due to increased social pressure to 'look good', his problems with eating have resurfaced. Rob sometimes uses sex to feel better about himself. He does not always enjoy the sex he has or feel particularly attracted to the men he has sex with, but casual sex gives him a temporary boost. He does not always feel confident about negotiating the type of sex he has or even condom use with his sexual partners. Rob is so focused on how he, and especially his body, is perceived by his sexual partners that condom use becomes secondary or even a non-issue in comparison. Having recently been diagnosed with chlamydia and gonorrhoea, Rob has heard about pre-exposure prophylaxis (PrEP) from the health advisor at his local sexual health clinic. He is thinking about it but in the meantime remains at significant risk of HIV.

Case Study 2: Karim, a British Pakistani Muslim Gay Man Living with HIV

Karim is a 27-year-old British Pakistani Muslim gay man living with HIV. He grew up in a close-knit Pakistani community in West London and was surrounded by his relatives and family friends as he grew up from whom he concealed his sexual orientation. Even as a child, Karim knew that he was attracted to men but did not know how to articulate this attraction to others and felt that it was wrong. He confided in a friend that he was attracted to men and faced a stigmatising response from him. Having lost that friendship, Karim decided never to reveal his sexual orientation to anyone in his own community because he believed that they too would reject him. Recently he has been meeting up with men from Grindr for casual sex but has not formed any strong friendships on the application. He sees himself as different from most other gay men. One of his Grindr acquaintances took him to a gay bar and introduced him to other gay men who appeared to be judgemental towards him because of his Muslim background. Karim anticipates homophobia from his ethnic community and racism on the gay scene. He feels isolated and lonely. Through Grindr, Karim has also started to attend chemsex sessions. Following an unusual illness, Karim was diagnosed with HIV. He did not really understand what this meant for his future but felt ashamed of his diagnosis because of common stereotypes about HIV. He has nobody to speak with or to confide in and is trying to forget all about this diagnosis. Karim continues to meet others for sex on Grindr, to attend chemsex sessions, and has started to drink alcohol and use substances. These activities help him forget about his diagnosis, which he never shares with his sexual partners. At home, he leads another life, attending the local mosque and making plans for an arranged marriage. He believes this might actually help him 'be normal'. Karim has stopped going to his sexual health clinic and is trying to put his HIV diagnosis to the back of his mind. Both his health and that of his sexual partners are at risk.

Prima facie, HIV may not seem a salient theme in these case studies. They invoke many seemingly unrelated issues—body image concerns, eating disorders, self-esteem, homophobia, sense of community, friendship, gay dating applications, identity issues, arranged marriage and others. In the chapters that follow, we argue that these and other social psychological themes are inextricably related to HIV risk and HIV clinical outcomes. Our combined empirical and clinical observations over the years demonstrate unequivocally that, in order for us to understand how to prevent HIV and to treat the condition effectively, we must also acquire a detailed understanding of the lives of gay men. The risk factors are multifarious and are intimately associated with the lived experience of being gay in a heteronormative society.

Rob has long-standing mental health issues, which appear to be associated with the concealment of his sexual orientation during childhood. Rob's preoccupation with his body image relegates HIV prevention to an inferior position in his list of priorities. He is more concerned about what his sexual partners think about his appearance than about his health. Rob is at risk of HIV and may not benefit from the highly effective prevention tools that are available because of this preoccupation. Karim's life-long struggle with the stigma surrounding his sexual orientation is clearly compounded by the stigma of his HIV diagnosis, which he refuses to accept. He is accustomed to denial, concealment and disengagement in relation to his sexual orientation and now replicates the same coping strategies in response to his HIV diagnosis. Though designed to protect psychological wellbeing, these strategies may have serious consequences for Karim's physical health. It is clear that the problems that both Rob and Karim face are deep-rooted—not only in their own experiences but also in the shared experience of many other gay men and in the pervasive societal stigma in relation to homosexuality and HIV. Some insight into the experience of being a gay man in contemporary Britain is useful.

Gay Men in Contemporary Britain

These case studies exemplify just some of the social and psychological challenges that gay men face. Empirical research shows that gay men are more likely than heterosexual men to have experienced sexual abuse, bullying and rejection from significant others in earlier life (Jaspal, 2019). Moreover, adult gay males are more susceptible than heterosexual males to experiencing intimate partner violence, negative body image and relationship problems (Finneran, Chard, Sineath, Sullivan, & Stephenson, 2012; Jaspal, 2019). It is noteworthy that, across the life course, gay men are exposed to heteronormativity and, often, overt homophobia, which in turn can result in the *internalisation* of stigma, that is, its uncritical acceptance in their self-definition. Consequently, many are psychologically motivated to conceal their sexual orientation from others, to feign heterosexuality and, consequently, may lack a sense of identity authenticity. It is easy to see how these 'situational stressors' (situations that can cause psychological stress) and the often ill-fated attempts to protect oneself from them (e.g. concealment) can result in poorer mental health outcomes among gay men—an empirical fact that has been observed in many studies (see Chap. 6).

In order to understand the origins of these situational stressors, psychological self-schemata and mental health outcomes, it is important to consider briefly the history of gay men. Gay men have faced stigma, persecution and criminalisation for many centuries, including capital punishment until the nineteenth century, imprisonment and 'conversion therapies' designed to change their sexual orientation (Cook, Mills, Trumbach, & Cocks, 2007). Their lives have been characterised by significant social, political and psychological change in the last few decades. The decriminalisation of homosexuality in the UK in 1967 paved the way for greater openness in relation to gay sexuality, identity and community. It enabled gay men to abandon fear of prosecution in favour of hope for the future. Gradually, social and institutional attitudes began to improve. For instance, in 1973, homosexuality was removed from American Psychiatric Association's register of mental illnesses. This in turn removed the scientific basis for pathologising attitudes towards homosexuality which constructed homosexuality as a sickness in need of 'cure'.

Britain held its first Pride Festival on 1 July 1972, in order to coincide with the Stonewall Riots in the US—widely believed to be the beginning of modern lesbian, gay, bisexual and transgender (LGBT) activism. This served to increase the visibility of LGBT people and enabled them to replace long-standing feelings of shame with a sense of pride. In the UK, the twenty-first century saw the repeal of Section 28 (which outlawed the 'intentional promotion' of homosexuality in schools but actively served to stifle any acknowledgement or discussion of sexual orientation diversity), the introduction of civil partnerships and then gay marriage, and the Equality Act 2010 protecting people from discrimination on the basis of their sexual orientation and other 'protected characteristics'.

Yet, centuries of oppression, persecution and criminalisation undoubtedly contributed to a sense of distinctiveness, activism and defiance among many gay men in the years that followed decriminalisation. There was a pervasive sense of sexual liberation among gay men who, for centuries before, had lived under repressive social and political conditions. Gay bars and nightclubs began to emerge. Gay saunas and bathhouses were frequented. Gay cruising spots were visited. Gay men used these spaces not only to seek casual sexual encounters but also to celebrate their newfound sexual freedom and to brandish a distinctive sexual identity from that of heterosexual people. Sex with multiple partners replaced the heteronormative ideal of monogamy and, for many, became a marker of gay identity. In many ways, sexualised spaces became central to gay identity, community and sexuality. When these spaces subsequently came under attack during the early phase of the AIDS epidemic, gay men construed the public health advice not to frequent gay saunas, bathhouses and cruising sites as an attack on their identity. Many defiantly refused to relinquish these spaces—emblematic of gay rights—without a fight.

When the first AIDS cases among gay men began to emerge in New York, San Francisco and London and suspicion grew that this was principally a *sexually transmitted infection*, these very spaces were recognised as vectors for HIV infection. Public health specialists hypothesised that, if gay saunas and sex shops were closed down and cruising grounds policed more effectively, they would be able to control the spread of HIV and reduce the number of AIDS cases. Policies such as this required the acknowledgement of gay men, their identities and, most importantly, their sexual behaviour. This was politically difficult for the Conservative government of Margaret Thatcher and the Republican administration of Ronald Reagan in the early 1980s. For several years, their government tiptoed around the issue of HIV, whom it affected and how it was spread, leading to political inertia, defiance and paralysis on all sides. This clearly contributed to the growth of the HIV epidemic and many more infections. (This is covered in more detail in Chap. 2.)

Throughout much of the 1980s, 1990s and early 2000s at least, condom use was vigorously promoted across all relevant social, community and institutional platforms. This was largely successful in creating a coercive social norm concerning condom use among gay men, which served conversely to stigmatise the non-use of condoms as 'reckless' (Shernoff, 2006). Yet, many gay men did not correctly or consistently use condoms and many subsequently became infected with HIV. The norm of condom use was simply rejected by some gay men who expressed a preference for sexual freedom. Some reported a preference to die, literally, rather than give up this freedom. Others were very fearful and expressed relief at their eventual diagnosis with HIV because it at least represented closure and removed the long-standing fear of infection.

As exemplified by the case studies above and in the chapters that follow, several social, psychological and technological factors have conspired to create the 'perfect storm' for increased HIV incidence among gay men in the UK. Since the early days of the epidemic, new factors have emerged. Social norms in the gay community, psychological issues and technological innovation are just some of the contributing variables. The advent of the Internet in the late twentieth century created unprecedented opportunity for gay men to find sexual partners. The subsequent innovation of geospatial mobile gay social networking applications, such as Grindr and Scruff, have enabled gay men to arrange instantaneous sexual encounters with others in their geographical vicinity. The emergence of 'chemsex', drug use in sexualised settings, has created ideal conditions for HIV to spread and thrive.

The history of gay men has been variously characterised by stigma, concealment and freedom. Social, legal and institutional factors have contributed to its vicissitudes. HIV represented a significant setback for gay men, their social development and their physical and psychological wellbeing. There remains an increased risk of infection in gay communities throughout Britain, despite the significant advances in HIV medicine (see Chap. 3). A key tenet of this volume is that the clinical and social psychological aspects of HIV are intimately entwined.

What Is Next for HIV?

The Joint United Nations Programme on HIV/AIDS (UNAIDS) has set ambitious targets in relation to the prevention and management of HIV. By 2020, it hoped to achieve the 90-90-90 target whereby 90% of people living with HIV would be aware of their HIV status, that 90% of those diagnosed would be in receipt of ART and that 90% of them would have a suppressed viral load. By 2030, UNAIDS hopes to achieve a target of 95-95-95, as well as the total elimination of AIDS, the late stage of untreated HIV. This ambition has underpinned the development of the UNAIDS Fast-Track strategy whose central object is the rapid scale-up of both prevention and treatment efforts throughout the world. There has been momentum and optimism behind the 90-90-90 targets, with some countries, such as Britain, having already achieved them. Yet, there are significant challenges in achieving these targets in both developed and developing countries—analyses have revealed a significant impact of social psychological, political and economic barriers (e.g. Levi et al., 2016; Maatouk & Jaspal, 2020a).

The story in Britain inspires confidence. In 2018, 93% of people living with HIV had been diagnosed, 97% of those diagnosed were in receipt of ART and 97% of those receiving ART had an undetectable viral load. Having exceeded the 90-90-90 target, Britain has now set itself an even more ambitious goal. In 2019, Matt Hancock, the Secretary of State for Health and Social Care, reiterated Britain's ambition of zero HIV transmissions by 2030. In the same year, leading HIV charities in the UK, the Terrence Higgins Trust and the National AIDS Trust, created the HIV Commission with UK government support, in order to facilitate evidence-based recommendations for achieving the 2030 target. The HIV Commission is chaired by Dame Inga Beale and is supported by a multi-sectoral and multidisciplinary Advisory Board, responsible for collating evidence in support of the zero-infections target.

In Britain, there is optimism that this ambitious goal can be achieved. There was of course a dramatic decline in HIV incidence at the end of 2016 and, since then, there has been a steady fall in new infections each year, and, among gay, bisexual and other men who have sex with men, there was a 71% decrease in HIV transmissions between 2012 and 2018 (O'Halloran et al., 2020). It is clear that we do now possess the clinical tools to achieve zero new transmissions—condom use, regular HIV testing, PrEP and treatment as prevention are all key components. In combination, they work effectively. However, it has also become clear that clinical and biomedical approaches to HIV prevention alone are unlikely to be successful. After all, gay men must be willing to use condoms, appraise their risk accurately and construe PrEP as personally beneficial. If they test positive for HIV, they must be able to incorporate their positive serostatus into identity, to engage with clinical services and to adhere to ART. Gay men will need to feel empowered to discuss HIV, to share their own HIV status and to negotiate safer sex with their partners. These are all quintessentially social psychological questions with significant clinical implications.

The crucial bridge between clinical medicine and social psychology constitutes the rationale for this volume. We do believe that it is possible to achieve the zero-infections target by 2030. However, we argue that an adequate understanding of the social psychological drivers of particular cognitions, emotions and behaviours among gay men will help us achieve it more quickly and effectively. If we can understand the social psychological 'blackbox' of risk behaviour, we will be better positioned to ensure that our clinical tools can be directed at those at risk of, and living with, HIV appropriately. If we understand the identities, histories and wellbeing of gay men, we might be able to predict who is likely to engage in risk behaviour and under which circumstances this will occur. In some ways, the moment of truth for HIV science has arrived—can we really end HIV transmissions and eliminate AIDS by 2030? We think that this is possible and, in the chapters that follow, explain the preconditions, commitments and actions that will be necessary for this ambitious goal to be achieved.

Why a Multidisciplinary Book on HIV among Gay Men?

HIV is unlike any other virus. It is biologically complex, targeting and hijacking the very cells intended to defend the human body. It is highly stigmatised given its associations with sex, promiscuity and mortality. And it has thrived amid such coercive societal stigma. It is evident that, in order to understand HIV, its impact and its future, a multidisciplinary approach will be necessary. In this volume, we provide such an approach, focusing on both the clinical and social psychological aspects of the disease. More specifically, we show how social and psychological factors, such as stigma and internalised homophobia, may discernibly impact on clinical outcomes, such as HIV infection, ART initiation and virological outcomes. We argue that the effectiveness of clinical innovations in HIV, such as ART and PrEP, can be predicted only if we understand their social psychological dimensions. We believe that it is impossible to eliminate HIV and to reduce its adverse impact on gay men if either the clinical or social psychological dimensions is neglected. This volume is an attempt to integrate these two crucial dimensions of HIV in research, clinical practice and policy debates. We do so by addressing three prime questions:

- What are the major clinical and social psychological challenges associated with HIV risk, prevention and treatment among gay men?
- How can theoretical, empirical and methodological tools from the clinical and social psychological sciences be bridged in order to address some of these challenges?
- What are the next steps for HIV research, theory and practice among gay men?

Every book has a target readership. Ours is a very diverse one. This book is of course intended to benefit academic research into HIV and particularly its clinical and social psychological dimensions. The theoretical innovations, summaries of empirical research and development of future research hypotheses are provided in an attempt to enhance academic debates about HIV. It is hoped that this volume will similarly benefit practitioners involved in the care of those at risk of, or living with, HIV. Academic research is most powerful when it can be used in a way that enhances clinical practice. The 'clinical snapshots' presented throughout this volume are provided principally for the benefit of the HIV clinical practitioner working with gay men. This volume is intended also to demystify HIV for the general reader who will be introduced to both the clinical and social psychological dimensions of HIV, its history and its future. HIV is a condition that concerns us all. Therefore, it is important that we are all informed about it.

Overview of the Book

In Chap. 2, the history, science and epidemiology of HIV are discussed in more detail, and the rationale for focusing on gay men as a key population in the epidemic is provided. Chapter 3 focuses on aspects of gay sexuality and HIV risk in gay men, exploring the biological, social and psychological risk factors for infection in this population. Chapter 4 outlines various methods for preventing HIV infection, including condom use, PrEP, post-exposure prophylaxis (PEP) and behavioural strategies, such as 'serosorting'. Both the clinical effectiveness and social psychological aspects of HIV prevention are examined. In Chap. 5, major developments in HIV diagnosis, management and prognosis are discussed, focusing particularly on HIV testing, the advent of ART and social psychological drivers of ART initiation and adherence. Chapter 6 examines one of the most significant comorbidities of HIV infection in the era of effective ART, namely, poor mental health. The chapter describes a reciprocal relationship between HIV and mental health, outlining both the role of poor mental health in increasing HIV risk and the adverse impact of HIV infection on mental health outcomes. In Chap. 7, the potential impact of complex intersecting identities on HIV is discussed through the case study of sexuality and ethnicity among Black, Asian and Minority Ethnic (BAME) gay men, a group at especially high risk of poor HIV outcomes. The implications for both HIV risk and HIV outcomes are considered. In the final chapter of this volume, we look towards the future of HIV in Britain and return to the three key questions posed in this introductory chapter. The feasibility of achieving the zero-infections target by 2030 in Britain is discussed, and a series of recommendations for researchers, practitioners and policymakers are offered. Theoretical, methodological and disciplinary flexibility characterise the ethos of this volume—we believe that both clinical science and social psychology should be key components of our strategy to end HIV transmissions and to eliminate AIDS by 2030. In the chapters that follow, we discuss how this ought to be done.

References

Cook, M., Mills, R., Trumbach, R., & Cocks, H. G. (2007). *A gay history of Britain: Love and sex between men since the middle ages.* Oxford: Greenwood World Publishing.

Finneran, C., Chard, A., Sineath, C., Sullivan, P., & Stephenson, R. (2012). Intimate partner violence and social pressure among gay men in six countries. *Western Journal of Emergency Medicine, 13*, 260–271.

Jaspal, R. (2019). *The social psychology of gay men.* London: Palgrave Macmillan.

Jaspal, R., & Breakwell, G. M. (Eds.). (2014). *Identity process theory: Identity, social action and social change.* Cambridge: Cambridge University Press.

Levi, J., Raymond, A., Pozniak, A., Vernazza, P., Kohler, P., & Hill, A. (2016). Can the UNAIDS 90-90-90 target be achieved? A systematic analysis of national HIV treatment cascades. *BMJ Global Health, 1*(2), e000010. https://doi.org/10.1136/bmjgh-2015-000010

Maatouk, I., & Jaspal, R. (2020a). Barriers to HIV treatment as prevention (TasP) in men who have sex with men in the Eastern Mediterranean Region. *Journal of Public Health.* https://doi.org/10.1093/pubmed/fdz186

Maatouk, I., & Jaspal, R. (2020b). Religion, male bisexuality and sexual health in Lebanon. In A. K. T. Yip & A. Toft (Eds.), *Bisexuality, spirituality and identity: Critical perspectives* (pp. 137–155). London: Routledge.

O'Halloran, C., Sun, S., Nash, S. Brown, A., Croxford S, Connor, N., … Gill, O. N. (2020). *HIV in the United Kingdom: Towards zero 2030.* London: Public Health England. Retrieved March 20, 2020, from https://assets.publishing.service.gov.uk/government/uploads/system/uploads/attachment_data/file/858559/HIV_in_the_UK_2019_towards_zero_HIV_transmissions_by_2030.pdf

Shernoff, M. (2006). *Without condoms: Unprotected sex, gay men & barebacking.* New York, NY: Routledge.

Shilo, G., & Savaya, R. (2012). Mental health of lesbian, gay, and bisexual youth and young adults: Differential effects of age, gender, religiosity, and sexual orientation. *Journal of Research on Adolescence, 22*(2), 310–325.

Tan, R. K. J., Lim, J. M., & Chan, J. K. W. (2020). "Not a walking piece of meat with disease": Meanings of becoming undetectable among HIV-positive gay, bisexual and other men who have sex with men in the U = U era. *AIDS Care, 32*(3), 325–329.

2

HIV: Its History, Science and Epidemiology

Introduction

The history of HIV/AIDS is a story of human suffering but also one of hope, human perseverance and scientific ingenuity. Many battles have been won, such as the identification of the virus, developing effective treatment and challenging societal prejudice. Another battle, which still rages in many parts of the world, is the reduction of stigma attached to what was thought of as the 'gay plague' by many for decades. HIV is indiscriminate in its ability to infect those of all ages, races, sexualities and nationalities. Unfortunately, as with many other viruses, it starkly reveals the usual fault lines of socio-economic inequality with a disproportionate burden falling on the most marginalised within society. Notable landmarks, such as the discovery of the virus itself and the development of effective ART, have been both life-saving and life-changing for millions who thought the diagnosis bought with it an inevitable death sentence.

© The Author(s) 2020
R. Jaspal, J. Bayley, *HIV and Gay Men*, https://doi.org/10.1007/978-981-15-7226-5_2

The Origins of HIV

Much of our human DNA consists of viruses we have adopted, evolved and integrated into our genome since the first *Homo sapiens* emerged from Central Africa over 200,000 years ago. Indeed, it has been estimated that up to 8% of our genome consists of ancient retroviruses integrated into ours (Belshaw et al., 2004). It appears that we have long been exposed to numerous microbial assaults over the course of our evolution—with varying degrees of successful adaptation. It is quite possible that humans will eventually adapt to HIV, but this specific virus is far too young, ever-changing, virulent and deadly for this to be an acceptable method of controlling it.

Our immunological mechanisms safeguard us against many pathogens, especially those from animal species. These zoonoses are usually unable to take hold in human populations, but occasionally we see the infection cross species—the devastating COVID-19 pandemic is an example of this. Unfortunately, rapidly replicating and evolving viruses, such as HIV, can work quickly to exploit and overcome our protective mechanisms leading to a translocation of the infection from animals to humans, who have little or no innate immunity to fight off these infections. Thus, despite our relatively complex and sophisticated immune system, these pathogens can disable our immunological safeguards leading to the establishment of infection in humans.

An example of this is the circumnavigation of these protective mechanisms; we can use a protein called tetherin (also called CD317) as a demonstration of the many safeguards made ineffective by HIV. Tetherin is a transmembrane protein which 'tethers' newly formed virus to each other and to the cell membrane. HIV has a potent anti-tetherin protein which inactivates this protective mechanism and facilitates efficient viral budding releasing new virus to infect other cells. This circumnavigation of our sophisticated immune system may be one of the many reasons that cross-species infection occurred (Sauter et al., 2009). Research continues to investigate how else HIV is able to evade our sophisticated immune system and establish infections, which will hopefully provide more detailed insight into the functionality of the virus and possible ways to defeat it.

SIV

The origin of the Simian Immunodeficiency Virus (SIV), the precursor of HIV, dates back as far as 30,000 years. SIV is a collection of lentiviruses with a single phylogenetic lineage directly related to HIV. Lentiviruses are defined as viruses that have long, slow periods of incubation ('lente' is Latin for slow) and are known to affect a number of mammals including horses, sheep and cats as well as humans. The fact that they incubate for such long periods without symptoms allows for their propagation and spread within populations. It is believed that some lentiviruses became embedded in the mammal's DNA many millions of years ago—in other words, the virus is incorporated into the host's genome and can then be transmitted to its offspring.

Many lentiviruses affect a number of monkeys, gorillas and chimpanzees living in East and Central Africa, with SIV having been discovered in the late 1980s and early 1990s in chimpanzees (Huet, Cheynier, Meyerhans, Roelants, & Wain-Hobson, 1990) and sooty mangabeys (Hirsch et al., 1989). Most primate species are infected with a single type of SIV. However, it is now accepted that strains of SIV found in chimpanzees are a cross-species recombinant virus from different species of monkeys infected with SIV over many thousands of years, resulting in a virus similar to HIV. These recombinant viruses within primates have led to two distinct HIV populations; the more common HIV-1 and less virulent HIV-2. HIV-1 accounts for 90% of all infections with HIV-2 being found mainly in West Africa. The origins of both can be traced to chimpanzees (HIV-1) and sooty mangabey monkeys (HIV-2) with distinct viral sequences for each type.

SIV from red-capped mangabey and the greater spot-nosed monkey have been shown to be the origin of SIV in chimpanzees (Bonn, 2003), the precursor of HIV-1 and the most likely source of cross-species infection. In their natural environment, chimps are known to hunt and eat other species of monkeys, which may explain how SIV could have jumped into different species of primates. This SIV is now thought to have been transmitted from chimpanzees to humans from either the butchering or eating of chimp meat.

Fieldwork in Gombe National Park, Tanzania, studied different groups of chimpanzees and revealed that linked SIV infections were found to be passed on through sexual intercourse. Analysis of these linked infections demonstrated similar rates of transmission to heterosexual humans (transmission per coital act: 0.0008–0.0015 in chimps versus 0.0011 in heterosexual humans) (Rudicell et al., 2010). Other routes of infection include vertical transmission (i.e. mother to child) and during aggressive exchanges/blood to blood contact.

It was widely believed that SIV was non-pathogenic in many mammals and researchers attempted to understand why these species were not immunocompromised by the virus, hoping that it would lead to the elusive cure for HIV. However, a study in *Nature* (Keele et al., 2009) revealed AIDS-like illnesses in wild chimpanzees with those infected with SIV being 10–16 times more likely to die compared to non-infected chimps. Post-mortem results showed parasitic infections and significant depletions in the CD4 cells mirroring the pathology found in human AIDS.

The First Human Infections

HIV has four separate lineages divided into groups, namely, M, N, O and P. Group M is the main virus that has caused the global spread of HIV, while the others constitute only a fraction of total infections. Phylogenetic analysis has shown that group M originated in Kinshasa (or Leopoldville, as it was then called), now in the Democratic Republic of the Congo, in the early twentieth century (Castro-Nallar, Crandall, & Pérez-Losada, 2012).

The first humans to be infected with HIV are thought to have been part of the Bantu tribe, which comprises 30% of Africa's population. There had been an unprecedented rise in lymphomas and Kaposi's sarcoma in Africa in this specific population in the first half of the twentieth century without any clear indications as to the cause (Oettle, 1962). Given that the Bantu tribes were in close contact with wild chimpanzees, cross-species HIV infection may be the reason for this sudden unexpected rise in these possible AIDS-defining illnesses. As the forces of colonialism and globalisation took hold, HIV was able to thrive and proliferate along transport routes and then be transported to Haiti, thought to be the main bridge of infection into the US. Many Haitians worked in Congo during this period as the Belgian colony was undergoing significant economic growth through the discovery and export of copper. The earliest retrospectively confirmed HIV case in humans was in 1959 in Zaire (now the Democratic Republic of the Congo), where SIV is believed to have crossed the species barrier (Nahmias et al., 1986). Using Western Blot analysis, scientists tested a blood sample taken from a Bantu male in Zaire in 1959 and found evidence of a HIV-like virus.

The first suspected case in the US was that of Robert Rayford in 1968, a 15-year-old African American who was admitted with disseminated chlamydia infection and subsequently died of pneumonia (Garry et al., 1988). Subsequent analysis of tissue samples revealed an earlier form of HIV—different from the form which predominates today. Rayford died three days after his 16th birthday with the source of his infection never having been identified. It is plausible that only a few cases of HIV were translocated into the US this early, with those affected never having been formally identified as having AIDS.

Throughout the 1970s, there were many cases of patients presenting with unusual symptoms suggesting immunosuppression with unusual opportunistic infections. Grethe Rask, a Danish surgeon who had been posted in Congo, returned to Denmark with a serious case of *Pneumocystis carinii* pneumonia (PCP), a fungal pneumonia, and subsequently died in 1977. The discovery of pneumocysts on her autopsy puzzled her colleagues and only later was it hypothesised that she may have contracted HIV whilst working near Kinshasa—an early reminder of how easy it is for HIV to cross international boundaries. In fact, it was impossible, at the time, to detect which part of the complex immune system was being destroyed by this mysterious condition as CD4 cells (a T-cell lymphocyte and the cell targeted by HIV) had yet to be discovered as part of the immune system.

Initial Medical Responses to HIV/AIDS

T-cell lymphocytes, the cellular host supplying the machinery for HIV replication, had only been discovered in the late 1970s, and when the AIDS crisis began, research into this new area of immunology was still in its infancy. The first person to discover the effect of HIV on CD4 cells (a subsection of T-cells) was Dr James Goedert of the National Cancer Institute in the US. He had developed a new diagnostic test called Fluorescent Activated Cell Sorting, a technique using fluorescent dyes to 'label' immune cells allowing CD4 counts to be calculated. A study from 1985 demonstrated severely depleted CD4 cells for the first time in gay men who had shown signs of immunosuppression (Goedert et al., 1985). In the early 1980s, this formed the only reliable diagnostic and reproducible test for HIV infection until the antibody test became available.

It was in the early 1980s that clinicians began to regard the mysterious illness as a distinct syndrome—for a few years they had been observing inexplicable cases of severe immunosuppression in otherwise young healthy men with homosexuality being the only common factor. Physicians in San Francisco saw increasing numbers of gay men attending their clinics with the pathognomonic purple skin lesions of Kaposi's sarcoma. The presence of this new aggressive form in gay men remained a mystery as it usually presented as an indolent skin cancer seen in elderly Jewish men. Kaposi's sarcoma lesions became one of the earliest herald lesions and visible stigmata of AIDS patients and became synonymous with inevitable death. Many US-based physicians used to treating gay men observed the lesions followed by a swift decline into immunosuppression and death. It was these physicians who alerted the medical community to a new pathogen circulating among gay men well before HIV was identified.

Kaposi's sarcoma was often a precursor of other more serious and often fatal opportunistic infections. *Pneumocystis carinii* pneumonia (PCP) (or *Pneumocystis jirovecii* pneumonia [PJP] as it is now known) is a ubiquitous fungus that was generally seen only in malnourished children in Eastern Europe during the Second World War and in severely immunosuppressed patients. Prior to AIDS, there were fewer than 100 cases of reported PCP in the US. The accepted treatment was, and remains, pentamidine, a potent antimicrobial.

Given that this was such an unusual treatment (and indeed because PCP itself was so rare), a technician at the Food and Drug Administration (FDA) was charged with the task of dispensing pentamidine and recording patient details when requests for the drug were received. It was the young FDA technician Sandra Ford who took the decision to alert her senior colleagues at the FDA after receiving several pentamidine requests for otherwise healthy young men (and multiple courses in some patients) who had no identifiable risk factors for immunosuppression. This was the first time that the authorities were made aware of this new disease observable mainly in young gay men. Sandra Ford was the first government official to take notice of this new syndrome and, thus, the catalyst for the start of the institutional response to the AIDS crisis.

Meanwhile, Michael Gottlieb, an Assistant Professor of Immunology at the University of California in Los Angeles Medical Centre, and Wayne Shandera, a public health doctor in Los Angeles, had encountered at least five cases of PCP in gay men and decided to submit a brief article describing their observations to the US Centre for Disease Control and Prevention (CDC) *Morbidity and Mortality Weekly Report*. This report, an alert system for medical professionals to share emerging information about new infections, was published on 5 June 1981 and is the first written scientific account of HIV/AIDS. The editors also erroneously attributed the cluster of this unusual disease to high levels of cytomegalovirus (CMV), a sexually transmissible infection that is highly prevalent in gay men. The working hypothesis at the time was that CMV had somehow overwhelmed the immune system, leading to profound immunosuppression.

This new syndrome attracted the attention of Dr Jim Curran, a public health physician who proceeded to establish the Kaposi's sarcoma and Opportunistic Infection Task Force to ascertain the aetiology of the immunosuppression observed in growing numbers of gay men.

At the time, there were three key hypotheses. It was thought that the syndrome may be attributable to (1) an infectious agent, which was as yet unidentified; (2) amyl nitrate (or 'poppers'), which is an inhaled form of nitrates used by gay men during sex as a muscle relaxant; or (3) CMV, which could be overwhelming the immune system and, thus, causing the immunosuppression. All three hypotheses were treated as equally plausible given the lack of reliable empirical data. The second and third hypotheses were gradually rejected as more evidence came to light. More specifically, many samples of amyl nitrates were analysed and found to have no effect on immune status. For the CMV hypothesis, it was known that it is a virus that infects between 60 and 70% of adults in developed countries and close to 100% of those in developing countries (Cannon, Schmid, & Hyde, 2010), but the cases appeared, at the time, to be limited only to gay men. When scientists first began to examine the blood of those who were immunosuppressed, they found extremely high levels of CMV. In fact, CMV lies dormant in the body after infection and only when the body is immunosuppressed does it 'reactivate', leading to the high levels seen in the gay men exhibiting immunosuppression.

Much of the initial understanding of AIDS was from the work of Selma Dritz, the Public Health Assistant Director for San Francisco, who had been interviewing gay men affected by this new syndrome. She had previously completed work on 'gay bowel syndrome' (a common presentation in the 1980s and usually due to amoebiasis and giardia from faeco-oral contact) and was familiar with the sexual norms and behaviours of gay men in San Francisco. She attempted to trace who had developed Kaposi's sarcoma and ascertained that many of the men affected were in fact connected—by sexual contact. This evidence constituted one of the missing pieces of the puzzle and was to be key to shaping the response to the AIDS crisis (Loewenberg, 2008).

Another significant development in the early epidemic was made by Arye Rubinstein, a paediatrician based in New York. He was alarmed when he began to observe cases of unexplained immunosuppression in newborn infants as early as December 1981. Many of these children were born to mothers from the Bronx, a deprived area of New York, who were also injecting drug users and were themselves showing the hallmarks of immunosuppression. He speculated that this might be linked to the syndrome observed in gay men, given the similarities. Transmission from mother to child was indicative of a bloodborne infectious agent as it appeared to follow a very similar pattern to that of the recent outbreak of hepatitis B.

In times of uncertainty, scapegoats are often used as a way of helping people direct anger or frustration at otherwise unfathomable circumstances. AIDS was no different. In the early days of the research, many of those affected had had sexual contact with one person, Gaeten Dugas, a Canadian airline steward. As he was part of some sexual networks, many believed he was personally responsible for the propagation of HIV across the US—the cities he flew to were heavily affected by AIDS. Dugas continued to be sexually active after his diagnosis with Kaposi's sarcoma, which shocked public health officials at the time. There was even talk of legally curtailing his sexual activities to reduce the spread of AIDS, setting a very dark precedent for many in the gay community. With hindsight, it is clear the 'patient zero' theory was inaccurate, and it has since been proven that HIV arrived in the US long before Gaetan Dugas was identified (Worobey et al., 2016).

A much more important catalyst for AIDS were the gay bathhouses in which many gay men at the time reported having condomless sex with multiple partners in a single visit. This undoubtedly led to an increase in the rate of new infections with HIV in the US and elsewhere. When it was understood that AIDS was associated with sexual behaviour, there were calls from public health officials and some within the gay community for the bathhouses to be closed. However, bathhouses represented a symbol of recently hard-won civil rights for gay men, and many refused to renounce the bathhouses despite the dangers that they clearly posed. Ultimately, the bathhouses were allowed to remain open provided they displayed posters about the risks associated with condomless sex. Attendance did fall in this period although the saunas and bathhouses continued to provide the perfect amplification apparatus for new transmissions in the gay community.

The search for the cause of AIDS was paramount not only to controlling its spread but also to generating possible treatment options for those affected. Given that T-cells were the potential target with a long period of infection before immunosuppression, a retrovirus was suspected. A known retrovirus, another human T-lymphocyte virus (HTLV) had already been identified and its clinical course seemed to fit this picture.

Two laboratories, one in the Pasteur Institute in Paris, France, and the other a government laboratory in Bethesda, US, worked with tissue and blood samples of known AIDS patients to ascertain the cause of what was initially called HTLV-III. Retroviral research at the time was painstakingly laborious and error-prone given the limited tools available at the time. A breakthrough came when the lymph node of a gay man was analysed in Paris and a new virus isolated, with both research groups publishing their findings in the same issue of *Science* in 1983 (Barre-Sinoussi et al., 1983; Gallo et al., 1983).

Once the pathogen had been identified, intense work began on how to identify whether someone had the infection. Often, clinicians use antibody tests to ascertain whether someone has been exposed to an infectious agent. Direct visualisation or isolation of the pathogen itself is time-consuming and technically difficult. The then recent test for hepatitis B had used a similar method for detecting previous infection, and this was translated into the first HIV antibody test in 1985—a huge step forward for patients to learn their HIV status in the early phase of infection (and prevent them from passing it onto sexual partners) and to help plan public health prevention strategies once the true prevalence had been ascertained in different communities.

Early AIDS Treatments

The early days of the HIV epidemic were characterised by fear, distress and uncertainty. Following the development of an antibody test, scientific discussions about HIV/AIDS turned to possible treatments, with the hope of enabling those diagnosed to survive. This optimism was sadly short-lived. Given the urgency of the situation, a large number of untested and largely ineffective antivirals and immune system 'boosters' appeared on the market. Many of these drugs (e.g. isoprinosine) had been used in the treatment of other viruses such as herpes and influenza, and it was hoped that would have a similar effect on HIV. Some other known drugs were able to stimulate the immune system to help control, or even resist, viral infections, such as interferon, a commonly used drug for hepatitis C. There were no data on the effectiveness of these drugs, but in the early clamour for survival, many searched for a glimmer of hope. The terrible side effects of many of these under-researched drugs were silently tolerated in the hope that they would have some effect on extending the life expectancy of those infected with HIV.

Yet, the only reliable means of reaching any scientifically viable conclusions is to compare new treatments to established therapy in clinical trials. As there were no 'gold standard' treatments at the time, an effective agent against HIV proved elusive for many years. Drug development is a lengthy and complicated process; medicines take an average of 17 years to get from the experimental stage to becoming available to patients (Morris, Wooding, & Grant, 2011).

The history of zidovudine (AZT)—the first proven drug to work against HIV—starts in 1964, when Joseph Horwitz, a cancer researcher at Michigan Cancer Foundation, developed the drug to cure certain types of leukaemia. It was found to be ineffective and the compound was shelved. Twenty years later, it was revived by the Wellcome Foundation—a charity on the cutting-edge of antiviral treatments at the time. AZT is a base analogue, that is, it resembles one of the naturally occurring building blocks of DNA found in most human cells. When this imposter is ingested, it is incorporated into the viral DNA and inhibits further transcription, thereby halting viral replication. A number of other HIV drugs work in a similar way. (This is covered in detail in Chap. 5.) After demonstrating that AZT had direct antiretroviral effects, a sample was sent to the FDA in 1984 for further analysis.

Having confirmed its action against HIV, the FDA now set out to test the tolerability of AZT in human subjects. The first clinical trial published in 1987 showed impressive drug efficacy—during the 24-week trial, 19 of the 137 patients in the placebo arm had died, compared to just 1 of the 145 patients taking AZT (Fischl et al., 1987). The results were so dramatic that the trial was stopped early and all of the study patients were given AZT. It later emerged that patients from both arms of the clinical trial were sharing drugs to reduce the chances of taking placebo—an understandable act of desperation by those living with HIV at the time.

Sadly, the optimism surrounding AZT was short-lived. The first antiretroviral (ARV) clinical trial, the CONCORDE study which looked at placebo versus AZT showed that, after 16 weeks, the mortality rate of those taking AZT was equal to placebo ('Concorde', 1994). AZT was found to be effective against HIV but only for a short period of time—when AZT was administered alone, HIV quickly developed resistance to the drug. Drug resistance was not properly understood at the time, but it was clear that this was a huge setback in the treatment of HIV. It was not until 1996 that effective combination therapy consisting of three drugs became a reality. The impact of highly effective ART cannot be underestimated and was a turning point in the fight against HIV.

HIV/AIDS in the UK

Although HIV incidence was far higher in the US than in the UK, gay communities in towns and cities throughout the UK were profoundly affected by the arrival of HIV, commonly referred to as the 'silent killer' on the gay scene. In 1982, Terrence Higgins, a 37-year-old gay man, was among the first individuals confirmed to die of an AIDS-related illness in the UK. In response to Terrence's death, several of his friends set up the Terry Higgins Trust to help gay and bisexual men who were living with, at risk of, and affected by HIV. Following a public meeting organised by the Gay and Lesbian Switchboard (now called Switchboard LGBT+), which provided much of the sexual health information to sexual minorities at the time, volunteers came together to support the newly established HIV charity. Hundreds of volunteers manned the telephones, answering questions and signposting callers to appropriate services. In the early days of AIDS, this was the only coordinated response.

The gay community mobilised and recognised the severity and impact of HIV long before the authorities did—publicly at least. Mel Rosen, a well-known HIV activist in the US, attended a meeting organised by the Gay and Lesbian Switchboard and recounted disturbing accounts of young, otherwise healthy men dying in their hundreds. Rosen discussed the steps being taken in San Francisco to assist those affected, such as a buddy scheme for daily tasks and for supporting people living with HIV when others had rejected them.

Following its renaming as the 'Terrence Higgins Trust', volunteers from the charity produced the first ever educational leaflet with practical advice on how to recognise symptoms and to reduce transmission. It also provided advice about how and where to seek treatment and, for gay men, stressed the importance of seeking a doctor aware of HIV and accepting of gay sexuality.

It is noteworthy that, at the time, HIV had not yet been discovered. AIDS was recognised only when individuals became symptomatic. Advice was at times contradictory and inaccurate. For instance, leaflets provided the following advice: 'Have as much sex as you want, but with fewer and healthy people'. However, it was unclear what 'fewer' meant and how one might identify 'healthy people'. It seems odd now that there was no mention of using condoms or trying to avoid the highest-risk sexual behaviours, such as condomless receptive anal sex. Talking openly about sex was not a socially acceptable method of health promotion in the early 1980s—a social impediment to HIV prevention that would continue for years and only increase the spread of HIV.

HIV entered the British public consciousness for the first time in 1983 when Horizon (a factual programme broadcast by the British Broadcasting Corporation [BBC]) first aired the documentary 'Killer in the Village'. The programme provided a detailed account of HIV, the risk factors and the experience of gay men living with, or at risk of, HIV. The media played a fundamental role in shaping public understanding of HIV/AIDS. Much of the reporting was simply inaccurate due to the lack of information. It also drew upon the prevailing anti-gay attitudes in 1980s Britain, further fuelling the stigma surrounding gay men and their lifestyle.

The publication of a study in *The Lancet* in 1984 highlighted the growing challenge of HIV in the UK (Cheingsong-Popov et al., 1984). The study had examined 2000 serum samples across distinct populations. At the time HIV was called both HTLV III and LAV (lymphadenopathy associated virus) so they set out to detect both—before the commercially available tests we see today. Using immunofluorescence looking for antibodies, they revealed that 30 out of 31 gay men who had AIDS were HTLV III- and LAV-positive. They also correctly deduced these two viruses were the same. In their study, 79% of patients had lymphadenopathy and 17% showed no symptoms, and it became clear that even someone with advanced disease could still 'look healthy'. However, it was still unknown whether those with positive antibody results would go on to develop AIDS. Given the prevalence shown in this early study, this now represented a very real public health emergency.

Yet, the initial political response to AIDS in the UK was ambivalent at best. Initially, AIDS was presumed to affect gay men and injecting drug users only, two of the most marginalised groups in society at the time. Despite fervent campaigning by activists and clinicians in the UK, the political response to the epidemic was slow, indecisive and laced with anti-gay social attitudes.

Despite mounting evidence of increasing numbers of AIDS cases in the UK, there was initially limited political attention to the AIDS crisis—the then Prime Minister Margaret Thatcher and Secretary of State for Health and Social Care, Norman Fowler, said very little about AIDS during its early stages. In 1983, Margaret Thatcher had swept to power promising 'back to family values' which clearly resonated with the British electorate who returned a 144-seat majority for the Conservatives. The discourse of HIV prevention (including the overt focus on sex) seemed to contradict the family values which Thatcher's government attempted to promote. Norman Fowler became a hugely important advocate for HIV prevention and, as a patron for the British HIV Association, remains a staunch supporter of HIV education and prevention to this day.

In 1985, Donald Acheson, the Chief Medical Officer at the time, had met with both clinicians on the front line of the AIDS crisis and volunteers from the newly formed Terrence Higgins Trust to understand how the condition was affecting people in the UK. Clinicians referred to an influx of patients with severe immunosuppression into hospitals which were largely unprepared—this was particularly acute in the London area where most of the first AIDS cases emerged. In the same year, the Expert Advisory Group on AIDS was set up consisting of 22 members of clinicians, researchers, politicians and voluntary sector workers. The principal aim of the Expert Advisory Group on AIDS was to advise the Chief Medical Officer on how to tackle the unfolding public health crisis.

The subsequent report 'HTLV-III infection, the AIDS epidemic and control of its spread in the UK' by Acheson (1986) clarified that AIDS posed a significant challenge to public health in the UK, affecting not only gay men and injecting drug users but also the general population. Dr Acheson wrote:

> heterosexual intercourse cannot be excluded as a possible means of transmission. Although the American data suggests that homosexual intercourse is the most important means of sexual spread of HTLV-III infection in our present state of knowledge, it would be wrong for policy to be based on the assumption that heterosexual intercourse will not in the long run assume a significant role.

Having fully understood the scale of the AIDS crisis, Norman Fowler advocated for a public health campaign with clear information about risky sexual practices. This was initially construed as distasteful and potentially harmful to the public and thus resisted by Margaret Thatcher. Though cautious about the language used in public health messaging, the government now realised that it was necessary to talk about sex openly in order to prevent HIV. The government allocated £2.5 million for a public health campaign to provide accurate information about HIV transmission.

There were no data on public awareness of AIDS in 1985 which would inform the public health campaign. In other words, it was unclear what the British public knew or thought about AIDS or how accurate their knowledge was. One US study in 1985 (Price, Desmond, & Kukulka, 1985) revealed high levels of AIDS awareness in adolescents who reportedly had acquired information from the mainstream media. The results showed that, despite high levels of awareness, only 27% of young people believed themselves to be at risk of infection. It seemed that AIDS was perceived to be a 'gay disease'—a representation also promoted by the mass media—and that anyone outside of this population was not at risk.

Another US survey (DiClemente, Zorn, & Temoshok, 1986) showed that only 66% of respondents knew that AIDS could not be transmitted through kissing or close non-sexual contact. In their London survey (with comparator groups in San Francisco and New York), Temoshok, Sweet, and Zich (1987) found that Londoners were the least worried about

AIDS, but also that those with the least AIDS knowledge thought that they were at much lower risk.

The First Public Health Campaign in the UK

The UK government opted for two separate national press advertisements—each full page for maximum impact—in all Sunday papers. The wording of the adverts was to become contentious as Margaret Thatcher resisted references to risky sex, noting in a Number 10 memo that 'Do we have to have the section on risky sex? I should have thought it could do immense harm if young teenagers were to read it'.[1]

The fact that the AIDS public health campaign was conducted from neither the Cabinet Office nor Number 10 directly suggests that the Prime Minister wished to distance herself from a public backlash which could be politically damaging. At one point, Margaret Thatcher questioned the legitimacy of using the term 'anal sex' and enquired about its consistency with the Obscene Publications Act—the term 'rectal sex' was finally agreed upon.

This highlighted one of the biggest barriers to the initial public health campaign, because of its association, in most cases, with sexual behaviour. This meant that HIV prevention in turn necessitated open discussions about sex and gay sexual behaviour, which was not openly discussed before. Due to pervasive conservative attitudes at the time and indeed a government that itself espoused a socially conservative ideology, this was challenging—political hesitation about engaging with HIV and sexual behaviour undoubtedly fuelled the epidemic.

The advertisements were finally published on 16 March 1986 and consisted of poorly presented dense text with no mention of high-risk sex, condoms or how to reduce the risk of infection. Both the Expert Advisory Group on AIDS and the Terrence Higgins Trust emphasised that a clearer message about AIDS and its risk factors was necessary for it to resonate among all members of the public and not only among those who were *believed* to be at risk. The government faced pressure from

---

[1] http://discovery.nationalarchives.gov.uk/details/r/C15189597.

those on the right of its party but, to its credit, proceeded with its HIV prevention campaign. £20 million was allocated to include a leaflet on HIV which was delivered to every household in the UK, a television advertisement, billboard posters and another newspaper campaign. The iconic 'tombstone' television advert, 'Don't Die of Ignorance', was deliberately unsettling and alarmist and drew on imagery of death for maximum impact.

The TV advert appeared to utilise fear as a catalyst for awareness, engagement and behaviour change. The aim of the campaign was to ensure that everyone had heard of AIDS, knew how it was transmitted and, crucially, knew how to reduce their own risk of infection. It is doubtful that all of these objectives were achieved due to the pressure to avoid discussions about sexual behaviour.

There is much debate about the value of fear in increasing awareness, engagement and behaviour change (Ruiter, Abraham, & Kok, 2001). Although some believed that the campaign marginalised certain groups and instilled unnecessary fear in those who were in fact at low risk of HIV infection, the campaign did have a profound effect on the British public and is still remembered by many today who witnessed it first-hand. The impact of the campaign on sexual health was nothing short of astonishing. The incidence of gonorrhoea, a useful proxy for condomless sex, decreased from 50,000 cases per year to 10,000 following the airing of the television advertisements (Mohammed et al., 2018). National interest was maintained when both the Independent Television (ITV) and BBC began a week-long series of programmes called 'AIDS Help!' in which politicians, activists and alternative comedians discussed HIV on television. The use of television, in addition to the print media, made a significant contribution to HIV education and myth-busting in the British public.

Gay men were the group most affected by HIV and at highest risk of infection. They were, however, a stigmatised group whose identities, lifestyles and health the government generally avoided acknowledging. Thus, there was no government-endorsed campaign to prevent HIV among gay men until 1989, which generated confusion, misinformation and, undoubtedly, further engagement in high-risk sexual behaviour. In the absence of an institutional campaign, community groups, such as the Terrence Higgins Trust and the National AIDS Trust (formed in 1987 with an emphasis on HIV policy development), provided grassroots education to ensure accurate information, dispel HIV myths and ultimately curb the spread of HIV in the gay community. The government understood that community organisations were best positioned to provide HIV education and that they would have the greatest impact on their respective communities. In 1989, David Mellor, the Minister for Health at the time, pledged increases in funding for HIV. £25 million was provided in 1988, which rose to £62 million and then to £132 million in 1989 and 1990, respectively. Of this, £62 million was set aside for HIV treatment and care with the rest allocated to education and support for both those at risk and patients already living with HIV.

The involvement of the UK government and the pledge of funding to support HIV education, advocacy and prevention undoubtedly saved many thousands of lives in the pre-ART era when HIV still constituted a life-limiting condition. It is important to note that this early political intervention was by no means common across Europe and, thus, in many other countries the virus devastated high-risk groups.

The late 1980s saw a gradual change in tone towards those living with HIV as understanding improved and the general public realised that it affected all groups indiscriminately. In 1987, Princess Diana, a trailblazing advocate of HIV education, was one of the first celebrities to be photographed touching and hugging people living with HIV. It must be remembered that many at the time thought that one could contract HIV from touching. These iconic images helped dispel some of the myths concerning HIV transmission and sought to normalise the condition for many across the world. Princess Diana continued her advocacy work until her death, which has subsequently been taken forward by her son Prince Harry.

In 1988, the first 'World AIDS Day' was created with an emphasis on testing and educating those who might not perceive themselves to be at risk. At this time, HIV was still largely thought of as the 'gay plague' and the result of lifestyle choices made by gay men.

Clinical Snapshot 1: Antiretroviral Therapy

The most significant turning point in the treatment of HIV came in July 1996 at the 11th Conference for AIDS in Vancouver, where it was shown that giving patients 3 drugs (i.e. combination therapy) with the use of the newly released protease inhibitors, led to significant reductions in AIDS deaths by 60–80%. These landmark findings revolutionised the treatment of HIV with patients no longer facing imminent death and led to the now accepted model of treating the majority of HIV patients in an outpatient setting, with early testing and treatment being the norm. Early HIV drugs were often toxic and required perfect adherence to be effective, but offered hope to thousands of people who were infected. The evolution of combination therapy has been rapid and now the emphasis is on quality of life, principally by reducing the side effects of antiretroviral therapy. As treatments continue to evolve, longer acting injectable drugs and implants will become the standard of care in the future, negating the need for daily oral therapy and improving patient satisfaction and adherence to medication.

The Slow March to Controlling the Virus

A huge shift in British social attitudes towards HIV occurred in 1990 when *Eastenders*, one of the most popular BBC soap operas in the UK, introduced its first HIV-positive character. Mark Fowler, an affable market trader, was a heterosexual man who had acquired HIV from his previous girlfriend. The show sought to challenge stereotypes about those living with HIV and demonstrated that everyone was at risk, not just gay men. With a viewership of up to 30 million, over half the country was able to witness the issues facing those living with HIV. The importance of this storyline cannot be underestimated. It dealt with relevant topics, such as the difficulties around HIV disclosure, use of third-sector organisations (he attended therapy at the Terrence Higgins Trust) and how people react to HIV based on their own lack of knowledge—which many gay men had experienced. This was followed by the death of Freddy Mercury, lead singer of *Queen*, in 1991 which, given the band's huge following worldwide, sought to highlight the need for testing and early diagnosis. At that time, more open discussions around sexual practices were taking place slowly, which began to challenge stigma and deeply held prejudices against gay men and HIV.

As HIV testing became standardised and more commonplace, more infections were detected. There was an increase in new HIV diagnoses in 1985, most likely reflecting improved testing rather than actual prevalence. After the public health campaigns and HIV education packages, the number of new HIV diagnoses in the late 1980s and early- to mid-1990s remained relatively stable at just under 2000 new diagnoses per year. With the advent of effective treatment in 1996, the number of people dying from AIDS- and HIV-related complications reduced dramatically. However, a side effect of this reduction in AIDS-related mortality was a creeping complacency within the gay community in relation to the disease. It was no longer a death sentence. In the UK, the drugs were effective, free and easily available. Younger gay men had not lived through the trauma of the AIDS crisis with many having a misplaced sense of security about the longer-term effects of living with HIV. As such, at the turn of the century HIV rates began to increase year on year for the next 15 years with 3480 new diagnosis in 2015, nearly double the figure from the 1990s (see Fig. 2.1).

During these years of a steady increase in new diagnoses, public health campaigns became more nuanced with the 'use a condom' message

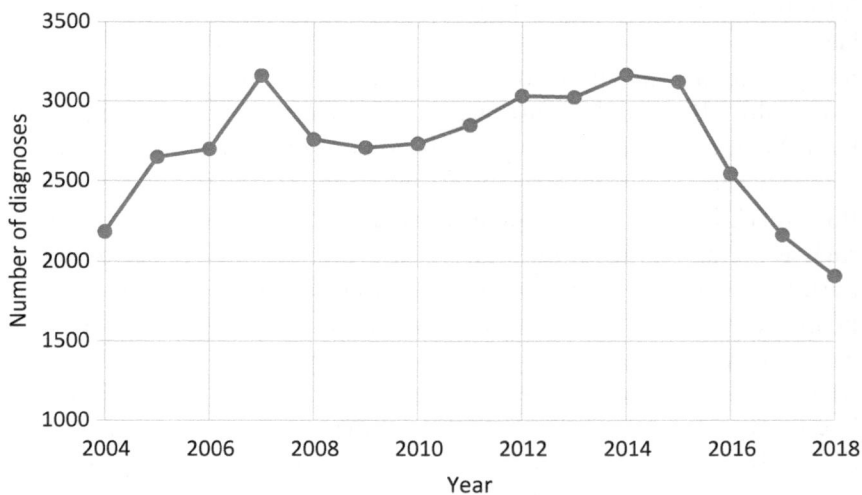

Fig. 2.1   Number of HIV diagnoses in the UK by year (2004–2018)

staying front and centre but also utilising more third-sector organisations to provide HIV education. Many of these organisations had the knowledge and prior experience of engaging certain communities at risk of HIV and took an approach which they knew would resonate with their target audience—and using colloquial language to demystify some of the technical terms that were used in other campaigns.

In 2004, the Blair Labour government published a white paper 'Choosing Health' which, for the first time, prioritised sexual health.[2] Much of the focus was on the rising rates of chlamydia in young people, but the paper was instrumental in setting standards for sexual health and improving access to testing, raising awareness of HIV and increasing funding for overstretched sexual health services. The New Labour model of introducing targets in healthcare were instrumental in improving HIV testing amongst all groups, not just gay men.

From 2010, there was an acceleration of new HIV infections in gay men due in part to the proliferation of smart phone location-based social networking applications (e.g. Grindr, Scruff) whereby gay men could find a sexual partner within minutes in their local area if desired (Jaspal, 2017). Prior to this, only computer-based applications, such as Gaydar, were available and lacked the speed and convenience of the newer smart phone applications. During this time, there was also an explosion of 'chemsex', that is, the use of drugs in sexualised settings. This is discussed further in Chap. 3.

Clinicians in the UK have struggled to fully understand the complexities of this new era of HIV risk behaviour. It is not uncommon to hear of someone taking crystal methamphetamine, being awake for many days and, with the use of Grindr, having dozens of sexual partners within a relatively short period of time. The identification and treatment of this subset of the gay population has been difficult and is contingent on the ability of clinicians and services to respond effectively to this challenge. As many gay men are now also injecting drugs (or 'slamming'), the standard injecting drug services have struggled to cope with the complex health issues in this population. As the landscape has shifted, so have the

---

[2] https://webarchive.nationalarchives.gov.uk/+/http://www.dh.gov.uk/en/Publicationsandstatistics/Publications/PublicationsPolicyAndGuidance/DH_4094550.

public health campaigns, and much work has been undertaken to understand the emerging risks associated with young gay men today. Some of these risks were summarised in Chap. 1.

In addition to the increasingly nuanced public health campaigns to improve HIV awareness, three significant developments since 2015 have turned the tide in HIV incidence in the UK. First, PrEP has enabled gay men to take control of their HIV risk by taking a pill on either a daily or intermittent basis to prevent their acquisition of HIV. As PrEP is only dispensed for three to six months at a time, users must attend sexual health services where testing can be performed and high-risk behaviours identified and addressed. PrEP is covered in more detail in Chap. 4 on HIV prevention. Second, there has been an increase in HIV testing, which is central to early HIV diagnosis. On the one hand, this facilitates the identification of those with undiagnosed HIV who may be transmitting the virus to others, and, on the other hand, it provides an opportunity for increasing patients' awareness and understanding of HIV and appropriate prevention approaches. Third, those who are living with HIV and on effective ART cannot transmit HIV to their sexual partners. This powerful U = U message (undetectable = untransmittable) has had a seismic impact on the lives and wellbeing of gay men and all those living with HIV. They no longer need to be in fear of onward transmission. Moreover, U = U has the potential to challenge social stigma surrounding HIV given that fear of infection constitutes a key component of stigma.

In view of these significant advances, between 2012 and 2018, HIV incidence in gay, bisexual and other men who have sex with men (MSM) in the UK decreased by 71% (O'Halloran et al., 2020). This sharp decline should be cause for celebration as gay men begin to utilise the various different forms of HIV prevention and adapt them to their own lifestyles and attitudes. Moreover, sexual health charities have developed innovative ways of reaching subgroups within the gay community which have historically been viewed as 'hard-to-reach'. However, there remains much work to be done.

HIV Today: An Epidemiological Snapshot

HIV prevalence in the UK is approximately 0.18% of the population aged between 15 and 59. Gay men constitute a relatively small minority group and are estimated to represent approximately 2% of the London population. Yet, Public Health England (2018) data show that, of the 103,800 people currently living with HIV, approximately 49,800 are gay, bisexual or other MSM. Moreover, it is estimated that 1 in 11 gay men in London is HIV-positive. HIV incidence in gay and bisexual men is reducing year on year due to a mixture of increased testing, availability of PrEP and treatment as prevention for those living with HIV.

There have been significant increases in most STIs in gay men from 2014 to 2018. A 61% increase in both chlamydia (from 11,760 to 18,892) and syphilis (from 3527 to 5681), and a 43% increase in gonorrhoea (from 18,568 to 26,574). The increase in STIs is multifactorial with many attributing this to reduced condom use due to PrEP and those living with HIV being unable to transmit the virus when on effective treatment. The fact remains that many gay men have never used condoms for a variety of reasons. If anything, this increase in STIs allows sexual health clinics to intervene in those who may need support around drug or alcohol use and may never have visited a sexual health clinic previously.

Overview

In this chapter, the socio-historical, scientific and epidemiological aspects of HIV were considered. Since the initial clinical observations of HIV, there have been significant scientific developments, which have resulted in a much improved disease prognosis for those diagnosed and treated early. Moreover, biomedical tools for preventing HIV are highly effective. These developments have not occurred in a social vacuum but rather they have been shaped by activism, society and politics. As demonstrated in this chapter, the stigma associated with both sex and the groups dispro-portionately affected by HIV at the start of the epidemic caused some political trepidation about discussing the disease openly. Moreover, there were challenges in addressing the possible drivers of infection in key pop-ulations, such as gay men. History demonstrates that, while silence may have facilitated short-term political victories for some, its implications for the progression of HIV/AIDS have been devastating. Where there is silence, there is decreased awareness, understanding and action against the virus. The fight against this invisible enemy was, and still is, a feat of human endurance against all odds. The human cost of HIV/AIDS would have been far higher unless the numerous community groups, activists, scientists, clinicians and politicians had stepped up and tackled not only the effects of the virus but also the insidious stigma of HIV. Their efforts have enabled the general population to acknowledge and understand the health of marginalised groups within our societies. Often, the groups most affected by HIV are unable to advocate in order to challenge the thinking of politicians and the general public. HIV would be an even more dangerous global threat if these people had not stepped in to help. To achieve the eradication of HIV, public health campaigns should be based on evidence and education to help those at risk understand how to have a healthy sex life without fear or prejudice. These campaigns must not be marred or impeded by politics. This chapter elucidates the central-ity of the socio-historical dimension of HIV in enabling us to control, curb and, ultimately, eradicate the virus.

References

Acheson, E. D. (1986). AIDS: A challenge for public health. *Public Health, 327*(8482), P662–P666.

Barre-Sinoussi, F., Chermann, J. C., Rey, F., Nugeyre, M. T., Chamaret, S., Gruest, J., … Montagnier, L. (1983). Isolation of a T-lymphotropic retrovi-rus from a patient at risk for acquired immune deficiency syndrome (AIDS). *Science, 220*(4599), 868–871.

Belshaw, R., Pereira, V., Katzourakis, A., Talbot, G., Pačes, J., Burt, A., & Tristem, M. (2004). Long-term reinfection of the human genome by endogenous retroviruses. *Proceedings of the National Academy of Sciences, 101*(14), 4894–4899.

Bonn, D. (2003). Chimp SIV could come from monkeys. *The Lancet Infectious Diseases, 3*(8), 457.

Cannon, M. J., Schmid, D. S., & Hyde, T. B. (2010). Review of cytomegalovirus seroprevalence and demographic characteristics associated with infection. *Reviews in Medical Virology, 20*(4), 202–213.

Castro-Nallar, E., Crandall, K. A., & Pérez-Losada, M. (2012). Genetic diversity and molecular epidemiology of HIV transmission. *Future Virology, 7*(3), 239–252.

Cheingsong-Popov, R., Weiss, R. A., Dalgleish, A., Tedder, R. S., Shanson, D. C., Jeffries, D. J., … Mitton, S. (1984). Prevalence of antibody to human T-lymphotropic virus type III in AIDS and AIDS-risk patients in Britain. *Lancet, 2*(8401), 477–480.

Concorde Coordinating Committee. (1994). Concorde: MRC/ANRS randomised double-blind controlled trial of immediate and deferred zidovudine in symptom-free HIV infection. *Lancet (London, England), 343*(8902), 871–881.

DiClemente, R. J., Zorn, J., & Temoshok, L. (1986). Adolescents and AIDS: A survey of knowledge, attitudes and beliefs about AIDS in San Francisco. *American Journal of Public Health, 76*(12), 1443–1445.

Fischl, M. A., Richman, D. D., Grieco, M. H., Gottlieb, M. S., Volberding, P. A., Laskin, O. L., … Schooley, R. T. (1987). The efficacy of azidothymidine (AZT) in the treatment of patients with AIDS and AIDS-related complex. A double-blind, placebo-controlled trial. *The New England Journal of Medicine, 317*(4), 185–191.

Gallo, R. C., Sarin, P. S., Gelmann, E. P., Robert-Guroff, M., Richardson, E., Kalyanaraman, V. S., … Popovic, M. (1983). Isolation of human T-cell leukemia virus in acquired immune deficiency syndrome (AIDS). *Science, 220*(4599), 865–867.

Garry, R. F., Witte, M. H., Gottlieb, A. A., Elvin-Lewis, M., Gottlieb, M. S., Witte, C. L., … Drake, W. L. (1988). Documentation of an AIDS virus infection in the United States in 1968. *JAMA, 260*(14), 2085–2087.

Goedert, J. J., Biggar, R. J., Winn, D. M., Mann, D. L., Byar, D. P., Strong, D. M., … Blattner, W. A. (1985). Decreased helper T lymphocytes in homosexual men. I. Sexual contact in high-incidence areas for the acquired immunodeficiency syndrome. *American Journal of Epidemiology, 121*(5), 629–636.

Hirsch, V. M., Edmondson, P., Murphey-Corb, M., Arbeille, B., Johnson, P. R., & Mullins, J. I. (1989). SIV adaption to human cells. *Nature, 341*(6243), 573–574.

Huet, T., Cheynier, R., Meyerhans, A., Roelants, G., & Wain-Hobson, S. (1990). Genetic organization of a chimpanzee lentivirus related to HIV-1. *Nature, 345*(6273), 356–359.

Jaspal, R. (2017). Gay men's construction and management of identity on Grindr. *Sexuality & Culture, 21*(1), 187–204.

Keele, B. F., Jones, J. H., Terio, K. A., Estes, J. D., Rudicell, R. S., Wilson, M. L., … Hahn, B. H. (2009). Increased mortality and AIDS-like immunopathology in wild chimpanzees infected with SIVcpz. *Nature, 460*(7254), 515–519.

Loewenberg, S. (2008). Selma Dritz. *The Lancet, 372*(9646), 1296.

Mohammed, H., Blomquist, P., Ogaz, D., Duffell, S., Furegato, M., Checchi, M., … Hughes, G. (2018). 100 years of STIs in the UK: A review of national surveillance data. *Sexually Transmitted Infections, 94*(8), 553–558.

Morris, Z. S., Wooding, S., & Grant, J. (2011). The answer is 17 years, what is the question: Understanding time lags in translational research. *Journal of the Royal Society of Medicine, 104*(12), 510–520.

Nahmias, A. J., Weiss, J., Yao, X., Lee, F., Kodsi, R., Schanfield, M., … Motulsky, A. (1986). Evidence for human infection with an HTLV III/LAV-like virus in Central Africa, 1959. *Lancet, 1*(8492), 1279–1280.

O'Halloran, C., Sun, S., Nash, S. Brown, A., Croxford S, Connor, N., … Gill, O. N. (2020). *HIV in the United Kingdom: Towards zero 2030*. London: Public Health England. Retrieved March 20, 2020, from https://assets.publishing.service.gov.uk/government/uploads/system/uploads/attachment_data/file/858559/HIV_in_the_UK_2019_towards_zero_HIV_transmissions_by_2030.pdf

Oettle, A. G. (1962). Geographical and racial differences in the frequency of Kaposi's sarcoma as evidence of environmental or genetic causes. *Acta—Unio Internationalis Contra Cancrum, 18*, 330–363.

Price, J. H., Desmond, S., & Kukulka, G. (1985). High school students' perceptions and misperceptions of AIDS. *Journal of School Health, 55*(3), 107–109.

Public Health England. (2018). *Prevalence of HIV infection in the UK in 2018.* Health Protection Report, 13(39). Retrieved May 5, 2020, from https://assets.publishing.service.gov.uk/government/uploads/system/uploads/attachment_data/file/843766/hpr3919_hiv18.pdf.

Rudicell, R. S., Holland Jones, J., Wroblewski, E. E., Learn, G. H., Li, Y., Robertson, J. D., … Wilson, M. L. (2010). Impact of Simian immunodeficiency virus infection on chimpanzee population dynamics. *PLoS Pathogens, 6*(9). https://doi.org/10.1371/journal.ppat.1001116

Ruiter, R. A. C., Abraham, C., & Kok, G. (2001). Scary warnings and rational precautions: A review of the psychology of fear appeals. *Psychology & Health, 16*(6), 613–630.

Sauter, D., Schindler, M., Specht, A., Landford, W. N., Münch, J., Kim, K.-A., … Kirchhoff, F. (2009). Tetherin-driven adaptation of Vpu and Nef function and the evolution of pandemic and nonpandemic HIV-1 strains. *Cell Host & Microbe, 6*(5), 409–421.

Temoshok, L., Sweet, D. M., & Zich, J. (1987). A three city comparison of the public's knowledge and attitudes about AIDS. *Psychology & Health, 1*(1), 43–60.

Worobey, M., Watts, T. D., McKay, R. A., Suchard, M. A., Granade, T., Teuwen, D. E., … Jaffe, H. W. (2016). 1970s and 'Patient 0' HIV-1 genomes illuminate early HIV/AIDS history in North America. *Nature, 539*(7627), 98–101.

3

Sexuality and HIV Risk in Gay Men

The Biology of HIV Risk

There are some biological determinants of HIV risk in gay men. Specific sexual behaviours carry different levels of HIV transmission risk. It is consensually accepted that receptive anal intercourse carries the highest risk of HIV transmission—in fact, the risk of transmission is estimated to be up to 15 times higher than receptive vaginal intercourse (Cresswell et al., 2016). Many gay men engage in anal intercourse—a practice which is more widespread in this population than among heterosexuals—which means that their risk of HIV infection is generally higher. There are several biological reasons that receptive anal sex poses a high risk. First, the rectal lining is thin, delicate and, thus, susceptible to tearing or injury during sexual intercourse, which in turn can provide HIV (present in blood, semen or pre-seminal fluids from the insertive partner) with direct access to the bloodstream. Of course, the risk of injury to rectal tissue during sexual intercourse can be reduced somewhat through the use of lubrication, but use of lubricants is not an effective prevention strategy in itself. Second, the surface area of mucosal membranes in the rectal area is large, which provides more potential entry points for HIV. Third, rectal

© The Author(s) 2020
R. Jaspal, J. Bayley, *HIV and Gay Men*, https://doi.org/10.1007/978-981-15-7226-5_3

tissue actually has a large concentration of CD4 cells which HIV directly targets in establishing an infection in the host (see Chap. 2).

One's sexual 'position' in anal sex also affects one's level of HIV risk—receptive anal intercourse carries a higher risk of transmission than insertive anal intercourse whose risk of transmission is comparable to that of insertive vaginal sex. The surface area of the mucosal membranes on the penis is smaller than the anus, and the virus can gain entry into the body only through a limited area. Anal secretions and blood from surrounding anal tissue render even insertive anal intercourse a high-risk activity for HIV infection. This risk is accentuated in uncircumcised men given that the surface area of the mucosal membranes and presence of 'target cells' for HIV within the foreskin will be greater in an uncircumcised penis than in a circumcised penis. Many gay men report a versatile sexual role, indicating that they engage in *both* receptive and insertive anal intercourse. This increases the risk of infection in gay male communities because a sexually versatile man is susceptible to acquiring HIV when he is sexually receptive (or 'bottom') and more likely to transmit it to his sexual partners when he is sexually insertive (or 'top'). Evidently, this level of HIV risk is not present in heterosexual couples in which men and women are generally restricted to specific sexual 'positions'.

HIV risk is further compounded by the fact that gay men tend to have a much higher number of sexual partners and to engage in a higher number of sexual encounters than the general population. Some of these issues are discussed in more detail in the subsection on sexual compulsivity below. However, suffice to say that the infection risk of one act of anal sex with an HIV-positive individual not on treatment is relatively low at approximately 0.1–3% (Cresswell et al., 2016). This risk obviously increases substantially at an individual level when one has a high frequency of receptive anal intercourse with multiple sexual partners or if the partner has a high viral load.

It is difficult to estimate the risk of HIV transmission during oral sex for two key reasons. First, there are few high-quality studies upon which to base a risk estimate, and, second, few people engage exclusively in oral sex which means that they are also at risk of exposure to HIV through other routes. Yet, a review which included just three studies with small samples of participants who reported oral sex as their only HIV risk behaviour showed no HIV transmissions (Baggaley, White, & Boily, 2008). Although it is impossible to claim, on the basis of these studies, that there is a zero HIV transmission risk, it is clear that the risk associated with oral sex is very low indeed. The advice remains that ejaculation in the mouth should be avoided if there are breaks or inflammation in the oral mucosa (such as a sore throat or bleeding gums). The risk of HIV infection may be greater for the individual who performs oral sex if they have an open wound in the mouth (e.g. a mouth ulcer, bleeding gums), and HIV present in seminal or vaginal fluid is able to gain access to the bloodstream. Yet, even this risk may be offset by the ability of saliva to disrupt the functioning of HIV (Baron, Poast, & Cloyd, 1999).

As outlined in Chap. 5, the key purpose of ART is to reduce the patient's HIV viral load to 'undetectable' levels (usually fewer than 40 copies of HIV per ml of blood). This reduces the risk not only of AIDS in the HIV-infected patient but also of onward HIV transmission. Although it has been estimated that receptive anal intercourse with an insertive sexual partner who is HIV-positive is relatively low, this risk is actually heavily dependent on the viral load of the source. A newly infected individual with a high viral load is significantly more likely to transmit HIV than an individual with middle-stage disease (Wawer et al., 2005). It is now generally accepted that an HIV patient who has had an undetectable viral load for the past six months cannot transmit HIV to their sexual partners (Rodger et al., 2019). Risk of HIV transmission is, thus, dependent on both biological and behavioural factors—the individual must be tested for HIV, diagnosed and treated, and they must initiate ART in order to achieve viral undetectability. These behavioural factors thus impact on the biological outcome of viral undetectability.

There is evidence that having concurrent STIs can increase the risk of HIV acquisition, which has been referred to as 'epidemiological synergy' (Cohen, Council, & Chen, 2019). Having a concurrent STI can increase the infectiousness of the HIV-positive individual because of increments in HIV viral concentration in genital secretions and viral phenotypical changes which facilitate transmission (see Chap. 4). For instance, it has been found that ulcerative STIs increase HIV shedding in the genital tract (Galvin & Cohen, 2004). Cohen et al. (2019) found higher concentrations of HIV in men with concomitant gonorrhoea, which reduced only several weeks after initiation of antibiotic treatment. Similarly, an STI in the HIV-negative person increases their vulnerability to HIV infection due partly to the presence of inflammation and ulcers which can reduce the physical 'barriers' between HIV and the bloodstream. STIs, or indeed any inflammation, cause an influx of CD4 cells (the target for HIV) in the genital region, which can also facilitate infection simply because there are more cells present for HIV to infect.

There are many other factors, aside from infections, that can cause inflammation in the gastrointestinal tract such as inflammatory bowel disease (IBD), namely, ulcerative colitis and Crohn's disease. There are limited data about the interaction between these two conditions, but the presence of ulceration in the rectum would serve to increase the risk of acquiring HIV (Serrero, Peyrin-Biroulet, & Grimaud, 2017). Some data even suggest that the resulting immunosuppression from HIV can reduce the inflammation seen in IBD, but further research is needed in this area. Interestingly, some STIs—especially LGV, a more pathogenic version of chlamydia—can mimic IBD, and these should be checked in all IBD patients deemed to be at risk (Gallegos, Bradly, Jakate, & Keshavarzian, 2012). This is especially important if immunosuppressive therapy for IBD is initiated as it can potentiate the effects of HIV.

Localised trauma is also a factor that influences HIV risk as the presence of breaks in the mucosa (for the HIV-negative person) and blood in the rectum (for the HIV-positive person) are all additive risk factors for acquiring HIV. Common causes of localised trauma include the use of sex toys, douches and fisting—these practices should be enquired about and behaviours modified if the patient is at high risk of HIV. Douches affect the microbiome of the rectal mucosa weakening the protective effect of the mucosal immune defences and can create lacerations if not used correctly—again increasing the risk of HIV. Fisting can be very traumatic, especially if pain thresholds are altered with the use of recreational drugs, and has been shown to increase the chances of HIV and other STIs. In one study (Rice et al., 2016), it was shown that those who engaged in fisting had an adjusted prevalence ratio of 4.75. Thus, education and risk reduction on how to reduce trauma from this practice should be integrated into gay men's sexual healthcare.

The Social Psychology of HIV Risk

At the outset, it is important to note that the debate on HIV prevention (which is the focus of Chap. 4) has focused largely on condom use. In many respects, this is understandable. After all, condoms are highly effective against not only HIV but also most other STIs. However, it must be acknowledged that the toolbox of HIV prevention options has grown significantly and that the personal HIV prevention strategies of gay men have similarly diversified. Many openly acknowledge their non-use of condoms but instead report serosorting, strategic sexual positioning and, increasingly, use of PrEP. None of these strategies are completely effective but they are all designed, and used by gay men, to reduce their risk of HIV infection. To the outside observer, some may seem dangerously ineffective, but to their proponents they reflect an awareness of HIV risk and an attempt to reduce it. In order to have a serious, insightful and progressive debate about HIV prevention, it is important to move beyond the sole focus of condom use to other more creative approaches to preventing infection.

It is generally accepted that HIV prevention campaigns have been highly effective in raising awareness and in enhancing public understanding of HIV. Campaigns have understandably focused on risk awareness in those communities at highest risk of HIV, such as gay men. For decades, gay bars, clubs and saunas have become foci for HIV prevention efforts, and it is difficult to enter these spaces without encountering an HIV prevention poster, information leaflet or complimentary pack of condoms. In short, HIV has been, and remains, visually present in gay spaces and psychologically present in the lives of gay men. Why then do gay men with high levels of HIV awareness continue to take risks? Why has risk awareness resulted not in a decline in HIV infections but, until 2015 at least, in rising incidence? What is the 'blackbox' of risk-taking behaviour?

The short answer to all of these questions is that awareness and understanding, though strong predictors of behaviour change, alone are not sufficient to promote long-term changes in behaviours. There is a tenuous relationship between attitudes and behaviours. Many social psychological factors can disrupt the relationship between risk awareness/ understanding and behaviour and lead people to engage in behaviours which, they know, could imperil their health and wellbeing. It is impossible to summarise every social psychological variable that plays a role in risk-taking, but, in this section, we discuss some of the factors that have been the focus of empirical research.

Attitudes Towards Condoms

Condoms have been the most significant component of our HIV prevention strategy since the beginning of the epidemic. Although condoms are generally very effective, not all gay men use condoms consistently simply because they have negative or ambivalent attitudes towards them (Shernoff, 2006). These attitudes may stem from the belief that condoms will reduce the quality of their sexual encounter or their own sexual performance, that they disrupt the sexual encounter by providing a distraction from the sensuality of the experience or that they impede sexual and emotional intimacy. The first two beliefs can be, and have been, challenged by interventions that aim to make available to individuals the correct type and size of condoms so that they feel more comfortable and, thus, are used more consistently, and by programmes to increase the sensuality and eroticism surrounding condom use.

Conversely, the belief that condoms reduce sexual and emotional intimacy has been more difficult to challenge—some gay men construe condoms not only as a physical barrier, which it of course is, but also as an emotional barrier that inhibits a sexual connection between two individuals. This can be attributed in part to the sensuality associated with 'skin-to-skin' contact but also to the psychological significance that semen can have for some gay men and the sexual arousal that can ensue from the exchange of semen (Jaspal, 2019). Vincke, Bolton, and De Vleeschouwer (2001) describe semen exchange as 'a means of showing devotion, belonging, and oneness' (p. 58). Semen is eroticised by many and perceived to strengthen the bond and unity of two individuals. Furthermore, in their early research into condom use among gay men, Flowers, Smith, Sheeran, and Beail (1997) found that gay men considered non-use of condoms with their primary partners as an expression of commitment, trust and love and that they therefore derived greater emotional intimacy when they did not use condoms. All of these factors can lead gay men to reduce their use of condoms.

Condom self-efficacy is also an important variable. Several theories of behaviour change, such as Social Learning Theory (Bandura, 1997) and the Theory of Planned Behaviour (Ajzen, 1991), highlight the importance of self-efficacy in engendering and sustaining behaviour change. Self-efficacy can be defined in terms of the individual's perceived control and competence to perform a behaviour, and, by extension, condom self-efficacy refers to the individual's perceived control and competence in sexual situations which enable them to use a condom if they wish to do so.

In some sexual situations, the individual may not have the confidence to initiate a conversation about condom use with their sexual partner and may instead wait for their partner to raise the topic. This may lead to engagement in condomless sex and, thus, increased HIV risk. Some gay men do not feel confident about negotiating condom use with their sexual partners and may feel compelled to acquiesce to the demands of their sexual partner, leading to behaviours that increase their risk of HIV acquisition. In some cases, the individual may believe that, by insisting on condom use, they will face rejection from their prospective sexual partner and, thus, miss the opportunity to engage in sex with them. This fear may be especially acute in individuals who habitually face stigma on the basis of their sexual or ethnic identities, for instance, or who have low levels of self-esteem. In Chap. 7, there is a discussion of the impact of gay racism on condom self-efficacy and, thus, HIV risk among ethnic minority gay men.

The Fear Factor

It is clear that fear was an important component of the HIV prevention strategy in the early days of the epidemic and, to a large extent, it was effective. The gay sexual liberation movement, described briefly in Chap. 1, was greatly curtailed as a result of HIV and the fear it induced in relation to condomless sex. Gay men did begin to reduce the number of sexual partners they had and, on the whole, they did begin to use condoms more consistently. This undoubtedly contributed to the control of HIV incidence but of course did not result in its eradication. Although fear was partially successful, there is empirical evidence that fear is limited in its capacity to promote long-term behaviour change (Ruiter, Kessels, Peters, & Kok, 2014). After a specific point, individuals begin to disengage as the 'fear factor' begins to wane or may deflect the hazard in order to avoid the negative emotional experience of fear. In short, people do not generally wish to live in fear and will evolve to lead a fear-free life. Moreover, some gay men resigned themselves to the 'fact' that they would eventually be infected with HIV, which could be attributed to the long-standing fear of infection that they experienced and the observation that others around them were infected. Indeed, even before the advent of ART and, thus, when HIV was still a life-limiting condition, some gay men diagnosed with HIV reported relief because the 'inevitable had happened' and they no longer needed to live in fear of infection.

Yet, there is another dimension to the fear factor in relation to HIV. There is of course a distinction between risk and hazard. The hazard is the harmful event or situation that is feared. Risk is the probability that the hazard will arise. In the early days of the epidemic, AIDS was clearly the hazard—the images of emaciated young men dying alone in hospitals around the country engendered fear in the gay community. In Western, industrialised societies with effective healthcare systems, we have now transitioned into a phase of the epidemic in which AIDS is seen less than it was during the first few decades of the crisis and most recover but some are left with long-term life-changing complications. AIDS is no longer construed as an omnipresent hazard in gay men's lives. In the era of effective ART, the risk of AIDS is deemed to be relatively low if one is diagnosed soon after infection.

Whether HIV infection is construed as a hazard is an interesting question—when HIV was closely associated with AIDS, it probably also represented a hazard in the minds of gay men. Today, its detachment from AIDS, its effective treatment and suppression to 'undetectable' levels and its gradual destigmatisation—in some sections of the population at least—have collectively decreased its construal as a hazard. Many healthcare practitioners no longer refer to AIDS, preferring to use the terms 'late-stage HIV' or 'advanced HIV infection'. In other words, some gay men may erroneously believe that AIDS does not exist. Moreover, they may believe that, because HIV is highly treatable, it is no longer life-threatening and, thus, no longer a hazard to be feared. As gay men increasingly observe others living and thriving with HIV, some even trivialise the condition and believe that the experience of living with HIV amounts to 'one pill a day'. This trivialisation of HIV has probably increased the acceptability of behaviours that in turn accentuate the risk of HIV infection and indeed the acceptability of HIV itself.

Sense of Invincibility

Some gay men simply perceive a sense of invincibility in relation to HIV. They believe that they will not be infected regardless of their sexual behaviour and therefore continue to engage in risk behaviour. Inaccurate risk appraisal is central to perceived invincibility. Essentially, some gay men are not appraising their HIV risk accurately, which contributes to the perception of invincibility in relation to HIV. Given the effectiveness of TasP, which refers to the function of ART to reduce the viral load of HIV patients, thereby rendering them uninfectious, there is growing confidence in HIV-negative gay men who are informed about HIV that their risk of infection is low. Yet, sole reliance on TasP is a problematic prevention strategy given that one's sexual partner may not be aware of their positive serostatus or fully adherent to ART and, thus, not virally suppressed.

Inaccurate risk appraisal can also be attributed to low levels of HIV knowledge. In their survey study of 538 ethnic minority gay and bisexual men, Jaspal and colleagues (2019) observed low levels of HIV knowledge in their sample, and found that those who perceived their sexual behaviour to be least risky had the lowest levels of HIV knowledge, suggesting that their risk appraisals were based on poor knowledge. Moreover, it has been found that psychological wellbeing predicts perceived HIV risk through the mediators of gay identification and sexual identity openness—that is, gay men who have high levels of psychological wellbeing are more able to construct a robust sexual identity which they feel comfortable displaying to others, and this in turn enables them to construe their HIV risk accurately (Jaspal & Lopes, 2020). This demonstrates that risk appraisal is a complex process, which is determined at least in part by psychological factors, such as knowledge and psychological wellbeing.

Some gay men may initially have believed that they were at risk of HIV, but numerous negative test results over the years may reinforce the belief that they will never be infected. Perceived invincibility may be the outcome of inertia and numbness after many years of fear in relation to HIV. Younger people who are also considered a high-risk group for HIV infection are more likely to have invincibility beliefs than other groups in society, which can be attributed to both physiological and social psychological causes (Shernoff, 2006).

There is also a convincing group-level explanation for the invincibility hypothesis. Of course, group identities function at distinct levels. Some gay men 'create' new identity categories and essentialise them, that is, they may come to view some 'types' of gay men as fundamentally different from others. For instance, Jaspal and Daramilas (2016) have found that those who 'do chemsex' (a subgroup of gay men) are perceived to be at higher risk of HIV infection than those who do not. Moreover, Goldenberg, Finneran, Sullivan, Andes, and Stephenson (2016) have found that some gay men perceive other non-gay identified men who have sex with men (another subgroup) as being at lower risk of HIV because they also have sex with women.

In some cases, the group-level explanation for HIV invincibility is based on pre-existing group identities, such as ethnicity or nationality. It has been observed that we tend to associate disease and adversity with outgroups and to perceive outgroup members to be more susceptible to them (Joffe, 2007). Conversely, we have a tendency to view ourselves as 'low risk' in comparison to outgroup members, which is why some people ask 'why me?' when they face disease or adversity. In his study of British South Asian gay men, Jaspal (2018) found that individuals tended to view HIV as a condition affecting White gay men, in particular, which led them to view their strategy of having sex with ethnic ingroup members as low risk. Individuals reported condomless sex with ethnic ingroup members but did not believe that this put them at risk of HIV. Moreover, Joffe (1995) has described the association of HIV with Black Africans, which leads some non-Black people to believe that HIV is irrelevant to them. Conversely, in some African countries, HIV is perceived as a 'White man's disease', which perpetuates the erroneous notion that one is immune to HIV due to one's group membership. Put simply, the misguided sense of HIV invincibility can put one at risk of infection.

Personality Traits

Personality is an important variable in explaining risk behaviours given that certain personality traits do appear to predispose people to behaviours that are risky. Traits such as extraversion, impulsivity and neuroticism all appear to be associated with higher engagement in sexual risk behaviour (Shernoff, 2006). Moreover, personal values (also considered to be personality traits), such as hedonism and stimulation, also appear to be related to engagement in risk behaviour (Goodwin et al., 2002). Yet, one of the most significant correlates of sexual risk behaviour is the personality trait of sensation-seeking, which has been defined as 'the seeking of varied, novel, complex, and intense sensations and experiences, and the willingness to take physical, social, legal, and financial risks for the sake of such experiences' (Zuckerman, 1994, p. 27).

In the pursuit of 'intense sensations' such as those afforded by condomless sex, the individual may readily take the risk of being infected with HIV. He may downplay the risk itself, convincing himself (and others) that the risk is not really as high as commonly believed. It is easy to see how this sense of invincibility and complacency might support sensation-seeking behaviour. Furthermore, awareness of the risk of HIV infection itself may provide the sensation-seeker with a thrill—knowing that one *could*, but may not, be infected with HIV may be psychologically gratifying for the sensation-seeker. Indeed, sensation-seeking has been used to explain the unusual practice of 'bugchasing' whereby one deliberately seeks to acquire or actively puts oneself at high risk of HIV infection (Jaspal, 2019).

In their review of empirical research into personality and sexual risk-taking, Hoyle, Fejfar, and Miller (2000) found that sensation-seeking predicted all forms of sexual risk behaviour. However, it must be noted that sexual risk behaviours are multifarious, and that some behaviours commonly thought to increase the risk of HIV infection may be practised relatively safely. For instance, in a study of 16,362 participants from 52 countries, Schmitt (2004) found that agreeableness and conscientiousness were negatively correlated with both relationship infidelity and sexual promiscuity and that the latter was positively associated with extraversion. Relationship infidelity and sexual promiscuity were conceptualised as risky sexual behaviour, but there is of course nothing inherently risky about these behaviours. It is quite possible to practice safer sex with partners that one's primary partner is aware of and to have sex with multiple partners using a condom or PrEP. In short, personality research may be telling us more about the types of behaviour one is more or less likely to adopt, rather than about HIV risk per se. It is therefore necessary to look at how personality functions in conjunction with other variables, such as social norms.

Social Norms

Social norms are collective representations of what is acceptable and appropriate behaviour in any given context. They differ from individual attitudes in that they are shared by members of a group, but they do tend to shape the individual beliefs and attitudes of group members. Social norms are significant because they have the power to shape, promote and constrain particular behaviours, and can be used to foster the acceptance and inclusion of those individuals who adopt the norms and the exclusion of those who do not. Like any other social group, gay men have developed social norms about 'appropriate' sexual attitudes, sexual behaviours and relationship types. At the height of the HIV epidemic, condom use became normative as massive efforts were enacted to promote the use of condoms among gay men. This norm was reflected and reinforced in pornographic films, in gay saunas and bathhouses and in everyday conversation between gay men. Indeed, non-use of condoms was widely regarded as reckless, irresponsible behaviour, which has also been described as 'slut shaming' (Spieldenner, 2016).

More recently, the social norm of condom use is changing. More gay men are 'coming out' as barebackers and are reaffirming their right to decide the level of HIV risk that they find acceptable. Many are using PrEP and other alternative HIV prevention methods. Many are using technology and frequenting specific contexts to seek like-minded others. In gay communities in Britain, the norm of condom use is waning, and several of the factors described above may be contributing to the cessation of this norm. For instance, the fear factor that has surrounded condomless sex has been replaced by feelings of safety among PrEP users and those aware of TasP. There is arguably now social pressure to forego condoms in sex, which has been developing since the advent of effective ART (Morin et al., 2003). In much gay pornography, condoms are no longer used, which too is contributing to the emerging counter-norm of condomless sex. Gay men who advocate, or insist on, condom use may be derided by others who lay claim to other HIV prevention methods. To return to our original definition of a social norm, it is increasingly the case that those gay men whose sole approach to HIV prevention is condom use are being positioned as 'outsiders' and that condomless sex is being represented as 'progressive'.

Identity Concerns

The role of identity in risk is significant. In response to the coercive norm of condom use among gay men, there has also been an emergence of a counter-norm of condomless sex. Some gay men who actively and purposefully engage in condomless sex refer to the practice as 'barebacking' and view themselves as 'barebackers'. Barebacking has developed into a social identity, since many gay men view themselves as having something in common with others who practice this sexual activity, perceive solidarity with one another and may deride gay men who do not share this sexual practice and who attempt to stigmatise it (Shernoff, 2006). The barebacking community provides a sense of belonging to some gay men who identify with it, and they are afforded feelings of acceptance and inclusion. Crucially, self-identified barebackers derive a sense of pride and self-esteem on the basis of their barebacking identity. As noted above, every social group has norms and so does the barebacking 'community'. Key norms include condomless sex and defiance towards the coercive norm of condom use. This community also has symbols and markers, such as the biohazard sign, to differentiate themselves from non-barebackers. Activists, pornstars and prominent gay men living with HIV, such as Scott O'Hara and Tony Valenzuela, openly 'came out' about their barebacking identity and became self-designated spokespersons for the barebacking community.

Identity process theory (see Chap. 6) postulates that identity processes are guided by the principles of self-esteem, continuity, distinctiveness, self-efficacy and coherence. We actively strive to maintain appropriate levels of these principles in thought and action, and feel 'threatened' when these principles are curtailed (for whatever reason). Vignoles and colleagues (Vignoles, Regalia, Manzi, Golledge, & Scabini, 2006) have shown that we tend to view as more central those identity elements (e.g. behaviours, representations) that provide us with appropriate levels of the identity principles. In the context of environmental behaviour, for instance, it has been shown that identity threat can impede behaviour change, especially when the identity element concerned is important to the individual (Murtagh, Gatersleben, & Uzzell, 2014). This is consistent with the hypothesis that, while negative emotions such as fear may be effective in the short term, it is unlikely to be a long-term solution to risk behaviour. When individuals face threats to identity, they experience negative affect, which can lead to deflection (e.g. denial, reconceptualisation, compartmentalisation) to protect identity.

As noted later in this chapter, some behaviours known to increase the risk of HIV, such as condomless sex and chemsex, may provide feelings of self-esteem, distinctiveness and so on. For some gay men, these high-risk activities may actually restore appropriate levels of identity principles which have previously been curtailed. For instance, many gay men experience poor self-esteem due to years of (internalised) homophobia, body image concerns and other adverse events, but in chemsex settings they may regain those lost feelings of self-esteem as they feel attractive to others and able to derive intimacy—sometimes for the first time (Jaspal,

2018). Furthermore, Shernoff (2006) has noted that the practice of 'bare-backing' can enable gay men to regain a sense of control over their HIV status amid the uncertainty, fear and perceived inevitability of their infection. In such cases, behaviours that increase HIV risk (i.e. barebacking and chemsex) can be said to enhance self-efficacy and other principles of identity. Therefore, it is easy to see why gay men may wish to maintain these behaviours despite their awareness that they may put them at risk of HIV infection. Indeed, as Pinkerton and Abramson (1992, p. 561) have indicated, engagement in risk behaviour may actually be rational in that 'the perceived physical, emotional, and psychological benefits of sex outweigh the threat of acquiring HIV'. In short, identity concerns may override risk awareness.

Poor mental health is a known risk factor for HIV with those suffering from depression and anxiety being more prone to sexual risk behaviours (Gerrard, Gibbons, & McCoy, 1993). Moreover, some mental health conditions can undermine the individual's ability to appraise risk effectively and to act rationally. In Chap. 6, we discuss the interface of mental health and HIV and outline evidence that poor mental health may lead some gay men to engage in behaviours that put them at risk of HIV infection. The social psychological antecedents, such as homophobia, of many mental health conditions among gay men are also outlined. That discussion will not be reproduced here. However, it is worth pointing out that, despite the observed role of poor mental health in HIV risk behaviour, it is important to avoid pathologising *all* instances of HIV risk behaviour as symptomatic of poor mental health.

Indeed, there are many seemingly 'rational' reasons underpinning gay men's engagement in high-risk behaviour. Some gay men feel that condom use impedes intimacy. Some believe that their risk of HIV is lower than that of other people. Some reach the conclusion that the psychological pros of the sexual risk behaviour outweigh the potential physical cons. Yet, outside observers may focus on the hazard (in this case, HIV, a lifelong incurable condition), disregard the extraneous variables that clearly disrupt the relationship between risk awareness and behaviour and, thus, conclude that the risk-taker is invariably suffering from some form of psychopathology. As highlighted in Chap. 6, it is likely that, in some cases, some sexual behaviours provide the individual (who may or may not be suffering from poor mental health) with psychological gratification. These sexual behaviours may well put the individual at risk of HIV infection. However, it is the psychological gratification, not the risk awareness, that drives this behaviour. In their study of 250 gay men, Halkitis and Wilton (2005) found that sex enhanced mood, reduced stress and safeguarded intimacy. It is of course foreseeable that those with reduced mood, compromised intimacy and high levels of stress might therefore seek out sexual experiences. For some, sex is quite simply a psychological escape—it provides temporary respite from the psychological ups and downs—a 'safe space' where one's troubles can be forgotten.

Risky Sexual Behaviours

Some sexual behaviours, which increase the risk of HIV infection, are prevalent and even normative among gay men. In this section, we describe some of these behaviours, including sexual compulsivity, the emergence of 'chemsex', and the use of geospatial gay mobile social networking applications and of public/commercial venues to find casual sexual partners. We focus on the social psychological underpinnings of these behaviours and their association with HIV risk.

Sexual Compulsivity

On the whole, gay men tend to have a higher number of sexual partners and report greater frequency of sexual behaviour than heterosexual men (Jaspal, 2019). Having a high number of sexual partners and a high frequency of sex is sometimes hastily labelled as sexual compulsivity, but this is misleading. How one defines 'too many' partners or encounters is a subjective matter—what one person considers to be 'normal' may be construed by someone else as 'excessive'. Sexual compulsivity refers to the frequent occurrence of sexual fantasies, urges and behaviours, over which the individual has little or no control, and which disrupts the individual's daily functioning. Thus, there is an element of subjectivity associated with sexual compulsivity—an individual may have multiple sexual partners every week but still have a positive self-image, have positive connections with others in his social environment and function adequately at work. Despite the number of sexual partners and the frequency of sexual encounters that he has, he may have an adequate level of psychological wellbeing and reject that he is sexually compulsive. It may be inaccurate, and even stigmatising, to label him as sexually compulsive when his sexual behaviour appears to have no adverse impact on his daily functioning. Conversely, another gay man may have a much lower number of sexual partners, but feel guilty about this number, prioritise his unsatisfactory sexual encounters over his relationships with significant others and over his work life, leading to poor social and occupational wellbeing. Although he may not initially accept the label 'sexual compulsivity', he acknowledges that his sexual behaviour is having an adverse impact on his daily functioning. One might reasonably label his behaviour as sexually compulsive.

Sexual compulsivity does appear to be more prevalent among gay men than among heterosexual men, and more prevalent in gay men living with HIV than among those who are HIV-negative (Coleman et al., 2010). The higher prevalence of sexual compulsivity in these populations may be attributed to the higher risk of psychological stress among individuals from these populations—sexual compulsivity may be considered a maladaptive coping response to such stress (Jaspal, 2018). In addition to its adverse effects on psychological wellbeing, sexual compulsivity can increase one's risk of HIV and other STIs—due to both the frequency of sexual encounters and the higher number of sexual partners. Furthermore, sexual compulsivity tends to be accompanied by an elevated state of sexual arousal which can result in decreased inhibitions and in reduced capacity to think and act rationally—one may forego condoms in such situations (Bancroft et al., 2003). Indeed, gay men with sexual compulsivity report a higher number of sexual partners than gay men with no sexual compulsivity, engage in more frequent condomless sex (including with HIV-positive partners or with those of unknown status) and are more likely to engage in chemsex (Grov, Parsons & Bimbi, 2010). It is also noteworthy that gay men living with HIV who have sexual compulsivity are less likely to disclose their HIV status to sexual partners, which in turn can undermine their individual health outcomes and public health outcomes, due to the increased risk of onward HIV transmission (Rosser et al., 2008).

There is an inverse relationship between self-esteem and sexual compulsivity (Chaney & Burns-Wortham, 2015). This suggests that gay men with sexual compulsivity tend to have a negative self-image, either because of sexual compulsivity or as a precursor to the practice. Furthermore, gay men with sexual compulsivity are more likely to report a history of childhood sexual abuse, depressive symptomatology and substance use (Parsons, Grov, & Golub, 2012), which suggests that sexual compulsivity may be part of a broader repertoire of risk behaviours as an overall escapist coping response. Moreover, the experience of proximal minority stress (e.g. internalised homophobia) and emotion dysregulation (the inability to manage the intensity and duration of one's emotions) are related to sexual compulsivity in gay men (Pachankis et al., 2015). This association can be attributed to homophobia pervasively experienced by many gay men who may internalise this stigma, feel obligated to conceal their sexual identities and cope individually with the negative emotions associated with homophobia.

Sexual compulsivity can be considered a coping response because it often represents an attempt to buffer the negative psychological effects of rejection, proximal minority stressors and emotion dysregulation. Some gay men engage in sexually compulsive behaviours in order to enhance identity proactively—they may do so to establish (transient) feelings of intimacy and connectedness with other people. Furthermore, sex is sometimes used as a means of assuaging anxiety, shame, guilt and other negative emotions, which are associated with stressful experiences. Regardless of the social psychological antecedents of sexual compulsivity, it is associated with increased risk of HIV infection.

Clinical Snapshot 2: Chemsex

Chemsex is the use of recreational drugs used in sexualised settings, namely, mephedrone, crystal methamphetamine and GHB (gamma hydroxybutyrate). In the last ten years, there has been an increase in the use of these drugs amongst gay men, especially in the cities of the UK. A more worrying trend has been the use (and subsequent sexualisation) of 'slamming' (injecting), with the risks inherent to this (especially needle sharing and transmis-

sion of HIV and hepatitis B and C). Identifying and dealing with this issue in clinic is difficult—many gay men are hesitant about acknowledging their chemsex behaviour due to stigma and shame in relation to injecting drugs. The clinician must not appear to be judgemental and must accept that not all of those identified will want to stop. Patients should be supported and risk reduction strategies implemented (e.g. needle exchange programmes or education about safer dosing of GHB). The patient should be signposted to culturally appropriate services for support and treatment. Sometimes, even though chemsex has been identified, it does not require immediate action. This can represent a dilemma for clinicians, and one's own prejudices must be challenged so that the clinician can work with the patient to ensure their safety and wellbeing.

Chemsex

The practice of chemsex, which refers to the use of psychoactive drugs in sexualised settings, has become increasingly widespread among gay men in large cities around the world. There is evidence that not only the prevalence is increasing even in small- to medium-sized cities in Britain and beyond but also the rates of injecting drugs, especially in gay men living with HIV. In one large survey (Frankis, Flowers, McDaid, & Bourne, 2018), only 3% of gay men had participated in chemsex in the preceding four weeks, but HIV-positive men were four times more likely to participate. Rates of injecting drug use is double those of who are HIV-negative—whether this increased risk is a direct result of adjusting to being diagnosed with HIV or to an altered risk appraisal in those living with HIV is difficult to say.

Chemsex participants tend to use mephedrone, γ-hydroxybutyrate (GHB), γ-butyrolactone (GBL) and crystallised methamphetamine in order to enhance sexual encounters—often in group settings—that can last for hours or days. The physiological impact of chemsex drugs vary—for instance, mephedrone raises sexual arousal in many, while GHB and GBL function as potent psychological disinhibitors, leading to engagement in novel and unusual sexual behaviours. It is easy to see how the practice of chemsex might increase one's risk of HIV infection.

It is difficult to ascertain unequivocally the prevalence of chemsex in Britain. First, it would be necessary to identify a definition of chemsex and for respondents to endorse that definition in studies relying on self-report data. Drug use in sexualised settings has existed for many, many years, but there is something novel and distinctive about the practice of chemsex. Many do not view themselves as 'doing chemsex'. Second, an accurate snapshot of chemsex would require a representative sample of gay men in Britain. Even the more significant surveys of gay men suffer from an element of sampling bias—in other words, some groups of gay men are more likely to complete the survey than others, and, thus, the prevalence of chemsex that we estimate may be inaccurate.

In any case, the available evidence suggests that chemsex is fairly widespread and that it is growing. The Chemsex Study (Bourne, Reid, Hickson, Torres Rueda, & Weatherburn, 2014) revealed that a fifth of the gay male survey respondents living in Lambeth, Southwark and Lewisham (three London boroughs with significant populations of gay men) reported chemsex in the last five years and that a tenth had engaged in the practice in the last month. Baseline data from the PROUD study, whose inclusion criteria focused on gay men at high risk of HIV infection, revealed that 44% of the 525 study participants reported chemsex in the last three months (Dolling et al., 2016). However, this study perhaps tells us less about the prevalence of chemsex in gay men than it does about the high risk of HIV in that particular setting.

There have been attempts to ascertain the prevalence of chemsex in studies conducted in clinical settings. In a retrospective case notes review study in two sexual health clinics in London, Lee et al. (2015) found that 59% of the gay male clinic attendees reported chemsex. Those who reported chemsex were more likely to be HIV-positive than those who did not. Indeed, a consistent finding across a growing number of empirical studies is that chemsex is especially prevalent among gay men living with HIV. In a study of HIV patients recruited from 30 UK HIV clinics in 2014 (Pufall et al., 2016), it was found that 29% of sexually active gay men had engaged in chemsex and that 10% had injected drugs in sexualised settings in the previous year.

Furthermore, survey data from 1484 HIV-negative or undiagnosed gay men recruited from 20 sexual health clinics in the UK revealed that over a fifth of respondents had engaged in chemsex in the last 3 months (Sewell et al., 2017). This suggests that a considerable proportion of gay men report regular and recent chemsex, and that this is a significant aspect of their lives. Pakianathan et al.'s (2018) retrospective case notes review study revealed that 16.5% of all gay men attending two London sexual health clinics during a 12-month period reported chemsex in the past, who in turn were more likely to report recent HIV infection. Recently diagnosed gay men who lack social support and who have not yet come to terms with their diagnosis may perceive chemsex as an attractive strategy for 'escaping' from the adverse social psychological aspects of their infection. This is consistent with the construal of chemsex as a form of escapism (Bourne et al., 2014). Moreover, this suggests that chemsex may be a context in which onward HIV transmission is not only possible but likely—especially if those recently diagnosed with HIV do not yet have an undetectable viral load.

The reasons underpinning chemsex behaviour are varied and complex. Chemsex participants tend to report better sexual experiences than they do when sober. This can be attributed to the tendency for some substances to reduce inhibitions and to increase sexual pleasure. It is possible that individuals who are dissatisfied with their current sexual experiences are more prone to chemsex than those who are satisfied, thereby suggesting a low 'baseline' of sexual satisfaction. Furthermore, in their seminal study of chemsex in Lewisham, Lambeth and Southwark London boroughs, Bourne et al. (2014) found that engagement in chemsex might decrease negative affect associated with adverse experiences, such as (internalised) homophobia, sexual rejection and HIV stigma, which in turn might protect their sense of self-esteem.

Conversely, the positive affect experienced during chemsex may lead to a form of psychological dependence on the practice, as some individuals may come to believe that the practice meets their sexual, social and psychological needs more readily than sober sex. Indeed, identity process theory postulates that events, beliefs and behaviours that are deemed to enhance identity processes are likely to be endorsed by the individual more readily than those that do not (Vignoles et al., 2006). Bourne et al.'s (2014) study has shown that chemsex participants may come to find sober sex unsatisfactory, leading to an inability to engage in sex outside of the chemsex environment.

In their overview of the possible causes of chemsex in gay men, Pollard, Nadarzynski, and Llewellyn (2017) suggest that stigma at multiple levels, minority stress and maladaptive coping strategies may contribute to the motivation to engage in chemsex. Furthermore, Weatherburn, Hickson, Reid, Torres-Rueda, and Bourne (2017) describe two distinct sets of motivations underlying chemsex. First, chemsex enables gay men to engage in the type of sex that they desire by increasing their sexual stamina and confidence and by decreasing inhibitions and, second, chemsex drugs enhance the quality of the sexual encounter by increasing interpersonal attraction and rapport (see also Bourne et al., 2014). Moreover, in chemsex settings, individuals report greater ability to engage in stigmatised sexual behaviours that might ordinarily be regarded as 'extreme' or 'high risk', such as transactional sex, group sex, fisting, sharing sex toys and HIV serodiscordant sexual relations (Lee et al., 2015).

Qualitative research has provided some insight into the reported motivations for engaging in chemsex. In the absence of experimental social psychological research, it is difficult to ascertain unequivocally the true causes of chemsex behaviour, other than that people find it a pleasurable activity. We can but speculate. Research into the correlates of chemsex provides a good empirical starting point for hypotheses concerning causality which can be tested in future research. Pufall et al. (2018) focused on HIV-positive gay men and found that engagement in chemsex was associated in part with diagnosed depression and anxiety. This suggests that, for some gay men at least, chemsex functions as a form of escapism because it enables them to distance themselves from social and psychological stressors which cause depression and anxiety. The practice may provide temporary respite from depressive symptomatology and obviate the practical obstacles that tend to emerge from it, such as avoidance, decreased self-confidence and low sex drive. Furthermore, in view of body image concerns that many gay men report, gay men who engage in chemsex may derive greater confidence about their physical appearance or sexual performance in this context than in sober settings. Gay men living with HIV tend to report that, in chemsex settings, positive HIV serostatus ceases to constitute a barrier for finding sexual partners or for establishing feelings of intimacy with partners.

Geospatial Gay Mobile Social Networking Applications

Geospatial gay mobile social networking applications (henceforth 'gay apps') play an important role in the lives of many gay men (Goedel & Duncan, 2015). Grindr, which was launched in 2009, is one of the most significant gay apps with over five million daily users in hundreds of countries.[1] Gay men use gay apps for a variety of purposes—to broaden their social circles, to establish romantic relationships but most commonly to seek casual sexual encounters. For many gay men, gay apps are a preferred method of communication with other gay men because one can control one's level of 'outness' and, thus, find sex without revealing one's identity or displaying a photograph. Prior to the advent of the Internet, gay men used various social and physical spaces to meet sexual partners, such as saunas/bathhouses and bars/clubs (Bérubé, 1996; Jaspal & Papaloukas, 2020). When the Internet became more widely available in the 1990s, it changed the ways in which gay men sought sexual partners—they were able to identify other gay men much more easily because their sexual orientation was no longer invisible on gay-related dating websites and then on gay apps. Moreover, some gay men feel safer meeting others online than in cruising grounds or in gay saunas where they may face rejection, harassment or even violence (Hennelly, 2010).

Although gay men do use gay apps for a variety of purposes, the search for casual sex is a key purpose. One survey revealed that 38% of Grindr users reported using Grindr to find new sexual partners and that, on average, they reported using the application 8 times per day and spending almost an hour and a half on the application per day (Goedel & Duncan, 2015). In their study of sexual partner-seeking among gay men, Grov, Breslow, Newcomb, Rosenberger, and Bauermeister (2014) found that Grindr users tended to have more sexual partners than those seeking sex in offline settings.

The proliferation of gay apps has facilitated social and sexual contact between gay men with implications for self-identity. Blackwell and Birnholtz (2015) have noted that Grindr enables gay men to connect

---

[1] https://www.statista.com/statistics/719621/grindr-user-number/.

with one another in ways that transcend geographical boundaries, thereby 'often blurring the boundaries around physical places and communities defined by shared interests in particular activities' (p. 17). This transcendence of physical space and 'communities' has implications for HIV risk. In their study of young gay men, Landovtiz et al. (2013) found that men recruited via Grindr were at especially high risk of HIV acquisition or transmission. Furthermore, in a study of 146 gay men recruited on Grindr, 20% of respondents had engaged in condomless sex with a sexual partner whom they had met on the application (Winetrobe, Rice, Bauermeister, Petering, & Holloway, 2014).

In his qualitative study of gay men who use Grindr, Jaspal (2017) found that users perceived a coercive norm of seeking casual sex on the application but also derived greater agency and self-efficacy in relation to their sexuality and sexual preferences on the application. Moreover, they felt more able to negotiate condom use prior to meeting with potential partners. This suggests that Grindr use may also be protective against HIV in that individuals feel more able to negotiate the type of sex they want, on the one hand, but it may also increase HIV risk in that it facilitates more sexual encounters with more sexual partners than other contexts, on the other hand. Yet, it must also be acknowledged that, like other HIV risk contexts, Grindr may be a feasible platform for HIV prevention, including awareness-raising and the distribution of HIV self-testing kits (e.g. Rosengren et al., 2016).

Gay Saunas

Gay saunas are a commercial space in which gay and other MSM can meet sexual partners. In this environment, it is possible to have relatively anonymous sexual encounters, sometimes with no verbal communication, in dyadic or group settings. When the first cases of AIDS were being discovered, gay saunas were fairly widespread in London, New York and other major cities and widely frequented by gay men (Bérubé, 1996). Gay saunas were quickly identified as a key site of HIV transmission, and attempts to close them were resisted by civil rights advocates in the early AIDS crisis only fuelling the epidemic further. However, it must also be acknowledged that gay saunas have since become an important context for raising awareness of safer sex and for enhancing HIV prevention efforts (Jaspal & Papaloukas, 2020).

Gay saunas are used for various purposes. Sex-seeking is a key purpose. Haubrich, Myers, Calzavara, Ryder, and Medved (2004) interviewed 23 users of a gay sauna in Toronto and found that they valued ease of access to sex in the sauna (in contrast to other venues), that anonymity was important to them and that they felt safer in the sauna than in other contexts. However, it is clear that the gay sauna can also perform functions for identity and psychological wellbeing. Bérubé (1996) notes that the gay sauna can enable gay men to overcome isolation to develop pride in their sexuality and to derive a sense of community with other gay men (see also Prior, 2009). Moreover, in their study of gay male sauna users, Jaspal and Papaloukas (2020) found that individuals derived feelings of identity authenticity and belongingness in that they felt able to express their sexualities authentically and to do so with the support of other gay men. In psychology, authenticity is conceptualised as 'the sense that one's life, both public and private, reflects one's real self' (George, 1998, p. 134). Belongingness is defined as the 'pervasive drive to form and maintain at least a minimum quantity of lasting, positive, and significant interpersonal relationships' which are characterised by 'affectively pleasant interactions' and by 'affective concern for each other's welfare' (Baumeister & Leary, 1995, p. 497).

In their survey of 134 gay sauna users in South West England, Horwood et al. (2016) found high rates of HIV risk behaviour, including higher numbers of casual sexual partners and higher frequency of condomless anal sex than in community samples of gay men recruited in other contexts. Moreover, it has been found that gay men who engage in unprotected anal intercourse are in turn more likely to report gay sauna attendance than those who do not, suggesting that sexual risk-takers are more likely to use this context to seek sexual partners (Binson, Pollack, Blair, & Woods, 2010). The work of Mazick et al. (2005) reiterates the prevalence of sexual risk-taking in gay sauna users—gay sauna attendance was a significant risk factor for hepatitis A infection and most of those infected had had sex in a gay sauna.

However, gay contexts can also be an effective context for the prevention of HIV. In their evaluation study, Ko et al. (2009) found that a structural intervention to increase condom use for anal sex among gay men was successful in producing this effect at the six-month follow-up. In recent years, there has been an increase in HIV testing in gay saunas in the US where approximately 75% of the saunas provide this service (Pollack, Woods, Blair, & Binson, 2014). There is evidence of high acceptability and effectiveness of HIV self-testing in gay saunas (Woods, Lippman, Agnew, Carroll, & Binson, 2016). Crucially, HIV prevention in gay saunas can target subgroups of gay men who might not ordinarily engage with sexual health services and who might therefore be missed through conventional HIV prevention routes (Debattista, 2015).

Gay Cruising

The practice of 'cruising' refers to the pursuit of, and interaction with, potential sexual partners, previously unknown to the individual, in public settings. There are usually specific locations which are informally known to be frequented by gay men in search of casual sex with other men. These may include parks, beaches, car parks, public toilets and alleyways. Unlike commercial sex venues, these public areas are of course not designed to facilitate sexual encounters but are used by those who cruise for this very purpose. Some men frequent venues known to be cruising venues, while others may seek sexual partners haphazardly in new areas. In these contexts, codified behaviours and non-verbal expression are habitually used to indicate and confirm sexual interest.

Cruising must be contextualised in the social and legal history of homosexuality in the UK (Jaspal, 2019). Homosexuality was of course illegal until the promulgation of the Sexual Offences Act 1967. Prior to that legislation, there were no official venues in which gay and bisexual men could meet openly, which led many to seek sexual partners using clandestine methods, such as in public places where they could remain relatively anonymous (Norton, 2007). Historically, venues known for gay cruising were policed, and arrests were indeed made, with even some significant political figures having to resign from their positions due to their apprehension. The reputational threat of social and legal sanction has also had to be managed alongside the physical threat of homophobic violence—indeed, in 2005 the young gay man Jody Dobrowski was brutally murdered on Clapham Common in London, a site known for gay cruising. Although the Sexual Offences Act 2003 continues to criminalise sex in public toilets, the law does not explicitly prohibit cruising in other venues, although individuals may be charged under the Public Order Act 1986, if their sexual act has been, or is likely to be, witnessed by a third party.

There have been claims that gay men engage in cruising because they are afraid of disclosing their sexual orientation to others and, thus, view this as the only acceptable means of meeting sexual partners, that those who cruise do so because of specific personality traits and that they are sexually compulsive (Shernoff, 2006). For some gay men who cruise, these claims are undoubtedly true. However, this is by no means true of all gay men who cruise—for instance, in their study of gay and bisexual college students who cruise for sex on campus, Reece and Dodge (2003) found that most participants were secure and open about their sexual orientation and were not sexually compulsive and perceived cruising as just one component of the broader repertoire of sexual behaviours within their sexual identity. Cruising is likely to provide sexual gratification to the sensation-seeker in pursuit of a 'thrill', and the risk of being seen by a passer-by or caught while having sex can be arousing for some.

Crucially, cruising is associated with HIV risk. Gay men who cruise for sex tend to be much more sexually active than those who do not—Frankis and Flowers (2006) found that almost a third of their sample of gay men recruited in cruising venues in Southern England had had over 50 sexual partners in the last year, that is, at least one new sexual partner every week. Similarly, in their study of gay men in Norway, Moseng and Bjørnshagen (2017) found that, on the whole, those who frequent cruising grounds have a much higher number of sexual partners than those who seek sex in other contexts and that a significant proportion has either never tested for HIV or last tested several months ago.

In their study of 580 gay men recruited on a popular geospatial gay social networking application in Paris, Al-Ajlouni et al. (2018) found that attendance at cruising venues was associated with condomless receptive anal sex, any kind of condomless anal sex, engagement in group sex, and sex with multiple partners. This was confirmed through an association between attendance at cruising venues and STI and HIV diagnoses. With the exception of group sex, none of these sexual risk behaviours was associated with sex-seeking in other contexts (such as at gay clubs or online), suggesting that cruising is an especially high-risk behaviour for gay men.

Similarly, Melendez-Torres, Hickson, Reid, Weatherburn, and Bonell (2016) studied the sexual encounters of gay men in England and found that, unlike encounters in sex-on-premises venues, those in cruising contexts were not associated with decreased odds of condomless anal sex. This could be attributed to the availability of condoms in sex-on-premises venues and the inconsistency of condom availability in cruising contexts. Binson et al. (2001) found that a quarter of the gay men who had engaged in cruising in their study reported having group sex and that a fifth of participants reported condomless sex with a casual partner. Berg, Tikkanen, and Ross (2013) studied the sexual behaviour of 3634 gay men in Nordic countries and found that those who reported condomless sex were more likely to have engaged in cruising in the preceding year and to have found their last sexual partner in a cruising venue.

Furthermore, Gesink et al. (2018) categorised gay men in accordance with their preferred context for sex-seeking and found that 'rovers' (those who have sex in cruising settings at least 80% of the time) exhibited the highest HIV prevalence (of 66%) of all other categories of gay and bisexual men. Similarly, in their study of 1011 gay men in Portugal, Gama et al. (2017) found an almost threefold higher prevalence of HIV in those who reported frequenting cruising venues compared to those who did not. Binson et al. (2001) found that 61.8% of HIV-positive gay men who participated in their study reported frequenting a cruising venue in the last 12 months. Gay men living with HIV who cruise are also less likely to use condoms than those who are HIV-negative (Frankis & Flowers, 2006).

Serosorting is by no means an effective strategy for reducing HIV risk since individuals may be unaware of, or unable to disclose, their actual HIV status. Yet, serosorting does often entail a discussion about HIV and risk reduction before a sexual encounter. It provides an opportunity for individuals to share their HIV status and, if positive, to behave in a manner that reduces the risk of HIV transmission. In their study of 881 gay men in France, Velter, Bouyssou-Michel, Arnaud, and Semaille (2009) found that, regardless of HIV status, gay men who cruised for sex were less likely to serosort than those who did not. This suggests that no discussion of HIV or risk reduction takes place, which in turn likely increases the risk of infection.

In short, cruising behaviour is associated with engagement in HIV risk behaviour. However, like gay saunas, cruising venues are an important context in which HIV prevention services can be offered and in which 'hard-to-reach' gay men, such as those who are foreign-born or of ethnic minority background, can be accessed (Strömdahl, Hoijer, & Eriksen, 2019).

Overview

In this chapter, it has been shown that biological and social psychological factors, collectively, determine the individual's risk of HIV infection. Although some sexual behaviours (such as condomless anal sex) do put gay men at higher risk of infection than others, social psychological considerations can also affect the level of risk. HIV risk awareness and understanding, for instance, are key social psychological considerations. In this chapter, the social psychological underpinnings of HIV risk were explored, including the role of fear, perceived invincibility, social norms, identity concerns and personality traits. These factors operate at different levels of human identity—some are social and group based, while others are individual factors. Moreover, it is clear that some behavioural trends in gay communities around the world are further fuelling the HIV epidemic. Sexual compulsivity, chemsex, use of geospatial gay social networking applications, gay saunas and gay cruising are just some examples. Their emergence can be attributed to many factors, including the long history of prejudice, which has led gay men to seek 'safe' and discreet spaces for seeking sexual partners, and to the desire to seek a sense of distinctiveness from heterosexuals by challenging norms and practices deemed to be heteronormative. The quest for a distinctive identity, of which gay men can be proud, has undoubtedly contributed to HIV risk. Biological, social and psychological drivers of risk must be explored and understood by researchers, practitioners and policymakers. This is critical for effective HIV prevention.

References

Ajzen, I. (1991). The theory of planned behavior. *Organizational Behavior and Human Decision Processes, 50*(2), 179–211.

Al-Ajlouni, Y. A., Park, S. H., Schneider, J. A., Goedel, W. C., Rhodes Hambrick, H., Hickson, D. A., ... Duncan, D. T. (2018). Partner meeting venue typology and sexual risk behaviors among French men who have sex with men. *International Journal of STD & AIDS, 29*(13), 1282–1288.

Baggaley, R. F., White, R. G., & Boily, M. C. (2008). Systematic review of oro-genital HIV-1 transmission probabilities. *International Journal of Epidemiology, 37*(6), 1255–1265.

Bancroft, J., Janssen, E., Strong, D., Carnes, L. C., Vukadinovic, Z., & Long, J. S. (2003). The relationship between mood and sexuality in heterosexual men. *Archives of Sexual Behavior, 32*, 217–230.

Bandura, A. (1997). *Self-efficacy: The exercise of control*. New York: W. H. Freeman.

Baron, S., Poast, J., & Cloyd, M. W. (1999). Why is HIV rarely transmitted by oral secretions? Saliva can disrupt orally shed, infected leukocytes. *Archives of Internal Medicine, 159*(3), 303–310.

Baumeister, R. F., & Leary, M. R. (1995). The need to belong: Desire for inter-personal attachments as a fundamental human motivation. *Psychological Bulletin, 117*(3), 497–529.

Berg, R. C., Tikkanen, R., & Ross, M. W. (2013). Barebacking among men who have sex with men recruited through a Swedish website: Associations with sexual activities at last sexual encounter. *Eurosurveillance, 18*(13), pii=20438. https://doi.org/10.2807/ese.18.13.20438-en

Bérubé, A. (1996). The history of gay bathhouses. *Journal of Homosexuality, 44*(3), 33–53.

Binson, D., Pollack, L. M., Blair, J., & Woods, W. J. (2010). HIV transmission risk at a gay bathhouse. *Journal of Sex Research, 47*(6), 580–588.

Binson, D., Woods, W. J., Pollack, L., Paul, J., Stall, R., & Catania, J. A. (2001). Differential HIV risk in bathhouses and public cruising areas. *American Journal of Public Health, 91*(9), 1482–1486.

Blackwell, C., & Birnholtz, J. (2015). Seeing and being seen: Co-situation and impression formation using Grindr, a location-aware gay dating app. *New Media & Society, 17*(7), 1117–1136.

Bourne, A., Reid, D., Hickson, F., Torres Rueda, S., & Weatherburn, P. (2014). *The Chemsex study: Drug use in sexual settings among gay & bisexual men in Lambeth, Southwark & Lewisham.* London: Sigma Research, London School of Hygiene & Tropical Medicine. Retrieved June 2, 2020, from https://www.lambeth.gov.uk/sites/default/files/ssh-chemsex-study-final-main-report.pdf.

Chaney, M. P., & Burns-Wortham, C. M. (2015). Examining coming out, loneliness, and self-esteem as predictors of sexual compulsivity in gay and bisexual men. *Sexual Addiction & Compulsivity, 22*(1), 71–88.

Cohen, M. S., Council, O. D., & Chen, J. S. (2019). Sexually transmitted infections and HIV in the era of antiretroviral treatment and prevention: The biologic basis for epidemiologic synergy. *Journal of the International AIDS Society, 22*(Suppl 6), e25355. https://doi.org/10.1002/jia2.25355

Coleman, E., Horvath, K. J., Miner, M., Ross, M. W., Oakes, M., Rosser, B. R., & Men's INTernet Sex (MINTS-II) Team. (2010). Compulsive sexual behavior and risk for unsafe sex among internet using men who have sex with men. *Archives of Sexual Behavior, 39*(5), 1045–1053.

Cresswell, F., Waters, L., Briggs, E., Fox, J., Harbottle, J., Hawkins, D., … Fisher, M. (2016). UK guideline for the use of HIV Post-Exposure Prophylaxis Following Sexual Exposure, 2015. *International Journal of STD & AIDS, 27*(9), 713–738.

Debattista, J. (2015). Health promotion within a sex on premises venue: Notes from the field. *International Journal of STD and AIDS, 26*(14), 1017–1021.

Dolling, D. I., Desai, M., McOwan, A., Gilson, R., Clarke, A., Fisher, M., … PROUD Study Group. (2016). An analysis of baseline data from the PROUD study: An open-label randomised trial of pre-exposure prophylaxis. *Trials, 17*, 163. https://doi.org/10.1186/s13063-016-1286-4

Flowers, P., Smith, J. A., Sheeran, P., & Beail, N. (1997). Health and romance: Understanding unprotected sex in relationships between gay men. *British Journal of Health Psychology, 2*, 73–86.

Frankis, J., Flowers, P., McDaid, L., & Bourne, A. (2018). Low levels of chemsex among men who have sex with men, but high levels of risk among men who engage in chemsex: Analysis of a cross-sectional online survey across four countries. *Sexual Health, 15*(2), 144–150.

Frankis, J. S., & Flowers, P. (2006). Cruising for sex: Sexual risk behaviours and HIV testing of men who cruise, inside and out with public sex environments (PSE). *AIDS Care, 18*(1), 54–59.

Gallegos, M., Bradly, D., Jakate, S., & Keshavarzian, A. (2012). Lymphogranuloma venereum proctosigmoiditis is a mimicker of inflammatory bowel disease. *World Journal of Gastroenterology, 18*(25), 3317–3321.

Galvin, S. R., & Cohen, M. S. (2004). The role of sexually transmitted diseases in HIV transmission. *Nature Reviews Microbiology, 2*(1), 33–42.

Gama, A., Abecasis, A., Pingarilho, M., Mendão, L., Martins, M. O., Barros, H., & Dias, S. (2017). Cruising venues as a context for HIV risky behavior among men who have sex with men. *Archives of Sexual Behavior, 46*(4), 1061–1068.

George, L. (1998). Self and identity in later life: Protecting and enhancing the self. *Journal of Aging and Identity, 3*, 133–152.

Gerrard, M., Gibbons, F. X., & McCoy, S. B. (1993). Emotional inhibition of effective contraception. *Anxiety, Stress & Coping: An International Journal, 6*(2), 73–88.

Gesink, D., Wang, S., Guimond, T., Kimura, L., Connell, J., Salway, T., … Grace, D. (2018). Conceptualizing geosexual archetypes: Mapping the sexual travels and egocentric sexual networks of gay and bisexual men in Toronto, Canada. *Sexually Transmitted Diseases, 45*(6), 368–373.

Goedel, W. C., & Duncan, D. T. (2015). Geosocial-networking app usage patterns of gay, bisexual and other men who have sex with men: Survey among users of Grindr, a mobile dating app. *JMIR Public Health and Surveillance, 1*(1), e4. https://doi.org/10.2196/publichealth.4353

Goldenberg, T., Finneran, C., Sullivan, S. P., Andes, K. L., & Stephenson, R. (2016). "I consider being gay a very high risk factor": How perceptions of a partner's sexual identity influence perceptions of HIV risk among gay and bisexual men. *Sexuality Research and Social Policy, 14*(1), 32–41.

Goodwin, R., Realo, A., Kwiatkowska, A., Kozlova, A., Luu, L. A. N., & Nizharadze, G. (2002). Values and sexual behaviour in central and eastern Europe. *Journal of Health Psychology, 7*(1), 45–56.

Grov, C., Breslow, A. S., Newcomb, M. E., Rosenberger, J. G., & Bauermeister, J. A. (2014). Gay and bisexual men's use of the Internet: Research from the 1990s through 2013. *Journal of Sex Research, 51*(4), 390–409.

Halkitis, P. N., & Wilton, L. (2005). The meanings of sex for HIV-positive gay and bisexual men: Emotions, physicality, and affirmations of self. In P. N. Halkitis, C. A. Gómez, & R. J. Wolitski (Eds.), *HIV+ sex: The psychological and interpersonal dynamics of HIV-seropositive gay and bisexual men's relationships* (pp. 21–37). American Psychological Association.

Haubrich, D. J., Myers, T., Calzavara, L., Ryder, K., & Medved, W. (2004). Gay and bisexual men's experiences of bathhouse culture and sex: 'looking for love in all the wrong places'. *Culture, Health & Sexuality, 6*(1), 19–29.

Hennelly, S. (2010). Public space, public morality: The media construction of sex in public places. *Liverpool Law Review, 31*(1), 69–91.

Horwood, J., Ingle, S. M., Burton, D., Woodman-Bailey, A., Horner, P., & Jeal, N. (2016). Sexual health risks, service use, and views of rapid point-of-care testing among men who have sex with men attending saunas: A cross-sectional survey. *International Journal of STD and AIDS, 27*(4), 273–280.

Hoyle, R. H., Fejfar, M. C., & Miller, J. D. (2000). Personality and sexual risk taking: A quantitative review. *Journal of Personality, 68*(6), 1203–1231.

Jaspal, R. (2017). Gay men's construction and management of identity on Grindr. *Sexuality & Culture, 21*(1), 187–204.

Jaspal, R. (2018). *Enhancing sexual health, self-identity and wellbeing among men who have sex with men: A guide for practitioners*. London: Jessica Kingsley Publishers.

Jaspal, R. (2019). *The social psychology of gay men*. London: Palgrave Macmillan.

Jaspal, R., & Daramilas, C. (2016). Perceptions of pre-exposure prophylaxis (PrEP) among HIV-negative and HIV-positive men who have sex with men. *Cogent Medicine, 3*, 1256850. https://doi.org/10.1080/2331205X.2016.1256850

Jaspal, R., & Lopes, B. (2020). Psychological wellbeing facilitates accurate HIV risk appraisal in gay and bisexual men. *Sexual Health, 17*(3), 288–295.

Jaspal, R., Lopes, B., Jamal, Z., Yap, C., Paccoud, I., & Sekhon, P. (2019). HIV knowledge, sexual health and behaviour among black and minority ethnic men who have sex with men in the UK: A cross-sectional study. *Sexual Health, 16*(1), 25-31.

Jaspal, R., & Papaloukas, P. (2020). Identity, social connectedness and sexual health in the gay sauna. *Sexuality Research & Social Policy*. https://doi.org/10.1007/s13178-020-00442-0

Joffe, H. (1995). Social representations of AIDS: Towards encompassing issues of power. *Papers on Social Representations, 4*(1), 29–40.

Joffe, H. (2007). Identity, self-control, and risk. In G. Moloney & I. Walker (Eds.), *Social representations and identity* (pp. 197–213). London: Palgrave Macmillan.

Ko, N. Y., Lee, H. C., Hung, C. C., Chang, J. L., Lee, N. Y., Chang, C. M., … Ko, W. C. (2009). Effects of structural intervention on increasing condom availability and reducing risky sexual behaviours in gay bathhouse attendees. *AIDS Care, 21*(12), 1499–1507.

Landovitz, R. J., Tseng, C. H., Weissman, M., Haymer, M., Mendenhall, B., Rogers, K., ... Shoptaw, S. (2013). Epidemiology, sexual risk behavior, and HIV prevention practices of men who have sex with men using Grindr in Los Angeles, California. *Journal of Urban Health: Bulletin of the New York Academy of Medicine, 90*(4), 729–739.

Lee, M., Hegazi, A., Barbour, A., Bavithra, N., Green, S., Simms, R., & Pakianathan, M. (2015). O11 Chemsex and the city: Sexualised substance use in gay bisexual and other men who have sex with men. *Sexually Transmitted Infections, 91*, A4. Retrieved from https://sti.bmj.com/content/91/Suppl_1/A4.2.info

Mazick, A., Howitz, M., Rex, S., Jensen, I. P., Weis, N., Katzenstein, T. L., ... Molbak, K. (2005). Hepatitis A outbreak among MSM linked to casual sex and gay saunas in Copenhagen, Denmark. *Eurosurveillance, 10*(4–6), 111–114.

Melendez-Torres, G. J., Hickson, F., Reid, D., Weatherburn, P., & Bonell, C. (2016). Drug use moderates associations between location of sex and unprotected anal intercourse in men who have sex with men: Nested cross-sectional study of dyadic encounters with new partners. *Sexually Transmitted Infections, 92*(1), 39–43.

Morin, S. F., Vernon, K., Harcourt, J. J., Steward, W. T., Volk, J., Riess, T. H., ... Coates, T. J. (2003). Why HIV infections have increased among men who have sex with men and what to do about it: Findings from California focus groups. *AIDS and Behavior, 7*(4), 353–362.

Moseng, B. U., & Bjørnshagen, V. (2017). Are there any differences between different testing sites? A cross-sectional study of a Norwegian low-threshold HIV testing service for men who have sex with men. *BMJ Open, 7*(10), e017598. https://doi.org/10.1136/bmjopen-2017-017598

Murtagh, N., Gatersleben, B., & Uzzell, D. (2014). Identity threat and resistance to change: Evidence and implications from transport-related behavior. In R. Jaspal & G. M. Breakwell (Eds.), *Identity process theory: Identity, social action and social change* (pp. 335–356). Cambridge: Cambridge University Press.

Norton, R. (2007). *Mother clap's molly house: The gay subculture in England, 1700–1830*. London: Chalford Press.

Pachankis, J. E., Rendina, H. J., Restar, A., Ventuneac, A., Grov, C., & Parsons, J. T. (2015). A minority stress—emotion regulation model of sexual compulsivity among highly sexually active gay and bisexual men. *Health Psychology: Official Journal of the Division of Health Psychology, American Psychological Association, 34*(8), 829–840.

Pakianathan, M., Whittaker, W., Lee, M. J., Avery, J., Green, S., Nathan, B., & Hegazi, A. (2018). Chemsex and new HIV diagnosis in gay, bisexual and other men who have sex with men attending sexual health clinics. *HIV Medicine.* https://doi.org/10.1111/hiv.12629

Parsons, J. T., Grov, C., & Golub, S. A. (2012). Sexual compulsivity, co-occurring psychosocial health problems, and HIV risk among gay and bisexual men: Further evidence of a syndemic. *American Journal of Public Health, 102*(1), 156–162.

Pinkerton, S. D., & Abramson, P. R. (1992). Is risky sex rational? *Journal of Sex Research, 29*(4), 561–568.

Pollack, L. M., Woods, W. J., Blair, J., & Binson, D. (2014). Presence of an HIV testing program lowers the prevalence of unprotected insertive anal intercourse inside a gay bathhouse among HIV-negative and HIV-unknown patrons. *Journal of HIV/AIDS & Social Services, 13*(3), 306–323.

Pollard, A., Nadarzynski, T., & Llewellyn, C. (2017). O13 'I was struggling to feel intimate, the drugs just helped'. Chemsex and HIV-risk among men who have sex with men (MSM) in the UK: Syndemics of stigma, minority-stress, maladaptive coping and risk environments. *Sexually Transmitted Infections, 93*, A5.

Prior, J. (2009). Experiences beyond the threshold: Sydney's gay bathhouses. *Australian Cultural History, 27*(1), 61–77.

Pufall, E., Kall, M., Shahmanesh, M., Nardone, A., Gilson, R., Delpech, V., ... the Positive Voices Study Group. (2016). Chemsex and high-risk sexual behaviours in HIV-positive men who have sex with men. In *Poster presented at the Conference on Retroviruses and Opportunistic Infections Conference, Hynes Convention Center, Boston, Massachusetts*, March 4–7, 2018. Retrieved August 13, 2017, from http://www.croiconference.org/sessions/%C2%93chemsex%C2%94-and-high-risk-sexual-behaviours-hiv-positive-men-who-have-sex-men.

Pufall, E. L., Kall, M., Shahmanesh, M., Nardone, A., Gilson, R., Delpech, V., ... Positive Voices study Group. (2018). Sexualized drug use ('chemsex') and high-risk sexual behaviours in HIV-positive men who have sex with men. *HIV Medicine, 19*(4), 261–270.

Reece, M., & Dodge, B. (2003). Exploring the physical, mental and social well-being of gay and bisexual men who cruise for sex on a college campus. *Journal of Homosexuality, 46*(1–2), 111–136.

Rice, C. E., Maierhofer, C., Fields, K. S., Ervin, M., Lanza, S. T., & Turner, A. N. (2016). Beyond anal sex: Sexual practices of men who have sex with men and associations with HIV and other sexually transmitted infections. *The Journal of Sexual Medicine, 13*(3), 374–382.

Rodger, A. J., Cambiano, V., Bruun, T., Vernazza, P., Collins, S., Degen, O., … PARTNER Study Group. (2019). Risk of HIV transmission through condomless sex in serodifferent gay couples with the HIV-positive partner taking suppressive antiretroviral therapy (PARTNER): Final results of a multicentre, prospective, observational study. *Lancet, 393*(10189), 2428–2438.

Rosengren, A. L., Huang, E., Daniels, J., Young, S. D., Marlin, R. W., & Klausner, J. D. (2016). Feasibility of using GrindrTM to distribute HIV self-test kits to men who have sex with men in Los Angeles, California. *Sexual Health, 13*, 389–392.

Rosser, B. R., Horvath, K. J., Hatfield, L. A., Peterson, J. L., Jacoby, S., & Stately, A. (2008). Predictors of HIV disclosure to secondary partners and sexual risk behavior among a high-risk sample of HIV-positive MSM: Results from six epicenters in the US. *AIDS Care, 20*(8), 925–930.

Ruiter, R. A., Kessels, L. T., Peters, G. J., & Kok, G. (2014). Sixty years of fear appeal research: Current state of the evidence. *International Journal of Psychology: Journal International de psychologie, 49*(2), 63–70.

Schmitt, D. P. (2004). The Big Five related to risky sexual behaviour across 10 world regions: Differential personality associations of sexual promiscuity and relationship infidelity. *European Journal of Personality, 18*, 301–319.

Serrero, M., Peyrin-Biroulet, L., & Grimaud, J.-C. (2017). IBD and HIV: 'Dangerous liaisons'. *Hepato-Gastro & Oncologie Digestive, 24*(1), 34–41.

Sewell, J., Miltz, A., Lampe, F. C., Cambiano, V., Speakman, A., Phillips, A. N., … Attitudes to and Understanding of Risk of Acquisition of HIV (AURAH) Study Group. (2017). Poly drug use, chemsex drug use, and associations with sexual risk behaviour in HIV-negative men who have sex with men attending sexual health clinics. *The International Journal on Drug Policy, 43*, 33–43.

Shernoff, M. (2006). *Without condoms: Unprotected sex, gay men & barebacking*. New York, NY: Routledge.

Spieldenner, A. (2016). PrEP whores and HIV prevention: The queer communication of HIV pre-exposure prophylaxis (PrEP). *Journal of Homosexuality, 63*, 1685–1697.

Strömdahl, S., Hoijer, J., & Eriksen, J. (2019). Uptake of peer-led venue-based HIV testing sites in Sweden aimed at men who have sex with men (MSM) and trans persons: A cross-sectional survey. *Sexually Transmitted Infections, 95*(8), 575–579.

Velter, A., Bouyssou-Michel, A., Arnaud, A., & Semaille, C. (2009). Do men who have sex with men use serosorting with casual partners in France? Results of a nationwide survey (ANRS-EN17-Presse Gay 2004). *Eurosurveillance, 14*(47), pii=19416. https://doi.org/10.2807/ese.14.47.19416-en

Vignoles, V. L., Regalia, C., Manzi, C., Golledge, J., & Scabini, E. (2006). Beyond self-esteem: Influence of multiple motives on identity construction. *Journal of Personality and Social Psychology, 90*(2), 308–333.

Vincke, J., Bolton, R., & De Vleeschouwer, P. (2001). The cognitive structure of the domain of safe and unsafe gay sexual behaviour in Belgium. *AIDS Care, 13*(1), 57–70.

Wawer, M. J., Gray, R. H., Sewankambo, N. K., Serwadda, D., Li, X., Laeyendecker, O., … Quinn, T. C. (2005). Rates of HIV-1 transmission per coital act, by stage of HIV-1 infection, in Rakai, Uganda. *The Journal of Infectious Diseases, 191*(9), 1403–1409.

Weatherburn, P., Hickson, F., Reid, D., Torres-Rueda, S., & Bourne, A. (2017). Motivations and values associated with combining sex and illicit drugs ('chemsex') among gay men in South London: Findings from a qualitative study. *Sexually Transmitted Infections, 93*(3), 203–206.

Winetrobe, H., Rice, E., Bauermeister, J., Petering, R., & Holloway, I. W. (2014). Associations of unprotected anal intercourse with Grindr-met partners among Grindr-using young men who have sex with men in Los Angeles. *AIDS Care, 26*(10), 1303–1308.

Woods, W. J., Lippman, S. A., Agnew, E., Carroll, S., & Binson, D. (2016). Bathhouse distribution of HIV self-testing kits reaches diverse, high-risk population. *AIDS Care, 28*(Suppl 1), 111–113.

Zuckerman, M. (1994). *Behavioral expressions and biosocial bases of sensation seeking.* Cambridge: Cambridge University Press.

4

HIV Prevention

The HIV Prevention Landscape

To date, approximately 75 million people have been infected with HIV globally and 32 million have died (UNAIDS, 2019). Countries in Sub-Saharan Africa have been disproportionately affected, which can be attributed, at least in part, to the lack of a coordinated political and institutional response to HIV in the early days of the epidemic. This is also true of developed Western, industrialised countries, such as the UK and the US, which similarly struggled to control the spread of HIV—especially in the most marginalised communities that were commonly affected. In these contexts, there was an additional layer of complexity, namely, prejudice against these minority communities, such as gay men, whose lifestyles were socially stigmatised and whose health and wellbeing were less of a policy priority for governments. As outlined earlier in this volume, this undoubtedly facilitated the spread of HIV, and with hindsight, it is now evident that much of the early spread could have been prevented with a more coherent governmental understanding of the infection and a more robust public health strategy to test and treat. The

R. Jaspal, J. Bayley, *HIV and Gay Men*, https://doi.org/10.1007/978-981-15-7226-5_4

present chapter focuses on this very question—how can HIV be prevented among gay men at risk of infection?

In order to understand HIV prevention among gay men in the UK, it is helpful to look at HIV in a global context. Globally, the tide does appear to be turning with a steady reduction in AIDS-related deaths over the last decade. In 2004, there were 1.7 million deaths, in 2010 the figure reduced to 1.2 million, and in 2018 to 770,000—this represents a 50% reduction in AIDS-related mortality in under 15 years.[1] This dramatic reduction can be attributed in part to better public health initiatives, improved HIV education programmes, increased awareness and understanding of HIV and its transmission routes in populations at risk and, crucially, the significant expansion of HIV treatment (including among pregnant women living with HIV). There must be effective knowledge exchange, with collaboration between governments, global health organisations and charities for prevention initiatives to work at a local level and to be sustainable. In the UK, the aim is to stop new HIV infections by 2030—an ambitious goal that is achievable now that the government has committed to implementing the recommendations of the HIV Commission (led by the Terrence Higgins Trust and the National AIDS Trust), utilising the expertise of clinicians and researchers, and working collaboratively with third-sector and voluntary organisations as well as key communities affected by HIV.

The history of HIV was outlined in Chap. 2. Here we consider the history of HIV prevention, in particular, focusing on the early efforts to control the spread of the virus. The initial responses to HIV in many Western countries were actually led by community groups which formed in response to the perceived lack of a coordinated institutional response to the growing epidemic. As described in Chap. 2, the Terrence Higgins Trust, one of the most significant UK charities focusing on HIV, later transformed into a charity with political lobbying, health advocacy and social support for those living with HIV. In conjunction with the Lesbian and Gay Switchboard and later the National AIDS Trust, they produced the first public health campaigns to prevent HIV in the UK with funding from the government.

---

[1] https://www.who.int/data/maternal-newborn-child-adolescent/monitor

Many of the earliest educational pamphlets from community organisations in the UK drew upon material from the Gay Men's Health Crisis organisation in the US. Other community groups across the globe also began to promote the use of condoms and to advocate reducing one's number of sexual partners. The 'Play Fair' leaflet released in 1982 by the Sisters of Perpetual Indulgence in San Francisco is a good example of the very first public health campaigns, aimed at educating and reducing anxiety within the gay community by giving direct and practical instructions on how to reduce risk by having sex with fewer partners. However, some gay community groups saw this as a curtailment of their recently hard-won civil rights and were opposed to advocating the use of condoms and to limiting one's number of sexual partners.

Initially, the US led the way in advocacy, with the original efforts originating from San Francisco and New York, two of the worst affected cities in the early phase of the AIDS crisis. It was to take until 1987 for the global community to take action when the World Health Organization (WHO) formulated the Global Program for AIDS which attempted to work with community groups and activists in a coordinated way for the first time. The central tenet of the programme was education for people in highly affected areas. Condom promotion was seen as the most important intervention as physical barrier methods had been shown to be effective in reducing HIV transmission. Recommendations for blood donations and needle exchange programmes were also put forward to support other at-risk groups.

A major impediment to HIV prevention at the time came in the form of growing 'anti-gay' sentiment in the UK. In 1987, the British Social Attitudes Survey demonstrated that three in four people viewed homosexual activity as 'always or mostly wrong', while only one in ten thought that it was never wrong.[2] Furthermore, Margaret Thatcher's government introduced Section 28, a hugely damaging piece of legislation which served not only to reinforce the prevailing anti-gay sentiment at both social and institutional levels but also to decrease social support for young gay men. Its purpose was to forbid local authorities, who oversaw schools

---

[2] https://www.bsa.natcen.ac.uk/latest-report/british-social-attitudes-30/personal-relationships/homosexuality.aspx

in the UK, to 'intentionally promote homosexuality or publish material with the intention of promoting homosexuality'. This legislation reinforced the stigmatising societal belief that homosexuality was chosen, could be encouraged and, thus, implicitly that it could be changed. Moreover, Section 28 caused confusion in local authorities and schools about what actually constituted 'intentional promotion', and, therefore, many simply avoided any acknowledgement of sexual diversity to the detriment of millions of young people growing up in the UK. Needless to say, this resulted in silence about many of the issues known to be related to HIV risk—safer sex knowledge, identity, psychological wellbeing and others (see Chap. 1). Until the repeal of Section 28 in 2003, the educational strand of HIV prevention policy was incapacitated, and it became virtually impossible to equip young gay men with knowledge about the dangers of HIV and how they might protect themselves.

On a more positive note, long-term projects overseen by nongovernmental organisations (and the WHO) have sought to de-politicise HIV/AIDS and to exert pressure on governments to take action and to support those most at risk of infection. For instance, the Global Program for AIDS went through many iterations firstly in 1996 to UNAIDS and was even discussed at the UN General Assembly 'Declaration of Commitment' in 2001, the first time a health issue had been scrutinised at a security council meeting. Furthermore, in 2003, there was a significant global development—the US President's Emergency Plan for AIDS Relief came into force, injecting $15 billion into HIV prevention over the next five years. The main objective was to increase access to HIV prevention in developing countries with the ABC method—Abstinence, Be faithful, Condoms. This narrow view of HIV prevention did not resonate with many at-risk groups, but countries welcomed the extra funding to bring their local epidemics under control. The fund transformed into the Global Fund to Fight AIDS, TB and Malaria, which now provides $4 billion per year in over 100 countries globally. It is believed to have saved 32 million lives, and of the 23 million people taking ART globally, 19 million are funded through this channel.[3]

---

[3] https://www.theglobalfund.org/en/financials/

Over the years, there has been a sustained focus on HIV prevention, which includes promoting condom use, increased HIV and STI testing, the use of PEP and PrEP, TasP and less common approaches, such as the use of microbicides and circumcision as prevention strategies. Alongside the promotion of a combination of these prevention tools, the search for an HIV vaccine has continued. In the remainder of this chapter, we consider each of these methods in turn and look at how they have impacted and shaped the HIV epidemic in gay men.

Adherence to the Norm of Condom Use

Condoms are a highly effective approach to preventing HIV and other STIs. However, their efficacy is determined, in large part, by correct and consistent usage. Accordingly, condom education constitutes a significant component of sexual health promotion globally—in various contexts, people are introduced to condoms, informed about how they can be used effectively and, in some cases, how they can be 'eroticised' so that the pleasure of sex is not in any way diminished (Shernoff, 2006). Although there has been a consistent emphasis on condom use in HIV prevention campaigns—a focus which remains even today—condom use among gay men has been decreasing over the last decade. There are several contributing factors to this behavioural decline—gay men may feel unable to negotiate their condom use in certain situations, face social pressures to engage in condomless sex, have impaired risk appraisal when using alcohol or substances in sexualised settings, experience erectile dysfunction and perceive a lack of 'closeness' or intimacy and reduced pleasure when condoms are used. The possible barriers to condom use were discussed in more detail in Chap. 3.

A significant longitudinal study has examined condom use among over 5000 gay men in 21 cities in the US between 2005 and 2014. Paz-Bailey et al. (2016) revealed a significant increase in condomless anal sex acts. There was a 12.3% increase among those living with HIV (34.2% in 2005 to 44.5% in 2014) and an increase of 11.8% among those who reported being HIV-negative (28.7% in 2005 to 40.5% in 2014). The most significant increase in condomless anal sex was detected in those aged 18–24 years, suggesting that this age group may be particularly vulnerable to HIV infection and, thus, should be a key focus of condom promotion interventions. Overall, numerous trials have shown that consistent condom use in gay men ranges from 40% to 60% (Leichliter, Haderxhanaj, Chesson, & Aral, 2013) with the latest data from a large sample of over 127,000 gay men in Europe indicating that only 40% of participants reported consistent condom use and that 10% reported never using condoms (Weatherburn et al., 2019).

Those gay men who do not use condoms consistently may attempt to adapt their sexual behaviour in order to reduce their risk of HIV infection. Some engage in the strategy of 'strategic positioning' whereby condoms are used only for those sex acts which are believed to be high risk. Receptive anal sex is by far the riskiest sex act with a 1–3% chance of acquiring HIV if the active partner has a detectable HIV viral load; and if the active (or insertive) partner is HIV-negative with an HIV-positive passive partner, the risk is much lower—around 0.1% (Cresswell et al., 2016). There are many other variables which affect the level of risk, such as whether or not the HIV-negative partner is circumcised, the viral load of the HIV-positive partner, bleeding caused during sex and many others. Yet, the *perception* of risk may be low and, thus, condoms may not be used.

Furthermore, some gay men engage in the practice of 'serosorting' which refers to the selection of sexual partners based on their *perceived* HIV status. This means that an HIV-negative individual will have sex only with an individual whom they believe also to be HIV-negative. How one reaches this conclusion is another interesting question—some people assume that their partner is HIV-negative because they have not proposed condom use or even because of their appearance or another characteristic, while others ask their partner's HIV status and then behave accordingly. Similarly, an HIV-positive individual who serosorts would restrict his condomless sexual encounters only to others who share his positive serostatus—a conclusion that can be reached in similar ways to HIV-negative individuals. Crucially, individuals who serosort often forego condoms.

Yet, there are significant problems with this prevention option, which is all too frequently used as a replacement for consistent condom use. The first is its lack of efficacy. The national recommendation in the UK is for high-risk gay men (i.e. those who engage in condomless anal sex) to be screened every three months for bacterial and viral STIs (chlamydia, gonorrhoea, HIV, syphilis and hepatitis B and C—depending on sexual behaviour). It is known that only one third of gay men in England frequently use sexual health services (Mercer et al., 2016). Thus, in a serosorting context, an individual may believe himself to be HIV-negative on the basis of their last HIV test (however long ago that may have been) but actually have acquired the infection since his last test and therefore be living with undiagnosed HIV.

Indeed, approximately 20% of people who acquire HIV will not exhibit symptoms during HIV seroconversion, and those who experience mild symptoms may misattribute them to a cold, influenza or even COVID-19. These issues are inextricably entwined with questions of risk perception, personality and healthcare engagement. However, they have decisive implications for HIV transmissions—in the early stages of HIV seroconversion, the individual's viral load is extremely high which translates into an extremely high risk of onward HIV transmission.

A second challenge concerns the stigma that is implicit in serosorting. The selection of sexual partners on the basis of their HIV status will include some and exclude others. This can fuel stigma against gay men living with HIV who may actually pose a lower risk than those claiming to be HIV-negative, given that those who are living with HIV but on effective ART with an undetectable viral load are not infectious (U=U [undetectable=untransmittable]). Yet, this scientific fact may be discarded by some gay men who serosort. Furthermore, the rejection of gay men living with HIV due to their HIV status may lead some to conceal it from others as a self-protection strategy, potentially leading to onward transmission to others. Indeed, a recurrent theme in this book is that HIV stigma is a key barrier to effective prevention. However, it must be noted that, despite the enormous advantage of U=U, condom use does appear to be waning among HIV-positive gay men with an undetectable viral load because they are increasingly aware that they are not infectious. This of course poses no risk to the HIV prevention agenda but is clearly contributing to the higher incidence of STIs observable in gay men.

Condom use among gay men continues to change as other methods of HIV prevention are emerging. In their study of 4388 gay men and transgender women, Traeger et al. (2018) found that PrEP use was significantly and positively associated with increases in rectal gonorrhoea, which is an indicator of *condomless* receptive anal intercourse. This suggests that PrEP users are less likely to use condoms consistently, which puts them at higher risk of STIs. Yet, it is perhaps due to social stigma towards gay men who do not use condoms that they are accused of recklessness when they do not use them. To contextualise, studies have found that rates of consistent condom use in heterosexual men in the UK are also approximately 40%, although they tend not to face the level of stigma that gay men report (Clifton et al., 2018). A key point is that gay men who, for whatever reason, do not consistently use condoms must be empowered to do so but also signposted to other effective prevention options, such as PrEP. Ultimately, the prime objective is to eradicate new HIV infections in those gay men at risk.

HIV Testing

HIV testing is key to prevention for at least two reasons: first, it enables people to know their HIV status and to modify their sexual behaviour accordingly, and, second, it provides an opportunity to acquire information about how one can limit one's risk of infection and the risk to others. The majority of sexual health clinics in the UK provide an 'opt-out' HIV testing service for patients who wish to be screened for STIs. In most clinics, a fourth-generation combined antigen/antibody HIV test is offered routinely with results usually available within 48–72 hours. Increasingly, rapid finger-prick HIV tests are being offered in community settings, such as LGBT charities, sexual health charities, LGBT nightclub venues and gay saunas. Many gay men prefer to test in these contexts (Thornton, Delpech, Kall, & Nardone, 2012). In addition, HIV self-testing has been legal in the UK since 2014. Self-testing kits can be purchased online and, at the time of writing, cost 29.95 UK pounds (approximately 40 US dollars). The individual personally conducts the test and receives the results within 15 minutes. No interaction with a healthcare professional is usually required. Given there are now a range of contexts in which one can test for HIV, it is crucial to understand attitudes towards them among gay men.

In previous research (e.g. Evangeli, Pady, & Wroe, 2016), several social and psychological barriers to regular HIV testing have been identified.

- Fear of mortality and illness as a result of HIV can lead some individuals to prefer not to know their HIV status (Lorenc et al., 2011).
- Some gay men do not view themselves as being at risk of HIV due, for instance, to low levels of awareness of HIV risk factors or because they do not self-identify as gay (Bond et al., 2015). People who perceive themselves to be at low risk of HIV are in turn less likely to test (Marcus, Gassowski, & Drewes, 2016).
- Endorsement of HIV-related stigma is negatively associated with HIV testing in gay men (Li, Gilmour, Zhang, Koyanagi, & Shibuya, 2012). Individuals may refrain from testing for HIV in order to avoid self-association with this stigmatised condition (Young, Nussbaum, & Monin, 2007).
- In the case of ethnic minority gay men, prejudice, such as homophobia and racism, is associated with decreased willingness to test for HIV (Bond et al., 2015).

Some of these barriers may be accentuated in some testing venues and attenuated in others. For instance, some gay men anticipate homophobia from healthcare professionals and, thus, avoid testing for HIV in sexual health clinics, while others may avoid testing in LGBT community settings due to fears of involuntary disclosure of their HIV status (Stutterheim et al., 2014). HIV testing in sexual health clinics can provide the opportunity for education and facilitation of behaviour change to reduce one's risk of acquiring HIV or of transmitting it to others. However, on the whole, gay men in the UK express satisfaction with sexual health services, and many regularly test for HIV in this context (Kurka, Soni, & Richardson, 2015).

Gay men may express ambivalence about testing in sexual health clinics due to concerns about stigma, loss of confidentiality and trustworthiness of healthcare professionals (St. Lawrence et al., 2015). Moreover, one's experience and satisfaction with sexual health services is likely to underpin future willingness to test in this context. Perceived discrimination and lack of empathy in healthcare settings can decrease willingness to test (Heijnders & Van Der Meij, 2006). Self-stigma can derive from perceived stigma in healthcare settings and may adversely affect engagement with health services, as well as HIV testing.

MacKellar et al.'s (2005) study of undiagnosed HIV and sexual risk behaviours among young gay men concludes with the recommendation that HIV testing should be expanded to gay bars, clubs and other social venues. The authors argue that the inclusion of testing in gay bathhouses and sex-on-premises venues would be effective in reaching gay men who are unaware of their positive serostatus. Rapid HIV testing in sexual health clinics and in bathhouse-based interventions appears to have high acceptability among gay men (Kendrick et al., 2005). Prost et al. (2007) conducted a study of gay men's perceptions of rapid HIV testing in social venues as a means of exploring the provision of testing in non-clinical settings. They found that men might refrain from testing in these settings due to (1) concerns about lack of privacy, (2) the perception that social venues are inappropriate spaces for learning one's HIV status, (3) concerns about a possible lack of post-test support and about the types of behaviour in which one might engage and (4) fears that the provision of HIV testing could have an adverse effect on the venues in which it is offered.

Furthermore, internalised homophobia can result in avoidance of HIV testing in LGBT community settings. HIV self-testing can obviate many of the obstacles that individuals perceive in relation to HIV testing in sexual health and community settings, and acceptability of HIV self-testing appears to be high among gay men (Figueroa, Johnson, Verster, & Baggaley, 2015). Convenience and confidentiality can facilitate HIV self-testing, while concerns around domestic confidentiality may impede it (Witzel, Rodger, Burns, Rhodes, & Weatherburn, 2016). Moreover, some people have experienced difficulties in utilising self-testing kits (Johnson et al., 2014)

It is clear that HIV testing is a key component of effective HIV prevention, but that there are several barriers to testing in specific contexts for gay men at risk of HIV. These barriers must be investigated, understood and removed in order to promote this vital prevention tool and to reap its full benefits. However, it is not only HIV testing, which is important—STI testing also plays a fundamental role.

Promoting STI Testing and Treatment

The synergy between HIV and STIs has been known for several decades but is only partially understood (Røttingen, Cameron, & Garnett, 2001). The role of rectal gonorrhoea as an indicator of condomless sex and therefore increased HIV risk has already been outlined. The most important group of STIs, that affect HIV transmission and acquisition, are those that cause genital ulceration, namely, syphilis and herpes simplex virus (HSV) in developed countries. Disruption of the mucosa, usually the first line of defence against pathogens, leads to an increase in the risk of HIV. It has been suggested that having symptomatic HSV, for example, increases one's risk of HIV acquisition three- to fivefold (Wald & Link, 2002), although it is difficult to demonstrate unequivocally the causal effect of HSV (Freeman et al., 2006). Accordingly, use of acyclovir to treat HSV and, as a consequence, to reduce HIV incidence has been considered. A large randomised control trial with over 3000 gay men (Connie Celum et al., 2008) demonstrated a reduction in genital ulcer disease and active herpes lesions for those taking acyclovir but no concurrent reduction in HIV incidence.

In addition to examining the risk of HIV acquisition, the impact of herpes on the *transmission* of HIV has been investigated. It has been shown in several studies that, in people who are living with HIV and have genital HSV-2 infections, the HIV viral load in genital secretions is two to four times higher than those with no HSV-2 infection (Galvin & Cohen, 2004). This increased shedding of virus stimulates the cell-mediated immune system, and attracts and activates CD4 cells, which in turn become an easy target for HIV entering the bloodstream (Biancotto et al., 2008; Root-Bernstein & Hobbs, 1993). This 'double whammy' of viral induction and propagation means that the genital tract will take up HIV more readily in those with HSV than those without.

A large trial examined whether treating HSV-2 with acyclovir in patients living with HIV and assessed HIV rates in their HIV-negative partners (Celum et al., 2010). The results of data from nearly 3500 couples showed that, despite reducing the prevalence of genital ulcers and HSV-2 outbreaks, it had no effect on reducing HIV transmission to one's partner. Interestingly, acyclovir did lead to a reduction in the level of HIV in the plasma (and most likely the genital tract) by an appreciable amount, but again was not found to be effective in reducing HIV transmission. The disappointing results of these clinical trials show the complexity of HIV transmission risk and, similarly, the complexities associated with developing effective prevention.

For the treatment of STIs overall, it seems sensible that reducing the frequency and latency time (by improved testing and detection) would lead to reduced incidence of HIV. To date, there have been four clinical trials looking at this, mainly based in Africa (Gregson et al., 2007; Grosskurth et al., 1995; Kamali et al., 2003; Wawer et al., 1999). Only the trial based in Tanzania demonstrated lowered HIV rates, with the other three showing lower levels of STIs as expected, but no discernible effect on HIV transmission. The rates of HIV were much lower in the successful study when compared to the others possibly indicating that the HIV epidemic was more established with fewer episodes of risky sexual behaviour and with fewer subsequent new HIV diagnoses.

Although controlling STIs does not appear to reduce HIV rates, a focus on STI prevention does stimulate patient engagement with sexual health services. It is very clear that engagement with sexual health services not only improves sexual efficacy and confidence but it also provides a perfect opportunity to educate and improve knowledge of how to have a safe healthy sex life and relationship. Improving understanding of one's sexual health alone is a good predictor of HIV prevention and allows clinicians to identify those who are having risky sex and to intervene preemptively with an acceptable and personalised behavioural and/or biomedical HIV prevention intervention.

The Emergence and Use of Post-exposure Prophylaxis

Post-exposure prophylaxis (PEP) is a biomedical approach to HIV prevention which is administered to patients after possible HIV exposure. In the UK, the treatment consists of a three-drug regimen—two non-nucleoside reverse transcriptase inhibitors (emtricitabine and tenofovir) and an integrase inhibitor (raltegravir). If initiated within 72 hours of possible exposure to HIV and taken for a period of 28 days, PEP is thought to be protective against permanent HIV infection (Cresswell et al., 2016). Although PEP was approved in 1988, it has remained a controversial prevention method for cases of sexual exposure to HIV. While supporters view it as an effective and, thus, important prevention tool, opponents fear that it can cause serious side effects, increase sexual risk-taking and undermine public health (Jaspal & Nerlich, 2016; Richens, 2005).

PEP has been in use since 1988, when the drug zidovudine was first used in healthcare workers potentially exposed to HIV in the workplace. There have been no randomised control trials in humans to determine the effectiveness of PEP due to the ethical problems of withholding a potentially effective prevention method from the control group. However, PEP is thought to be an effective prevention approach. An early retrospective study among healthcare workers who might have been exposed to HIV in the workplace estimated that PEP reduced the risk of infection by 81% (with a confidence interval of 48–94%) (Cardo et al., 1997). Furthermore, there have been several animal studies which show high efficacy—one animal trial revealed that HIV infection was prevented in all of the macaque monkeys who had been intravenously inoculated with HIV, when PEP was administered within 24 hours of exposure and for 28 days continuously (Tsai et al., 1995).

PEP is not guaranteed to inhibit HIV infection. Its effectiveness depends in part on the following factors:

- *The length of time between the exposure and start of treatment*: PEP is most likely to be successful if it is initiated as soon as possible after initial exposure, preferably within four hours. It is not usually prescribed after 72 hours since it is no longer thought to be effective beyond this point (Roland et al., 2005).

- *Adherence to the medication*: The available evidence suggests that PEP must be taken consistently for a period of 28 days after initial exposure. In a systematic review of 97 studies (Ford et al., 2014), it was shown that only 56.6% of individuals eligible for PEP (reporting a range of types of exposure) actually completed the full course. This may be attributed partly to side effects, a subjective reappraisal of HIV risk and stigma.
- *Drug resistance*: An individual may be exposed to a strain of HIV which is resistant to the drugs used as part of PEP. Though rare, this renders PEP ineffective (Beltrami, Luo, de la Torre, & Cardo, 2002).

In view of the apparent effectiveness of PEP in preventing infection in healthcare workers and its proven effectiveness in animal trials, PEP was considered as a possible prevention tool in the context of sexual exposure to HIV in the early 1990s. In 2006, the British Association of Sexual Health and HIV and the British HIV Association published guidelines on the appropriate use of PEP for non-occupational exposure. The guidelines outline the circumstances in which PEP is recommended, considered and not recommended (see Table 4.1).

In 2006, the then Chief Medical Officer for England, Sir Liam Donaldson requested that local NHS agencies make PEP available to those thought to have been exposed to HIV through sexual contact. Accordingly, patients were able to access PEP at NHS sexual health clinics and at Accident and Emergency Departments following suspected HIV exposure, subject to medical approval. It has been shown that not all health practitioners are fully aware of PEP (Benn et al., 2011) which suggests that not all patients potentially exposed to HIV will be offered it (Spence, 2003).

As outlined in Chap. 3, some gay men have a sense of invincibility in relation to HIV, which some critics believe could be accentuated in the context of PEP, and increase sexual risk-taking and the incidence of HIV and other STIs (Richens, 2005). Indeed, there is an emerging social representation in the era of ART that HIV is no longer a serious illness, which may increase condom fatigue among gay men (Shernoff, 2006). It must be noted, however, that empirical studies have generally found little

Table 4.1 Situations in which post-exposure prophylaxis (PEP) is considered

HIV status of source	HIV+ Viral load detectable	HIV+ Viral load undetectable	Status unknown from high prevalence group/ area	Status unknown from low prevalence group/ area
Receptive anal sex	Recommend	Not recommended	Recommend	Not recommended
Insertive anal sex	Recommend	Not recommended	Consider	Not recommended
Receptive vaginal sex	Recommend	Not recommended	Consider	Not recommended
Insertive vaginal sex	Consider	Not recommended	Consider	Not recommended
Fellatio with ejaculation	Not recommended	Not recommended	Not recommended	Not recommended
Fellatio without ejaculation	Not recommended	Not recommended	Not recommended	Not recommended
Splash of semen into eye	Not recommended	Not recommended	Not recommended	Not recommended
Cunnilingus	Not recommended	Not recommended	Not recommended	Not recommended
Sharing of injecting equipment	Recommended	Not recommended	Consider	Not recommended
Human bite	Not recommended	Not recommended	Not recommended	Not recommended
Needlestick from a discarded needle in the community	N/A	N/A	Not recommended	Not recommended

Cresswell et al. (2016)

evidence that PEP increases sexual risk-taking and most users of PEP do not request it repeatedly (Donnell et al., 2010).

It is important to understand the acceptability of PEP in order to determine its effectiveness in preventing HIV. In their Australian study of PEP users, Körner et al. (2003) found that PEP had an empowering effect for users and enabled them to regain feelings of control over their sexual health. Furthermore, in interviews with 15 gay men who were using PEP following sexual exposure, Sayer et al. (2009) found that, while participants had high awareness of PEP, they did not really understand it, but stated that the experience of taking PEP had led them to engage in less anal sex with casual partners (see also Körner et al. 2003). In short, although there is some awareness of PEP among gay men, due in part to its visibility in gay social contexts as a relevant health-related issue (de Silva, Miller, & Walsh, 2006), *understanding* of PEP (and particularly of the circumstances in which it is most effective) remains low.

Jaspal and Nerlich (2016) examined representations of PEP in the British print media, a key source of information regarding health, science and medicine, between 1997 and 2015. They identified three key social representations of PEP. In some articles, PEP was represented as a straightforward 'morning-after pill' which can prevent HIV, and in others, it was represented as posing risks to individual and public health and yielding uncertain outcomes. A third representation positioned healthcare workers as deserving recipients of PEP and gay men as being less ideal candidates for the prevention tool. The authors argued that media representations of this kind—devoid of technical information about PEP and its mechanisms—might lead to polarised perceptions of PEP, stigma of users and decreased PEP acceptability among both those who prescribe it and those who can benefit from it.

The Advent of Pre-exposure Prophylaxis

Pre-exposure prophylaxis (PrEP) is a biomedical HIV prevention tool that has shaped the HIV prevention landscape over the last decade by helping countless patients reduce their risk of HIV while enjoying a fulfilling sex life, with or without condoms. Its role in reducing HIV is

> ### *Clinical Snapshot 3: Pre-exposure Prophylaxis*
>
> *The advent of PrEP has been a game changer for many gay men. A signifi-cant minority have found it difficult to use condoms, be it due to reduced pleasure, personal choice or erection difficulties. Also, many gay men have been in a situation where condoms fail (i.e. break or slip off during sex) leading to stressful episodes of worry and attending clinic for PEP. This 'HIV anxiety' syndrome is a well-trodden path for many. PrEP not only protects against HIV but also reduces this level of anxiety leading to more enjoyable sex and fewer visits to the clinic or the Accident and Emergency Department in search of PEP. It can be compared to hormonal contraception in women in the 1960s (but protecting against HIV not pregnancy)—with similar soci-etal backlash about 'promoting' condomless sex when that was introduced. PrEP can also increase gay men's engagement with sexual health services and this in turn can help identify other issues (e.g. other STIs, substance misuse). This is especially true for younger gay men who may be unaware of the risks surrounding HIV and provides multiple opportunities to increase education and risk reduction strategies. It should also be noted that the uptake of PrEP is strongly associated with education level (i.e. those with higher level of educational attainment are more likely to access PrEP) and ethnicity (i.e. White gay men have better access) and work should also focus on marginalised groups. Most importantly, PrEP must be made available to all who perceive themselves to be at risk.*

unequivocal and, accordingly, it has been referred to as the 'game changer' of HIV prevention (Jaspal & Nerlich, 2016). Though clinically effective, it has not been fully available, or acceptable, to all patients at risk of HIV.

The Clinical Aspects of PrEP

As outlined earlier, it can take up to 17 years for a drug to be made avail-able to patients after initial drug discovery. This is also true of PrEP. In November 1995, a team of US researchers explored the use of tenofovir as a treatment for HIV and as a possible prevention tool (Tsai et al., 1995). Their study, published in *Science*, described the effect of tenofovir versus placebo on HIV infection in macaque monkeys who had been inoculated with HIV. For those treated with tenofovir either before or after exposure for four weeks, HIV infection was prevented in 100% of the macaques. This seminal research paved the way for both PEP and PrEP.

The first real-world study of PrEP in gay men materialised several years later. The iPrEx (preexposure prophylaxis initiative) randomised control trial in 2010 recruited almost 2500 gay men and transgender women at high risk of HIV infection (Grant et al., 2010). They received either placebo or Truvada (containing tenofovir and emtricitabine), which they were instructed to take daily. The trial demonstrated, for the first time, that daily Truvada reduced HIV incidence in the experimental group by 44%, an impressive reduction with significant public health ramifications. A strong indicator of effectiveness was the amount of drug in the blood of the participants—with high levels showing a strong correlation between drug adherence and protection against HIV. The iPrEx trial was a significant step forward for gay men at risk of HIV infection since it added another effective prevention method to the HIV prevention toolbox. HIV incidence in gay men had been on the rise, and it had become clear that the social norm of condom use was beginning to wane (Shernoff, 2006).

Following the promising results of the iPrEx trial, two additional clinical trials were conducted in the UK and in France—the PROUD (McCormack et al., 2016) and iPERGAY (Molina et al., 2015) studies, respectively. These trials set out to examine not only the effectiveness of PrEP but also the degree of risk compensation among PrEP users, that is, whether rates of condom use would decrease, in turn leading to increased STI rates. Moreover, the trials aimed to address the additional questions that had been raised in the iPrEx study, such as whether gay men would adhere to daily PrEP and what the alternatives to daily PrEP might be; whether gay men would acquire a false sense of protection against HIV despite poor adherence, leading to HIV infection; and how sexual health clinics might incorporate and manage PrEP within their existing services.

As in the iPrEx study, PROUD trial participants were randomly allocated to taking immediate PrEP or deferring PrEP for the first year and then taking Truvada daily. The results of the study were very encouraging, and when it became evident that PrEP worked, the trial was stopped early and all participants were offered PrEP immediately. The trial showed that

PrEP reduced HIV incidence by 86% although it must be noted that some participants in the experimental group did not adhere to the drug, which suggests that the efficacy rate may have been higher if adherence had been better.

Meanwhile, the French research group released data for iPERGAY (Molina et al., 2015), which had tested the efficacy of the same Truvada formulation as PrEP, but with a different dosage. Participants in the trial were instructed to take PrEP before and after sex (two tablets 2–24 hours before, followed by one tablet 24 hours later and a fourth tablet 48 hours later). The iPERGAY trial demonstrated an 86% reduction in HIV in participants, showing that intermittent dosage worked as effectively as daily PrEP.

Understandably there were concerns about the possible side effects of PrEP. Truvada had been used to treat HIV since the FDA in the US approved its use in 2004. Therefore, a great deal was known about its toxicity profile before it was licensed for use as PrEP. The main short-term side effects were found to include nausea, diarrhoea and headaches, which usually settle in the first few weeks. However, in practice, these are relatively uncommon. Long-term side effects include renal complications and a modest reduction in bone density. One of the main clinical concerns in relation to Truvada was renal injury observed in HIV patients when administered with other HIV drugs. However, for those taking Truvada alone, it was thought this renal damage may also be an issue. A large meta-analysis (Pilkington, Hill, Hughes, Nwokolo, & Pozniak, 2018) of over 15,000 people did not show increased rates of serious kidney damage for those taking PrEP, and thus yearly kidney monitoring is deemed to be sufficient.

The iPREX-OLE (open label extension) showed between a 0.5% and 1% loss of bone density in the hip and spine, respectively. In HIV negative patients, who are otherwise fit and well, this slight decrease in bone density is unlikely to lead to a higher risk of fracture. It is important to counsel patients about this risk, but with reassurances that it should not prevent them from taking PrEP if the benefits outweigh the possible risks.

The initial exorbitant cost of branded Truvada led many to acquire it from non-NHS settings (i.e. ordered online from other countries). Clinicians in the UK were concerned about advocating the use of non-branded Truvada from pharmaceutical companies based mainly in India and Canada. In particular, clinicians expressed concern about non-approval of the drugs by the European Medicines Agency and the possibility that the formulations did not contain the correct drugs or dosage. However, a study with those taking these non-branded drugs found that the drugs contained the same active ingredients as branded Truvada, eliminating this concern (Wang et al., 2019).

Social and Political Aspects of PrEP

In view of the convincing evidence regarding the impact of PrEP on HIV incidence, physicians and many in the gay community assumed that PrEP would be commissioned on the NHS. As pressure mounted on the government to provide PrEP to all, NHS England declined to fund the drug, stating that this was the responsibility of local authorities who currently fund sexual and reproductive healthcare in line with the Health and Social Care Act in 2012. The argument of NHS England was that it was responsible solely for HIV treatment (i.e. the treatment of those living with HIV) and that local authorities should fund HIV prevention from within their own budgets. In the era of austerity in the UK since the financial crash of 2009, budgets for public health were radically affected, with reductions of up to 40% in some boroughs. It was therefore unrealistic to expect local authorities to fund PrEP in their respective jurisdictions.

There was a significant community response with individuals and third-sector agencies taking on the responsibility of raising awareness of PrEP and how to access it. In the absence of a national commissioning strategy, activists and clinicians took the lead in ensuring this new prevention tool could become available to the many who needed it. Community activists set up a website[4] with information about PrEP and the option to purchase a generic version of PrEP at a fraction of the cost compared to Truvada. At the time, Gilead Sciences who had developed Truvada held the cost of a 30-day supply of PrEP at approximately £400, which was of course unaffordable for most people at risk of HIV. Given the complexities of drug patents, the US and Europe were unable to access generic PrEP (i.e. the same drugs as Truvada, but manufactured by other pharmaceutical companies at a lower cost). However, in the UK, Greg Owen (an activist living with HIV) and Dr Mags Portman (a consultant physician in HIV medicine) facilitated access to generic PrEP to many of those at risk (especially those in the gay community) and helped prevent thousands of new HIV infections.

The National AIDS Trust led the campaign to have the decision of NHS England not to fund PrEP overturned by the UK High Court in August 2016. After the successful High Court ruling, NHS England released a press statement, which began 'PrEP is a measure to prevent HIV transmission, particularly for men who have high-risk condomless sex with multiple male partners'.[5] The statement served to emphasise the benefits of PrEP to one group only—gay men—when it has been shown to be equally as effective in women, and to associate the prevention tool with 'high risk condomless sex with multiple male partners'. It is easy to see how this might have paved the way for polarised thinking and stigmatising perceptions not only of gay men but also PrEP.

However, in 2017, NHS England finally capitulated and instructed Public Health England to investigate the possibility of commissioning PrEP in England. This led to a second clinical trial—the IMPACT study—which, in many respects, replicated the work of the PROUD study eight years earlier. At the time of writing, the trial was still recruiting participants. However, in March 2020, Matt Hancock, the Secretary of State for Health and Social Care, announced that PrEP would be made available on the NHS free of charge to those at risk of HIV. Although PrEP was due to be made available in April of that year, the outbreak of

---

[4] www.iwantprepnow.co.uk
[5] https://www.england.nhs.uk/2016/08/august-update-on-the-commissioning-and-provision-of-pre-exposure-prophylaxis-prep-for-hiv-prevention/

COVID-19 (and the subsequent measures taken to curb its spread) has delayed this.

The media make important contributions to perceptions of PrEP in the general population. Jaspal and Nerlich (2017) found that media reporting of PrEP in the UK was polarised in that it represented PrEP either as a 'magic bullet' or as posing severe risks to individual and public health. Much of the reporting in the latter theme was characterised by social stigma—of HIV, of gay men and of PrEP itself.

In addition, as an 'expert community', healthcare professionals are of course key to the development of societal perceptions of PrEP. They have the ability to influence both public policy and patient engagement. In a survey of 328 healthcare professionals in the UK, Desai et al. (2016) found that just 54% of those surveyed endorsed PrEP for patients outside of the clinical trial and raised concerns about the current evidence base, patient adherence to PrEP and the potential for increased sexual risk-taking in patients. It is important to examine how healthcare profession-als think and talk about PrEP—especially with patients—because their approach to PrEP is likely to influence that of patients. Indeed, in previ-ous research, it has been noted that stigmatisation from both healthcare professionals and other gay men was a common experience for partici-pants in a qualitative study of PrEP users (Schwartz & Grimm, 2019). It is easy to see how stigma can challenge self-esteem among patients and, thus, inhibit access to PrEP and also interfere with adherence to the drug, which itself can reduce its effectiveness (Vaccher, Kaldor, Callander, Zablotska, & Haire, 2018). It has also been found that perceived stigma from healthcare professionals can decrease engagement with sexual healthcare (Williamson, Papaloukas, Jaspal, & Lond, 2019).

Although PrEP is clinically effective, its effectiveness depends on its acceptability among potential users. Given that gay men are one of the groups in society that are disproportionately affected by HIV, it is neces-sary to assess perceptions and acceptability of PrEP in this group. There have been several studies of PrEP awareness, understanding and accept-ability among gay men (Williamson et al., 2019; Jaspal, Lopes, Bayley, & Papaloukas, 2019). A survey study of 386 HIV-negative gay men revealed that just a third of respondents had heard of PrEP but that over half would be willing to utilise it if it were available (Frankis, Young, Flowers,

& McDaid, 2016). Those who tested for HIV every six months were more likely to be aware of PrEP. In their survey study of gay men in Leicester, Jaspal et al. (2019) found socio-economic inequalities in HIV knowledge and HIV testing, both of which are important predictors of PrEP acceptability. More specifically, it was found that gay men who have high levels of HIV knowledge and perceived HIV risk and who test for HIV regularly are most likely to perceive PrEP to be of personal benefit. Their findings indicated that one must first view oneself as being at risk of HIV (possibly through consultation with a healthcare professional) in order to accept PrEP as a viable HIV prevention method for oneself. In a US study, Raifman et al. (2019) examined awareness of PrEP among gay men presenting at a sexual health clinic from 2013 to 2016 and found that awareness increased over time, although Hispanic and Black gay men manifested consistently lower PrEP awareness than White gay men. Furthermore, Elopre et al. (2018) studied perceptions of PrEP among Black gay men and found that interviewees perceived a multi-faceted stigma in relation to their Black, gay and Southern identities, a lack of discussion regarding HIV prevention in the Black community and low HIV risk perception (Elopre et al., 2018).

This research suggests that societal perceptions of PrEP are developing and being disseminated to people at risk of HIV, such as gay men, but that there are some subgroups of gay men that have less access to this knowledge. Furthermore, it has been shown that gay men who participate in the gay community are more likely to be aware of PrEP than those who do not (Zarwell, Ransome, Barak, Gruber, & Robinson, 2019). Several empirical studies (e.g. Jaspal, 2019; Jaspal & Cinnirella, 2010) have revealed that ethnic minority gay men are less likely to be open about their sexual identity and less involved in the gay community. This can mean that they are less aware of issues that affect the gay community, such as HIV and PrEP. They may not be exposed to discussions about PrEP that ordinarily take place in gay social contexts. Furthermore, in order to protect self-esteem, individuals may avoid exposure to stigma, thereby reducing access to PrEP.

In addition to awareness, complex psychosocial factors like risk appraisal and perceived stigma also shape PrEP acceptability in gay men. Frankis, Young, Flowers, and McDaid (2014) found that few of the gay men they interviewed regarded themselves as candidates for PrEP because of low perceived risk of HIV and existing HIV prevention strategies that they were utilising. In view of the low uptake of PrEP in groups at high risk of HIV, Dubov, Galbo, Altice, and Fraenkel (2018) conducted semi-structured interviews with 43 HIV-negative gay men to explore their perceptions and experiences of stigma in relation to PrEP use. They found that interviewees experienced stigma from potential and actual sexual partners and reported being stereotyped as 'high risk'. Participants associated PrEP stigma with HIV stigma. In a qualitative interview study of Latino gay male PrEP users in Los Angeles, Brooks, Nieto, Landrian, and Donohoe (2019) found that perceptions that PrEP users engage in sexual risk behaviours and that they are in fact HIV-positive underpinned the stigma that participants faced. Moreover, interviewees described the risk of difficulties in relationships as a result of their PrEP use. Given the higher levels of internalised homophobia and motivation to conceal their sexual identity, ethnic minority gay men at risk of HIV may express concerns about involuntary disclosure of their sexual orientation and about potential exposure to HIV stigma as a result of PrEP use. Avoidance may constitute a strategy for coping with threats to self-esteem associated with potential or actual stigma.

In a qualitative interview study, Jaspal and Daramilas (2016) explored perceptions and understandings of PrEP among 20 HIV-negative and HIV-positive gay men, focusing on their beliefs about the potential impact of PrEP on their own lives and behaviours. They found three themes: uncertainty and fear, managing relationships with others and stigma and categorisation. HIV-negative participants appeared to manifest uncertainty and fear in relation to PrEP as they believed that it would not be completely effective and that it would leave them feeling uncertain due to the 'invisibility' of PrEP once it is taken (versus a condom which can be examined physically to ensure that it has remained intact during sex). Conversely, HIV-positive gay men were generally of the view that PrEP would reduce uncertainty and fear (primarily of onward HIV transmission to HIV-negative partners). It is possible that this might provide a sense of self-efficacy in that individuals feel more empowered to prevent onward transmission than they previously did with condoms as their sole prevention approach. There was a stark difference in how HIV-negative and HIV-positive men perceived the potential impact of PrEP on their relationships with others—while HIV-negative gay men felt that their use of PrEP could induce social stigma, HIV-positive men foresaw an improvement in relations with serodiscordant partners who they believed might feel less anxious about sex given the advent of PrEP.

Although both cohorts acknowledged the possible benefits of PrEP, they nonetheless manifested stigma in relation to the prevention tool, which led some HIV-negative gay men to reject PrEP for personal use. It is clear that social stigma underpins attitudes towards PrEP both at social (i.e. in the media) and individual levels. The prevalence of social stigma appears to have infiltrated thinking at an individual level, which has led individuals who may benefit from PrEP to reject it as an HIV prevention tool that people 'at high risk' might utilise. It is important that potential beneficiaries of PrEP are able to understand the benefits of this approach in preventing HIV and to access it. It is likely that social and political factors may inhibit this.

Clinical Snapshot 4: U=U

The release of the HPTN-052 and PARTNERS studies showed unequivocally that those taking effective ART cannot pass HIV on to their partners. Clinicians rarely deal in absolutes—however, the data surrounding U=U are clear and unambiguous. This certainty allows clinicians to relay this important information to their patients. In practice, this message is one of the most powerful for a number of reasons. Those living with HIV have often lived with the anxiety of possibly passing HIV on to their partners and loved ones—an anxiety that can cause shame and/or damage to relationships. The U=U message has important ramifications not only for reducing HIV transmissions but also for anxious patients. The reaction to this message in clinical practice is often one of relief and should be part of every HIV consultation—and reiterated as some patients take time to adjust to the relief of this news. The ability to have sex with a partner without anxiety is a significant step towards enhancing the quality of life of those living with HIV.

Treatment as Prevention

One of the greatest advancements in the fight against HIV has undoubtedly been TasP, which refers to the treatment of HIV (using ART) in those who have the infection. Essentially, effective ART reduces the individual's viral load to undetectable levels, which in turn reduces their risk of HIV transmission to zero. The most successful early case of TasP involved the use of AZT in pregnancy which was shown to reduce HIV transmission from HIV-positive mothers to their infants by up to two thirds (Connor et al., 1994). In 2000, a large study of 415 serodiscordant (i.e. one partner with HIV and one without it) heterosexual couples in Rakai, Uganda, showed that, over a period of 30 months, just over 20% of the HIV-negative individuals acquired HIV with a strong correlation between viral load and risk of HIV transmission (Quinn et al., 2000). Furthermore, there were no HIV transmissions when the HIV-positive individual's viral load was less than 1500 copies per millilitre.

The next seminal moment came in 2011 when the HIV Prevention Trial Network, a global coalition of clinicians and researchers published the results of the HPTN 052 study (Cohen et al., 2011). The study included 1763 serodiscordant couples, of which 97% were heterosexual, in South America, Africa and Asia. The HIV-positive partner in each couple was assigned to either 'delayed' treatment (i.e. waiting until the CD4 count had dropped to less than 200 cells/mm^3) or 'immediate' treatment (i.e. start treatment when the CD4 was between 350 and 550 cells/mm^3). Out of the 28 transmissions, 27 were from those who had delayed treatment with only one from the group on treatment. In other words, those on treatment were 96% less likely to transmit HIV than those who had deferred treatment. Such compelling results are rarely seen in such large clinical trials, given that human behaviour and chance often obfuscate the true effects of interventions. The results exceeded expectations and were hailed as a landmark in the history of HIV prevention.

As this was a study of heterosexual couples, the findings could not be easily generalised to gay men. Relevant data arrived five years later in the form of the PARTNER study (Rodger et al., 2016) which included a significant subsample of men who were in gay relationships. The trial results revealed *zero* linked transmissions of HIV if one partner was on effective HIV treatment and undetectable. This added to the evidence base that HIV transmission was impossible whilst taking effective HIV treatment—this time in gay couples. This evidence was reinforced with an extension of the original trial for only gay couples—in over 76,000 acts of condomless anal sex, there were zero linked HIV transmissions

(Rodger et al., 2019). Since one of the main psychological challenges faced by people living with HIV concerns the management of risk of onward transmission, this finding was life-changing for many. Clinicians across the globe could now say with certainty that there was no risk of HIV transmission for gay men living with HIV who are taking effective treatment.

These data underpinned the simple and powerful public health message of U=U. This message has since been the focus of a global effort to reduce anxiety among and reduce stigma towards those who are living with HIV. Community groups, activists and clinicians have been vociferous in their support for this message. U=U has been the most powerful (and emotional) message relayed to patients who often report feeling relieved and empowered as a result.

Other Prevention Options: Microbicides and Circumcision

In addition to the major components of combination HIV prevention, namely, condom use, HIV testing, PrEP and TasP, other prevention options that might complement these approaches are being explored. Interesting possible approaches include the use of microbicides and male circumcision. Much of the research into these approaches has focused on heterosexual populations but may also be transferable to gay men.

Some interest has been shown in the possibility of using topical preparations of anti-HIV drugs, mainly tenofovir disoproxil, to reduce the risk of HIV. The CAPRISA 004 study (Abdool Karim et al., 2010) evaluated the effectiveness of a vaginal gel containing 1% tenofovir which led to a 39% reduction in HIV infections when compared to placebo. However, adherence to the gel was poor. Another trial has focused on nonoxynol-9, a commonly used spermicide (which appears to be moderately protective against HIV and most STIs), in a vaginal gel (Van Damme et al., 2002). However, its use led to higher rates of genital ulceration and may in fact have increased the risk of HIV acquisition. It is possible that use of gels in the rectum also cause mucosal damage, thereby undermining their effectiveness as HIV prevention tools. Although some gay men have expressed interest in rectal gels, many prefer to use oral Truvada (Carballo-Diéguez et al., 2017). Yet, rectal gels may provide another tool for prevention and may suit gay men who find oral PrEP unacceptable. However, no commercial gel is, as yet, available.

The impact of circumcision on HIV risk in gay men has also been considered (Yuan et al., 2019). The procedure entails the surgical removal of the foreskin—often for cultural, religious and medical reasons. During the early days of the epidemic, it was noted that men who were uncircumcised (i.e. their foreskin remained intact) appeared to be at higher risk of acquiring HIV than those who were circumcised. An African study revealed an eightfold increase in HIV risk in uncircumcised men (Cameron et al., 1989) which subsequently led to research into whether male circumcision might constitute a feasible and cost-effective HIV prevention method, especially in developing countries. There have since been several large trials in Africa (Auvert et al., 2005; Bailey et al., 2007; Gray et al., 2007) which have generally shown a reduction of almost 60% in circumcised men compared to uncircumcised men. Evidently, circumcision is clinically effective but it has varying degrees of cultural and individual acceptability.

It is noteworthy that the aforementioned trials were all designed for heterosexual men who perform the insertive role in sex. However, sexual behaviour among gay men tends to vary between insertive and receptive sexual practices. A large meta-analysis (Yuan et al., 2019) examined the effectiveness of circumcision in gay men after two previous meta-analyses had shown no effect in this population (Millett, Flores, Marks, Reed, & Herbst, 2008; Wiysonge et al., 2011). The meta-analyses included data from over 100,000 gay men from low-, middle- and high-income countries and demonstrated 23% protection overall. However, the protective effect was stronger in gay men in low- and middle-income countries, those who mainly had insertive anal sex and those under the age of 29 years. It might be advantageous to examine the acceptability of circumcision in the UK population, especially given its clear contribution to HIV prevention. However, given the effectiveness of other prevention methods, circumcision remains an under-developed method of HIV prevention in the UK.

The Search for a Vaccine

In 1984, Margaret Heckler, the then US Secretary of State of Health, declared that 'a vaccine will be ready for testing within 2 years'. This assertion was based on successful development of vaccines for the feline leukaemia virus (FLV) and for hepatitis B in the early 1980s. However, it was not yet anticipated that developing a vaccine would be so challenging that, almost 40 years after its first clinical observations, there is still no effective vaccine for HIV.

The journey towards developing an effective preventive HIV vaccine has been long and arduous with numerous failures and a few modest successes. Viral vaccinology dictates that introduction of the whole or part of the virus in vectors (usually inert viruses which help to deliver the antigen to the body's immune system) will induce an antibody response from the patient's own immune system that then prevents future infection if challenged with the infective agent. A modern example of this is the hugely successful vaccination for Human Papillomavirus (HPV) whereby yeast cells are used to grow the external viral envelope proteins to form 'virus-like particles' which have a strong immunogenic reaction and produce high levels of protective antibodies. However, this method has thus far proven futile for HIV. Numerous vaccine trials have shown that using proteins from the surface of HIV (usually gp120 or gp160) do stimulate antibodies to HIV but that they do not appear to inactivate it. One of the biggest challenges is the heterogeneity, or variability, of HIV itself which undergoes millions of natural mutations during replication, as well as the different structures of viral subsets, or clades.

A notable trial in the search for a preventative vaccine was the much anticipated Step trial which began in 2004 (Buchbinder et al., 2008) and recruited gay and bisexual men from the Caribbean region. The trial used an adenovirus-type vaccine—shown to be the most immunogenic for anti-HIV CD4 responses—which coded for three HIV surface proteins (*gag, pol* and *nef*) in the hope the antibodies produced would protect against HIV. Sadly, the trial was terminated early after it was discovered that many of the vaccinated men who had previously been naturally exposed to adenovirus had higher rates of HIV acquisition when compared to placebo. The exact reason why those who were seropositive for adenovirus exhibited a higher rate of infection is unknown but proved a disappointment for HIV research.

There has also been another line of HIV vaccination science, focusing on combinations of immune responses, rather than on one aspect. This was tested in the Thai RV 144 study (Karasavvas et al., 2012), one of the few success stories of HIV vaccines, albeit a modest one. This vaccine used a 'prime boost' method, where two vaccines were given in succession—the first to stimulate cell-mediated immunity (via a canarypox vector), followed by another surface protein (recombinant gp120) to stimulate the antibody response to neutralise HIV. The study recruited over 16,000 adults in Thailand but only had a modest effect in reducing HIV acquisition by 31% overall, despite showing a 60% reduction at 12 months. The level of protection provided by this vaccine means it is unlikely to be adopted in the real world given that, with such low levels of protection, vaccinated individuals may acquire a false sense of security of being 'immune' to HIV with subsequent increased sexual risk.

Given that this was one of the only effective HIV vaccines, researchers went on to develop another vaccine with a 'prime boost' model using a similar method with slight alterations to the constituents. The HVTN 702 study[6] recruited nearly 5000 adults (half receiving placebo, the other half the vaccine) in 2016 but was stopped early in February 2020 after showing no success in reducing HIV acquisition. The cost of the trial was over $100 million, showing how resource-intensive these vaccination trials can be, but they enable researchers to discard some vaccination methods in favour of potentially more fruitful methods. The search for an effective vaccine continues.

The work of HIV vaccination science is also focusing on broadly neutralising antibodies (bNAb). These antibodies were found in 20% HIV-positive patients who develop them against their own HIV. These bNAb are able to inhibit a broad range of HIV mutations and clades. The AMP

---

[6] https://www.clinicaltrials.gov/ct2/show/NCT02968849

trial (HVTN 704/HPTN 085)[7] has recruited over 4000 adults and delivers monoclonal antibodies in an infusion every eight weeks by disrupting a protein involved in the attachment of HIV to the CD4 cell so the HIV is not allowed to enter. At the time of writing, the results of this exciting new HIV prevention strategy were not yet available.

Overview

In this chapter, the HIV prevention landscape in the UK has been outlined. While condom use has been a long-standing norm among gay men, it is clear that this norm is now waning. This has paved the way for other innovative approaches to HIV prevention, such as PrEP and TasP. Moreover, emerging prevention approaches, such as circumcision and microbicides, have shown some promise. A recurrent theme in this chapter is that, although significant advances have been made in developing effective prevention tools, there are varying levels of patient acceptability of these distinct approaches. It is important to explore their acceptability among gay men in distinct contexts and to attempt to remove any potential barriers to accessing them. Condoms may be an effective stand-alone prevention tool for some gay men but unacceptable to others who may require PrEP. Moreover, the science underpinning TasP must be effectively communicated to gay men—both HIV-negative and HIV-positive. Public health campaigns are instrumental in educating and raising awareness of the risks of HIV, but without sustained behaviour change, the effects of these campaigns will be short-lived. The condom use message of the 1980s and 1990s had some positive effect, especially alongside the potent 'tombstone' television adverts, but HIV incidence in gay men continued to increase. To ensure that HIV is eliminated by 2030, the emphasis and funding must be weighted towards prevention, that is, driving down the number of new infections. However, it is also essential to equip gay men with knowledge concerning sex, risk and STIs so that they can take informed decisions about the most effective prevention tool for them.

---

[7] https://clinicaltrials.gov/ct2/show/NCT02716675

References

Abdool Karim, Q., Abdool Karim, S. S., Frohlich, J. A., Grobler, A. C., Baxter, C., Mansoor, L. E., ... CAPRISA 004 Trial Group. (2010). Effectiveness and safety of tenofovir gel, an antiretroviral microbicide, for the prevention of HIV infection in women. *Science, 329*(5996), 1168–1174.

Auvert, B., Taljaard, D., Lagarde, E., Sobngwi-Tambekou, J., Sitta, R., & Puren, A. (2005). Randomized, controlled intervention trial of male circumcision for reduction of HIV infection risk: The ANRS 1265 Trial. *PLoS Medicine, 2*(11), e298. https://doi.org/10.1371/journal.pmed.0020298

Bailey, R. C., Moses, S., Parker, C. B., Agot, K., Maclean, I., & Krieger, J. N. ... Ndinya-Achola, J. O. (2007). Male circumcision for HIV prevention in young men in Kisumu, Kenya: A randomised controlled trial. *Lancet, 369*(9562), 643–656.

Beltrami, E. M., Luo, C.-C., de la Torre, N., & Cardo, D. M. (2002). Transmission of drug-resistant HIV after an occupational exposure despite postexposure prophylaxis with a combination drug regimen. *Infection Control and Hospital Epidemiology, 23*(6), 345–348.

Benn, P., Fisher, M., Kulasegaram, R., & BASHH, & PEPSE Guidelines Writing Group Clinical Effectiveness Group. (2011). UK guideline for the use of post-exposure prophylaxis for HIV following sexual exposure (2011). *International Journal of STD & AIDS, 22*(12), 695–708.

Biancotto, A., Iglehart, S. J., Vanpouille, C., Condack, C. E., Lisco, A., Ruecker, E., ... Grivel, J.-C. (2008). HIV-1 induced activation of CD4+ T cells creates new targets for HIV-1 infection in human lymphoid tissue ex vivo. *Blood, 111*(2), 699–704.

Bond, K. T., Frye, V., Taylor, R., Williams, K., Bonner, S., Lucy, D., ... Straight Talk Study Team. (2015). Knowing is not enough: A qualitative report on HIV testing among heterosexual African-American men. *AIDS Care, 27*(2), 182–188.

Brooks, R. A., Nieto, O., Landrian, A., & Donohoe, T. J. (2019). Persistent stigmatizing and negative perceptions of pre-exposure prophylaxis (PrEP) users: Implications for PrEP adoption among Latino men who have sex with men. *AIDS Care, 31*(4), 427–435.

Buchbinder, S. P., Mehrotra, D. V., Duerr, A., Fitzgerald, D. W., Mogg, R., Li, D., ... Step Study Protocol Team. (2008). Efficacy assessment of a cell-mediated immunity HIV-1 vaccine (the Step Study): A double-blind, randomised, placebo-controlled, test-of-concept trial. *Lancet, 372*(9653), 1881–1893.

Cameron, D. W., Simonsen, J. N., D'Costa, L. J., Ronald, A. R., Maitha, G. M., Gakinya, M. N., … Brunham, R. C. (1989). Female to male transmission of human immunodeficiency virus type 1: Risk factors for seroconversion in men. *Lancet, 2*(8660), 403–407.

Carballo-Diéguez, A., Balán, I. C., Brown, W., Giguere, R., Dolezal, C., Leu, C.-S., … Cranston, R. D. (2017). High levels of adherence to a rectal microbicide gel and to oral Pre-Exposure Prophylaxis (PrEP) achieved in MTN-017 among men who have sex with men (MSM) and transgender women. *PloS One, 12*(7), e0181607. https://doi.org/10.1371/journal.pone.0181607

Cardo, D. M., Culver, D. H., Ciesielski, C. A., Srivastava, P. U., Marcus, R., Abiteboul, D., … Bell, D. M. (1997). A case-control study of HIV seroconversion in health care workers after percutaneous exposure. Centers for Disease Control and Prevention Needlestick Surveillance Group. *The New England Journal of Medicine, 337*(21), 1485–1490.

Celum, C., Wald, A., Hughes, J., Sanchez, J., Reid, S., Delany-Moretlwe, S., … HPTN 039 Protocol Team. (2008). Effect of aciclovir on HIV-1 acquisition in herpes simplex virus 2 seropositive women and men who have sex with men: A randomised, double-blind, placebo-controlled trial. *Lancet, 371*(9630), 2109–2119.

Celum, C., Wald, A., Lingappa, J. R., Magaret, A. S., Wang, R. S., Mugo, N., … Partners in Prevention HSV/HIV Transmission Study Team. (2010). Acyclovir and transmission of HIV-1 from persons infected with HIV-1 and HSV-2. *The New England Journal of Medicine, 362*(5), 427–439.

Clifton, S., Mercer, C. H., Sonnenberg, P., Tanton, C., Field, N., Gravningen, K., … Johnson, A. M. (2018). STI risk perception in the British population and how it relates to sexual behaviour and STI healthcare use: Findings from a cross-sectional survey (Natsal-3). *EClinicalMedicine, 2–3*, 29–36.

Cohen, M. S., Chen, Y. Q., McCauley, M., Gamble, T., Hosseinipour, M. C., Kumarasamy, N., … Fleming, T. R. (2011). Prevention of HIV-1 infection with early antiretroviral therapy. *New England Journal of Medicine, 365*(6), 493–505.

Connor, E. M., Sperling, R. S., Gelber, R., Kiselev, P., Scott, G., O'Sullivan, M. J., … Balsley, J. (1994). Reduction of maternal-infant transmission of human immunodeficiency virus type 1 with zidovudine treatment. *New England Journal of Medicine, 331*(18), 1173–1180.

Cresswell, F., Waters, L., Briggs, E., Fox, J., Harbottle, J., Hawkins, D., … Fisher, M. (2016). UK guideline for the use of HIV post-exposure prophylaxis following sexual exposure, 2015. *International Journal of STD and AIDS, 27*(9), 713–738.

de Silva, S., Miller, R. F., & Walsh, J. (2006). Lack of awareness of HIV post-exposure prophylaxis among HIV-infected and uninfected men attending an inner London clinic. *International Journal of STD & AIDS, 17*(9), 629–630.

Desai, M., Gafos, M., Dolling, D., McCormack, S., Nardone, A., & PROUD study (2016). Healthcare providers' knowledge of, attitudes to and practice of pre-exposure prophylaxis for HIV infection. *HIV Medicine, 17*(2), 133–142. https://doi.org/10.1111/hiv.12285

Donnell, D., Mimiaga, M. J., Mayer, K., Chesney, M., Koblin, B., & Coates, T. (2010). Use of non-occupational post-exposure prophylaxis does not lead to an increase in high risk sex behaviors in men who have sex with men participating in the EXPLORE trial. *AIDS and Behavior, 14*(5), 1182–1189.

Dubov, A., Galbo, P., Altice, F. L., & Fraenkel, L. (2018). Stigma and shame experiences by MSM who take PrEP for HIV prevention: A qualitative study. *American Journal of Men's Health, 12*(6), 1843–1854.

Elopre, L., McDavid, C., Brown, A., Shurbaji, S., Mugavero, M. J., & Turan, J. M. (2018). Perceptions of HIV pre-exposure prophylaxis among young, Black Men who have sex with men. *AIDS Patient Care and STDs, 32*(12), 511–518.

Evangeli, M., Pady, K., & Wroe, A. L. (2016). Which psychological factors are related to HIV testing? A quantitative systematic review of global studies. *AIDS and Behavior, 20*(4), 880–918.

Figueroa, C., Johnson, C., Verster, A., & Baggaley, R. (2015). Attitudes and acceptability on HIV self-testing among key populations: A literature review. *AIDS and Behavior, 19*(11), 1949–1965.

Ford, N., Irvine, C., Shubber, Z., Baggaley, R., Beanland, R., Vitoria, M., … Calmy, A. (2014). Adherence to HIV postexposure prophylaxis: A systematic review and meta-analysis. *AIDS (London, England), 28*(18), 2721–2727.

Frankis, J., Young, I., Flowers, P., & McDaid, L. (2014). Understanding the acceptability of pre-exposure prophylaxis (PrEP) for HIV prevention amongst gay and bisexual men in Scotland: A mixed methods study. Retrieved from https://researchonline.gcu.ac.uk/en/publications/understanding-the-acceptability-of-pre-exposure-prophylaxis-prep-

Frankis, J., Young, I., Flowers, P., & McDaid, L. (2016). Who will use pre-exposure prophylaxis (PrEP) and why?: Understanding PrEP awareness and acceptability amongst men who have sex with men in the UK—A mixed methods study. *PLoS One, 11*(4). https://doi.org/10.1371/journal.pone.0151385

Freeman, E. E., Weiss, H. A., Glynn, J. R., Cross, P. L., Whitworth, J. A., & Hayes, R. J. (2006). Herpes simplex virus 2 infection increases HIV acquisition in men and women: Systematic review and meta-analysis of longitudinal studies. *AIDS, 20*(1), 73–83.

Galvin, S. R., & Cohen, M. S. (2004). The role of sexually transmitted diseases in HIV transmission. *Nature Reviews Microbiology, 2*(1), 33–42.

Grant, R. M., Lama, J. R., Anderson, P. L., McMahan, V., Liu, A. Y., Vargas, L., … Glidden, D. V. (2010). Preexposure chemoprophylaxis for HIV prevention in men who have sex with men. *New England Journal of Medicine, 363*(27), 2587–2599.

Gray, R. H., Kigozi, G., Serwadda, D., Makumbi, F., Watya, S., Nalugoda, F., … Wawer, M. J. (2007). Male circumcision for HIV prevention in men in Rakai, Uganda: A randomised trial. *Lancet, 369*(9562), 657–666.

Gregson, S., Adamson, S., Papaya, S., Mundondo, J., Nyamukapa, C. A., Mason, P. R., … Anderson, R. M. (2007). Impact and process evaluation of integrated community and clinic-based HIV-1 control: A cluster-randomised trial in Eastern Zimbabwe. *PLoS Medicine, 4*(3). https://doi.org/10.1371/journal.pmed.0040102

Grosskurth, H., Mosha, F., Todd, J., Mwijarubi, E., Klokke, A., Senkoro, K., … Ka-Gina, G. (1995). Impact of improved treatment of sexually transmitted diseases on HIV infection in rural Tanzania: Randomised controlled trial. *Lancet, 346*(8974), 530–536.

Heijnders, M., & Van Der Meij, S. (2006). The fight against stigma: An overview of stigma-reduction strategies and interventions. *Psychology, Health & Medicine, 11*(3), 353–363.

Jaspal, R. (2019). *The social psychology of gay men.* London: Palgrave Macmillan.

Jaspal, R., & Cinnirella, M. (2010). Coping with potentially incompatible identities: Accounts of religious, ethnic and sexual identities from British Pakistani men who identify as Muslim and gay. *British Journal of Social Psychology, 49*(4), 849–870.

Jaspal, R., & Daramilas, C. (2016). Perceptions of pre-exposure prophylaxis (PrEP) among HIV-negative and HIV-positive men who have sex with men. *Cogent Medicine, 3,* 1256850. https://doi.org/10.1080/2331205X.2016.1256850

Jaspal, R., Lopes, B., Bayley, J., & Papaloukas, P. (2019). A structural equation model to predict pre-exposure prophylaxis acceptability in men who have sex with men in Leicester, UK. *HIV Medicine, 20*(1), 11–18.

Jaspal, R., & Nerlich, B. (2016). A 'morning-after' pill for HIV? Social representations of post-exposure prophylaxis for HIV in the British print media. *Health, Risk & Society, 18*(5–6), 225–246.

Jaspal, R., & Nerlich, B. (2017). Polarised reporting about HIV prevention: Social representations of pre-exposure prophylaxis (PrEP) in the UK press. *Health: An Interdisciplinary Journal for the Social Study of Health, Illness and Medicine, 21*(5), 478–497.

Johnson, C., Baggaley, R., Forsythe, S., van Rooyen, H., Ford, N., Napierala Mavedzenge, S., ... Taegtmeyer, M. (2014). Realizing the potential for HIV self-testing. *AIDS and Behavior, 18*(Suppl 4), S391–S395. https://doi.org/10.1007/s10461-014-0832-x

Kamali, A., Quigley, M., Nakiyingi, J., Kinsman, J., Kengeya-Kayondo, J., Gopal, R., ... Whitworth, J. (2003). Syndromic management of sexually-transmitted infections and behaviour change interventions on transmission of HIV-1 in rural Uganda: A community randomised trial. *The Lancet, 361*(9358), 645–652.

Karasavvas, N., Billings, E., Rao, M., Williams, C., Zolla-Pazner, S., Bailer, R. T., ... de Souza, M. S. (2012). The Thai Phase III HIV Type 1 Vaccine Trial (RV144) regimen induces antibodies that target conserved regions within the V2 loop of gp120. *AIDS Research and Human Retroviruses, 28*(11), 1444–1457.

Kendrick, S. R., Kroc, K. A., Withum, D., Rydman, R. J., Branson, B. M., & Weinstein, R. A. (2005). Outcomes of offering rapid point-of-care HIV testing in a sexually transmitted disease clinic. *JAIDS Journal of Acquired Immune Deficiency Syndromes, 38*(2), 142–146.

Körner, H., Ellard, J. M., Hendry, O., Kippax, S. C., Grulich, A. E., & Hodge, S. R. (2003). Taking post-exposure prophylaxis: Managing risk, reclaiming control. National Centre in HIV Social Research, Sydney.

Kurka, T., Soni, S., & Richardson, D. (2015). Sexual health services for men who have sex with men (MSM): Are they acceptable? *Sexually Transmitted Infections, 91*, A51. https://doi.org/10.1136/sextrans-2015-052126.150

Leichliter, J. S., Haderxhanaj, L. T., Chesson, H. W., & Aral, S. O. (2013). Temporal trends in sexual behavior among men who have sex with men in the United States, 2002 to 2006–10. *Journal of Acquired Immune Deficiency Syndromes (1999), 63*(2), 254–258.

Li, J., Gilmour, S., Zhang, H., Koyanagi, A., & Shibuya, K. (2012). The epidemiological impact and cost-effectiveness of HIV testing, antiretroviral treatment and harm reduction programs. *AIDS, 26*(16), 2069–2078.

Lorenc, T., Marrero-Guillamón, I., Llewellyn, A., Aggleton, P., Cooper, C., Lehmann, A., & Lindsay, C. (2011). HIV testing among men who have sex with men (MSM): Systematic review of qualitative evidence. *Health Education Research, 26*(5), 834–846.

MacKellar, D. A., Valleroy, L. A., Secura, G. M., Behel, S., Bingham, T., Celentano, D. D., … Young Men's Survey Study Group. (2005). Unrecognized HIV infection, risk behaviors, and perceptions of risk among young men who have sex with men: Opportunities for advancing HIV prevention in the third decade of HIV/AIDS. *Journal of Acquired Immune Deficiency Syndromes (1999), 38*(5), 603–614.

Marcus, U., Gassowski, M., & Drewes, J. (2016). HIV risk perception and testing behaviours among men having sex with men (MSM) reporting potential transmission risks in the previous 12 months from a large online sample of MSM living in Germany. *BMC Public Health, 16*(1), 1111. https://doi.org/10.1186/s12889-016-3759-5

McCormack, S., Dunn, D. T., Desai, M., Dolling, D. I., Gafos, M., Gilson, R., … Gill, O. N. (2016). Pre-exposure prophylaxis to prevent the acquisition of HIV-1 infection (PROUD): Effectiveness results from the pilot phase of a pragmatic open-label randomised trial. *The Lancet, 387*(10013), 53–60.

Mercer, C. H., Prah, P., Field, N., Tanton, C., Macdowall, W., Clifton, S., … Sonnenberg, P. (2016). The health and well-being of men who have sex with men (MSM) in Britain: Evidence from the third National Survey of Sexual Attitudes and Lifestyles (Natsal-3). *BMC Public Health, 16*(1), 525. https://doi.org/10.1186/s12889-016-3149-z

Millett, G. A., Flores, S. A., Marks, G., Reed, J. B., & Herbst, J. H. (2008). Circumcision status and risk of HIV and sexually transmitted infections among men who have sex with men: A meta-analysis. *JAMA, 300*(14), 1674–1684.

Molina, J.-M., Capitant, C., Spire, B., Pialoux, G., Cotte, L., Charreau, I., … Delfraissy, J.-F. (2015). On-demand preexposure prophylaxis in men at high risk for HIV-1 infection. *New England Journal of Medicine, 373*(23), 2237–2246.

Paz-Bailey, G., Mendoza, M. C. B., Finlayson, T., Wejnert, C., Le, B., Rose, C., … NHBS Study Group. (2016). Trends in condom use among MSM in the United States: The role of antiretroviral therapy and seroadaptive strategies. *AIDS, 30*(12), 1985–1990.

Pilkington, V., Hill, A., Hughes, S., Nwokolo, N., & Pozniak, A. (2018). How safe is TDF/FTC as PrEP? A systematic review and meta-analysis of the risk of adverse events in 13 randomised trials of PrEP. *Journal of Virus Eradication, 4*(4), 215–224.

Prost, A., Sseruma, W. S., Fakoya, I., Arthur, G., Taegtmeyer, M., Njeri, A., … Imrie, J. (2007). HIV voluntary counselling and testing for African communities in London: Learning from experiences in Kenya. *Sexually Transmitted Infections, 83*(7), 547–551.

Quinn, T. C., Wawer, M. J., Sewankambo, N., Serwadda, D., Li, C., Wabwire-Mangen, F., ... Gray, R. H. (2000). Viral load and heterosexual transmission of human immunodeficiency virus Type 1. *New England Journal of Medicine, 342*(13), 921–929.

Raifman, J., Dean, L. T., Montgomery, M. C., Almonte, A., Arrington-Sanders, R., Stein, M., ... Chan, P. A. (2019). Racial and ethnic disparities in HIV pre-exposure prophylaxis awareness among men who have sex with men. *AIDS and Behavior, 23*(10), 2706–2709.

Richens, J. (2005). Can the promotion of post-exposure prophylaxis following sexual exposure to HIV (PEPSE) cause harm? *Sexually Transmitted Infections, 81*(3), 190–191.

Rodger, A. J., Cambiano, V., Bruun, T., Vernazza, P., Collins, S., Degen, O., ... PARTNER Study Group. (2019). Risk of HIV transmission through condomless sex in serodifferent gay couples with the HIV-positive partner taking suppressive antiretroviral therapy (PARTNER): Final results of a multicentre, prospective, observational study. *Lancet, 393*(10189), 2428–2438.

Rodger, A. J., Cambiano, V., Bruun, T., Vernazza, P., Collins, S., van Lunzen, J., ... PARTNER Study Group. (2016). Sexual activity without condoms and risk of HIV transmission in serodifferent couples when the HIV-positive partner is using suppressive antiretroviral therapy. *JAMA, 316*(2), 171–181.

Roland, M. E., Neilands, T. B., Krone, M. R., Katz, M. H., Franses, K., Grant, R. M., ... Martin, J. N. (2005). Seroconversion following nonoccupational postexposure prophylaxis against HIV. *Clinical Infectious Diseases: An Official Publication of the Infectious Diseases Society of America, 41*(10), 1507–1513.

Root-Bernstein, R. S., & Hobbs, S. H. (1993). Does HIV 'Piggyback' on CD4-like surface proteins of sperm, viruses, and bacteria? Implications for co-transmission, cellular tropism and the induction of autoimmunity in AIDS. *Journal of Theoretical Biology, 160*(2), 249–264.

Røttingen, J. A., Cameron, D. W., & Garnett, G. P. (2001). A systematic review of the epidemiologic interactions between classic sexually transmitted diseases and HIV: How much really is known? *Sexually Transmitted Diseases, 28*(10), 579–597.

Sayer, C., Fisher, M., Nixon, E., Nambiar, K., Richardson, D., Perry, N., & Llewellyn, C. (2009). Will I? Won't I? Why do men who have sex with men present for post-exposure prophylaxis for sexual exposures? *Sexually Transmitted Infections, 85*(3), 206–211.

Schwartz, J., & Grimm, J. (2019). Stigma communication surrounding PrEP: The experiences of a sample of men who have sex with men. *Health Communication, 34*(1), 84–90.

Shernoff, M. (2006). *Without condoms: Unprotected sex, gay men & barebacking.* New York, NY: Routledge.

Spence, J. M. (2003). Should emergency departments offer postexposure prophylaxis for non-occupational exposure to HIV? *CJEM, 5*(01), 38–45.

St. Lawrence, J. S., Kelly, J. A., Dickson-Gomez, J., Owczarzak, J., Amirkhanian, Y. A., & Sitzler, C. (2015). Attitudes toward HIV voluntary counseling and testing (VCT) among African American men who have sex with men: Concerns underlying reluctance to test. *AIDS Education and Prevention, 27*(3), 195–211.

Stutterheim, S. E., Sicking, L., Brands, R., Baas, I., Roberts, H., van Brakel, W. H., … Bos, A. E. R. (2014). Patient and provider perspectives on HIV and HIV-related stigma in Dutch health care settings. *AIDS Patient Care and STDs, 28*(12), 652–665.

Thornton, A. C., Delpech, V., Kall, M. M., & Nardone, A. (2012). HIV testing in community settings in resource-rich countries: A systematic review of the evidence. *HIV Medicine, 13*(7), 416–426.

Traeger, M. W., Schroeder, S. E., Wright, E. J., Hellard, M. E., Cornelisse, V. J., Doyle, J. S., & Stoové, M. A. (2018). Effects of pre-exposure prophylaxis for the prevention of human immunodeficiency virus infection on sexual risk behavior in men who have sex with men: A systematic review and meta-analysis. *Clinical Infectious Diseases: An Official Publication of the Infectious Diseases Society of America, 67*(5), 676–686.

Tsai, C. C., Follis, K. E., Sabo, A., Beck, T. W., Grant, R. F., & Bischofberger, N. … Black, R. (1995). Prevention of SIV infection in macaques by (R)-9-(2-phosphonylmethoxypropyl)adenine. *Science, 270*(5239), 1197–1199.

UNAIDS. (2019). Global HIV & AIDS statistics—2019 fact sheet. Retrieved May 27, 2020, from https://www.unaids.org/en/resources/fact-sheet.

Vaccher, S. J., Kaldor, J. M., Callander, D., Zablotska, I. B., & Haire, B. G. (2018). Qualitative insights into adherence to HIV pre-exposure prophylaxis (PrEP) among Australian gay and bisexual men. *AIDS Patient Care and STDs, 32*(12), 519–528.

Van Damme, L., Ramjee, G., Alary, M., Vuylsteke, B., Chandeying, V., Rees, H., … COL-1492 Study Group. (2002). Effectiveness of COL-1492, a nonoxynol-9 vaginal gel, on HIV-1 transmission in female sex workers: A randomised controlled trial. *Lancet, 360*(9338), 971–977.

Wald, A., & Link, K. (2002). Risk of human immunodeficiency virus infection in herpes simplex virus type 2-seropositive persons: A meta-analysis. *The Journal of Infectious Diseases, 185*(1), 45–52.

Wang, X., Nutland, W., Brady, M., Green, I., Boffito, M., & McClure, M. (2019). Quantification of tenofovir disoproxil fumarate and emtricitabine in generic pre-exposure prophylaxis tablets obtained from the internet. *International Journal of STD & AIDS, 30*(8), 765–768.

Wawer, M. J., Sewankambo, N. K., Serwadda, D., Quinn, T. C., Paxton, L. A., Kiwanuka, N., … Gray, R. H. (1999). Control of sexually transmitted diseases for AIDS prevention in Uganda: A randomised community trial. Rakai Project Study Group. *Lancet (London, England), 353*(9152), 525–535.

Weatherburn, P., Hickson, F., Reid, D. S., Schink, S. B., Marcus, U., Schmidt, A. J., & European Centre for Disease Prevention and Control, Sigma Research (London School of Hygiene and Tropical Medicine), & Robert Koch-Institut. (2019). EMIS-2017: The European men-who-have-sex-with-men Internet survey: Key findings from 50 countries. Retrieved from http://publications.europa.eu/publication/manifestation_identifier/PUB_TQ0319440ENN

Williamson, I., Papaloukas, P., Jaspal, R., & Lond, B. (2019). 'There's this glorious pill': Gay and bisexual men in the English midlands navigate risk responsibility and pre-exposure prophylaxis. *Critical Public Health, 29*(5), 560–571.

Witzel, T. C., Rodger, A. J., Burns, F. M., Rhodes, T., & Weatherburn, P. (2016). HIV self-testing among men who have sex with men (MSM) in the UK: A qualitative study of barriers and facilitators, intervention preferences and perceived impacts. *PLoS One, 11*(9), e0162713. https://doi.org/10.1371/journal.pone.0162713

Wiysonge, C. S., Kongnyuy, E. J., Shey, M., Muula, A. S., Navti, O. B., Akl, E. A., & Lo, Y.-R. (2011). Male circumcision for prevention of homosexual acquisition of HIV in men. *The Cochrane Database of Systematic Reviews, 6*, CD007496. https://doi.org/10.1002/14651858.CD007496.pub2

Young, S. D., Nussbaum, A. D., & Monin, B. (2007). Potential moral stigma and reactions to sexually transmitted diseases: Evidence for a disjunction fallacy. *Personality and Social Psychology Bulletin, 33*(6), 789–799.

Yuan, T., Fitzpatrick, T., Ko, N.-Y., Cai, Y., Chen, Y., Zhao, J., ... Zou, H. (2019). Circumcision to prevent HIV and other sexually transmitted infections in men who have sex with men: A systematic review and meta-analysis of global data. *The Lancet Global Health, 7*(4), e436–e447. https://doi.org/10.1016/S2214-109X(18)30567-9

Zarwell, M., Ransome, Y., Barak, N., Gruber, D., & Robinson, W. T. (2019). PrEP indicators, social capital and social group memberships among gay, bisexual and other men who have sex with men. *Culture, Health & Sexuality, 21*(12), 1349–1366.

5

HIV Diagnosis, Management and Prognosis

HIV: Its Effects and Treatment

Antiretroviral therapy (ART) is one of the most significant success stories of modern medicine. It has saved millions of lives and prevented countless HIV transmissions. The advent of effective ART in 1996 was to herald a new phase of hope in the fight against HIV. Treatment brings about suppression of HIV, which in turn allows the immune system to function normally without being impeded by viral replication. CD4 cells, part of the immune system and the main target for HIV, are destroyed when HIV uses their internal machinery to produce new copies of itself, thereby destroying the host's own immune cells and ensuring the propagation of new viral particles to infect other CD4 cells. This process is repeated until eventual destruction of all CD4 cells.

In uncontrolled HIV, it thought that up to ten billion copies are produced each day which slowly depletes the level of functioning CD4 cells, leading to profound immunosuppression and increased susceptibility to opportunistic infections which a competent immune system would neutralise easily. On average, the process of being immunocompetent to becoming immunosuppressed takes approximately ten years, but this time frame

© The Author(s) 2020
R. Jaspal, J. Bayley, *HIV and Gay Men*, https://doi.org/10.1007/978-981-15-7226-5_5

can be highly variable. Use of ART and restoration of immune function are key to living well with HIV. Opportunistic infections can be fatal or leave patients with significant morbidity, especially if the central nervous system is affected. This is entirely avoidable with early diagnosis and treatment.

Of course, access to treatment is not equitable with some groups having decreased levels of engagement with specialist HIV services which can lead to poorer outcomes in the long term. Adherence to ART has improved for most as the side effect profiles of the newer drugs are infinitely better than the first generation of drugs from the 1990s. Looking ahead, injectable ART and sub-dermal implants of HIV drugs will supplant the need to take tablets every day further improving adherence and lessening the impact that HIV has on one's life.

HIV Virology and Patient Prognosis

HIV is an extremely effective virus. Not only does it manage to evade our immune system, one of the most sophisticated on the planet, but it also uses our very own cells to replicate and produce more viruses. This leads to the double whammy of destroying our immune system that usually protects us from viruses whilst releasing billions of copies of new HIV every day to infect other cells, if untreated. The resulting immunosuppression leaves us open to numerous opportunistic infections—ranging from mild, transient symptoms to often fatal conditions with significant morbidity if one does survive.

HIV cannot replicate on its own. It needs to utilise the host's cellular machinery to be able to replicate and establish infection. HIV must first circumnavigate the immune defence on the exposed mucosal surface, be it anal or vaginal mucosa if sexually transmitted. However, in cases where immune cells are present, they can also be used as an entry point for the virus. These 'target cells' for HIV are then presented to the immune system in preparation to be destroyed. HIV overwhelms the immune cells and causes an acute infection (otherwise known as seroconversion) which is discussed later.

There are many different types of immune cell, some of which kill pathogens immediately (natural killer cells); some which 'present' pathogens to other parts of the immune system for subsequent destruction (T cells); and some which have memory for previous infections (B cells) and if re-challenged produce antibodies—protective proteins that help to reduce repeat infections of the same pathogen. The main immune cells involved in HIV are CD4 cells, a T lymphocyte: CD standing for 'cluster of differentiation', named after its specific receptor on its surface to differentiate it from the 400 or so other cells within the immune system.

The viral capsid, or outer coat, of HIV is rich in glycoproteins which are perfectly adapted to attach to our CD4 receptors on the T-cell's surface. To gain entry into the CD4 cell, however, another co-receptor is needed. The co-receptor is usually CCR5, but the CXCR4 receptor is used if HIV infection has been established for many years.

Once the HIV is attached to the CD4 cell, it leads to fusion of the HIV capsid to the T-cell injecting the 'core virus' into the cytoplasm. The viral RNA is then translated into DNA by the reverse transcriptase enzyme (Jayappa, Ao, & Yao, 2012). The DNA then moves into the nucleus of the cell where it integrates or splices with our DNA and begins its replication cycle.

After this, the viral RNA is configured into new virions as the outer shell or viral capsid is constructed around the viral RNA by cellular processes from the host cell—HIV cannot complete this without the help of the host cell's own machinery. The outer layer of the virion is a lipid layer taken directly from the host's CD4 cell as it buds from the cell. These immature virus-like particles are then processed further to form an infectious new virion, which is then capable of infecting other CD4 cells. The CD4 cell does not survive this process. The process repeats until CD4 counts are eventually depleted.

Innate Immunity

Approximately 1% of the world population are naturally immune to HIV. As discussed, two receptors are needed for HIV to enter a CD4 cell, the CD4 receptor and either a CCR5 or CXCR4 receptor. If a mutation occurs in the CCR5 receptor, this does not allow HIV to enter the cell—rendering oneself immune. Nearly every mammal has two matching chromosomes, one from each parent; the two different genes on each chromosome are called alleles. If the alleles are the same, we are homozygous for that gene, if different, heterozygous. The gene that codes for the CCR5 receptor sometimes has a deletion (or a mutation) which changes the shape of the receptor and does not allow HIV to enter the CD4 cell. When just one of the alleles contains the mutation and the other is normal (heterozygous), only some of the receptors will allow HIV to enter, reducing the risk of HIV entering the CD4 cell. If both chromosomes contain the same mutation (homozygous), one is essentially immune to HIV as all of the receptors are mutated and do not allow HIV to enter the CD4 cell. The prevalence of this mutation is related directly to geographical latitude with those in higher latitude countries (i.e. Scandinavian countries) having higher levels of mutations of the CCR5 receptor and therefore a lower risk of HIV infection (Ni, Wang, & Wang, 2018). The role of the CCR5 receptor is not fully understood, but it is thought to interact with other immune cells involved in the regulation of immune response. Interestingly, this mutation is the reason why two patients have been 'cured' following bone marrow transplants—after destruction of the immune system by chemo- and radiotherapy, the transplanted immune cells were selected to have CCR5 mutation, residual HIV was unable to infect the new immune cells, and a total cure was achieved. Given the dangerous nature of bone marrow transplants, this is unlikely to become a practical modality for HIV cure in the future.

HIV Seroconversion

Seroconversion, or very early infection, appears about two to four weeks after initial exposure to the virus and is characterised by a flu-like illness, sore throat, muscle aches and rash—not unlike many other common viral exanthems such as COVID-19, making it difficult to distinguish clinically. During early infection, the immune system is overwhelmed by HIV, and levels of virus in the blood are extremely high as the immune system tries to control its unrelenting replication. A corollary of this is that these patients are also extremely infectious during this period. Once the seroconversion period is over, a 'viral set point' is established with equilibrium between the immune system and HIV itself, that is, the immune system manages to gain control over HIV replication. The higher the viral set point, the quicker it takes to overwhelm the immune system leading to earlier onset immunosuppression (Geskus et al., 2007).

After seroconversion, viral replication continues, but at a more controlled rate than early infection. The viral set point is a good indicator of how long it will take to develop AIDS—defined as a CD4 <200 cells/mm^3 plus an AIDS-defining illness (Stein, Korvick, & Vermund, 1992). AIDS-defining illnesses are still commonly seen by HIV doctors who work on medical wards caring for hospitalised patients—the most commonly seen infections are PCP (or PJP as it now called), TB, progressive multifocal leucoencephalopathy (PML) and toxoplasmosis. One of most well-known of the AIDS diagnoses was the pathognomonic violaceous skin lesions of Kaposi's sarcoma—a skin cancer driven by a HSV that often heralded a diagnosis of AIDS in the early days. These lesions are still seen today and can affect skin and other organs needing intensive chemotherapy with unfavourable long-term side effects.

Most of us will have a CD4 count of above 500 cells/mm^3 and this constitutes a 'normal' immune system. This can be transiently increased by exercise but also temporarily depleted by any viral illness, such as the common cold or influenza. When we talk about immunocompromise, clinicians usually refer to a CD4 count of less than 200 cells/mm^3 where the chances of acquiring an opportunistic infection are greatly increased.

Patients may have up to ten years of latent infection before the CD4 count drops to dangerously low levels—with some never progressing to full immunosuppression, so-called elite controllers. The rate at which the CD4 count drops is variable, but observational data suggest that this can range from 35 to 60 cells/mm^3 per year (Verma, 2014; Wolbers et al., 2010). The slope of the decline does not accurately predict the time taken to progress to AIDS, but being older and having a lower CD4 count at diagnosis (especially <350 cells/mm^3) are associated with a more rapid decline in immune function.

In clinical practice, CD4 counts were the main HIV surrogate marker and were measured at every clinic visit (2–3 times a year for stable patients). These days HIV viral load (the amount of virus in each drop of blood) is a much better marker of whether treatment is working. CD4 counts are now only measured once a year, or less, if people are stable on treatment. CD4 count was used as a marker to determine when to initiate treatment with ART, as directed by the relevant national guidelines. For the UK, the British HIV Association (BHIVA) guidelines are the gold standard and updated regularly to reflect new data and commissioning changes.

Nowadays, HIV treatment is started immediately after diagnosis, regardless of CD4 count. However, this was not always the case. Generally, a CD4 count of between 200 and 350 cells/mm^3 was the recommended starting point for many years in most guidelines across the world. This involved waiting for the patient's immune system to reach these levels if they had a high CD4 at diagnosis. Exceptions were fairly common and those who were symptomatic, diagnosed with an AIDS-defining illness, or had a strong desire to start treatment were initiated on ART outside the recommendations of the guidelines. However, this began to change as new data from the SMART and START studies indicated that early initiation of ART, even while CD4 counts were still relatively high, yielded better clinical outcomes.

The SMART study (Strategies for Management of Antiretroviral Therapy (SMART) Study Group et al., 2006), funded by the National Institute of Allergy and Infectious Diseases in the US, sought to address the impact of drug holidays (the voluntary cessation of ART to minimise side effects) in a clinical trial focusing on continuous versus intermittent treatment. The trial was halted early as it was shown that intermittent treatment was associated with a 2.6 higher chance of dying than when taking continuous therapy. Unexpectedly, rates of non-AIDS-defining illnesses, such as cardiovascular, renal and hepatic complications were also greatly increased in those taking intermittent treatment. The assumption before the trial was that, given the sometimes harmful side effects of ART, health complications would reduce with drug holidays—the opposite was found to be true indicating a very strong protective factor when taking continuous ART.

Nine years later, the START study (INSIGHT START Study Group et al., 2015) further demonstrated the benefits of effective ART by comparing ART initiation at a CD4 of over 500 cells/mm^3 and less than 350 cells/mm^3. Incredibly, immediate treatment (i.e. CD4 >500 cells/mm^3)

led to a 57% reduction in all serious illnesses, whether related to AIDS or not. There was also a reduction in serious AIDS-related events of over 70%. These significant reductions in adverse outcomes has meant that the START study was one of the most influential HIV treatment studies in the last decade and that it has transformed how clinicians deliver HIV care. Prior to this, many physicians would wait for the CD4 count to fall, but on publication of these data, national guidelines were updated almost immediately and recommended immediate treatment for all, regardless of CD4 count.

With these data came the realisation that HIV not only depletes CD4 cells but that unchecked viral replication was causing widespread inflammation. The heart, kidney and brain especially were being subjected to damage from the very mechanism designed to protect the body from such assaults. Clinicians soon began to start HIV treatment immediately for all patients, challenging the central dogma of using CD4 thresholds as a treatment guide. This also led to a novel pathway for HIV research, namely, chronic inflammation caused by replicating virus.

Chronic Inflammation and HIV

Data from both the SMART and START trials demonstrated that cardiovascular and renal complications were much lower in those taking ART due to lower levels of immune activation in this cohort. It is now known that even this level of immune activation can lead to severe complications through a variety of mechanisms (Zicari et al., 2019).

For example, during the seroconversion illness, a large proportion of the memory immune cells, which usually reside in specialised tissue in the gastrointestinal tract (gastrointestinal-associated lymphoid tissue), are destroyed by HIV. This usually occurs within the first six months of infection and cannot be restored by ART, even if initiated relatively early. The destruction of this specialised gut tissue leads to a disruption in how pathogens are processed and leads to higher levels of inflammation within the gut with important consequences for the microbiome of the gut, or the balance of 'good' and 'bad' bacteria. Disruptions of the microbiome of the gut have been linked to depression, anxiety and a whole host of other conditions. There are significant differences in the microbiome of the gut in those living with HIV versus the general population (Dillon, Frank, & Wilson, 2016).

Some studies have shown increased levels of pro-inflammatory bacteria, such as *Prevotella* spp., which can lead to gut inflammation and overall increased immune activation (Dillon et al., 2014). Destruction of the gut immune tissue also impairs the ability to stop microbes from entering the bloodstream. This microbial translocation from the gut to the bloodstream activates the immune system, which recognises them as invaders and releases cytokines, or inflammatory messengers, into the blood leading to prolonged chronic inflammation which begins to exhaust the immune system over time. Known effects of this are a reduction in the function of the thymus gland (where T-cells are matured and released) and sclerosis of the immune lymphatic system. It also affects the intricate blood clotting system leading to the release of pro-coagulants which increases the risk of thrombosis, or blood clots, leading to higher rates of myocardial ischaemia (i.e. heart attacks) and strokes. Treatments that counter this unchecked inflammation have so far been inconclusive. Much hope is being placed on the anti-inflammatory effects of statins, anti-cholesterol drugs in a large trial called REPREIVE which aims to reduce inflammation seen in HIV and reduce negative health outcomes associated with chronic inflammation, such as cardiac events.

HIV Treatment

A key responsibility of HIV clinicians is to construct an effective combination of antiretroviral drugs, which is tailored to individual patients. Relevant factors to consider when starting ART include the patient's age, gender, immune status, renal function and the presence of other chronic diseases. Clinicians must also consider bone health, other medicines being taken, recreational drugs, HIV viral load, side effect profiles of each drug and the size of the tablets themselves (some are quite large and can be difficult to swallow). A key *psychological* factor is whether the patient is actually ready and willing to initiate life-long ART—if this part of the puzzle is missing, successful treatment is hard to maintain over long periods.

The patient's lifestyle is a key consideration. For example, a young gay man who participates in chemsex would not be initiated on a protease-based ART regimen, as ritonavir may boost (or potentiate) the drugs used in chemsex (i.e. GHB). Indeed, there have been many cases of HIV-positive gay men (on a protease-based regimen) who have taken GHB and ended up in hospital in a life-threatening condition. Another example is the patient who works night shifts regularly who may find that efavirenz (a commonly used non-nucleoside reverse transcriptase inhibitor [NNRTI]) gives him severe dizziness and disorientation during his night shift.

Moreover, clinicians must be mindful of the costs associated with particular ART regimens. The prescription of more expensive drugs is monitored closely, and they are often saved for those who are treatment-experienced with multiple class resistance (i.e. resistance to multiple classes of ART). In London, there is a collaboration of clinicians, policy-makers and academics who publish guidance on the most cost-effective treatments available at the time. For more expensive drugs to be prescribed, regimens must be discussed on a case by case basis at local team meetings to rationalise the use of expensive drugs.

It is useful to discuss briefly the drugs by class with common considerations given as to why they would be used.

Nucleoside Reverse Transcriptase Inhibitors

Nucleoside reverse transcriptase inhibitors (NRTI or 'nukes') are the backbone of the vast majority of HIV drug regimens. The basic building blocks of DNA, and therefore life, are the bases adenosine, cytosine, thymidine and guanine. These are the smallest building blocks in DNA which go on to form proteins, ubiquitous organic molecules vital to human function and survival. Each NRTI drug is essentially a copy of the corresponding base and similar to the naturally occurring bases found in almost all cells.

AZT is a copy (or analogue) of thymidine, tenofovir to adenosine, abacavir to guanine and so on. Structurally, they are nearly indistinguishable from naturally occurring bases (apart from a few extra phosphate groups), so will be fully utilised by HIV enzymes to form the DNA needed to produce new virus. Once these mimics are incorporated into the viral DNA, the added phosphate group leads to inhibition of the enzyme reverse transcriptase and stops further HIV replication by not allowing further bases to be added to the genetic material.

Each NRTI has its own side effect and pharmacological profile. However, this class of ART is generally well tolerated in most people. When HIV drugs were in their infancy, the older NRTIs did have significant longer-term side effects, such as lipodystrophy (abnormal accumulation of fat tissue), one of the most visible side effects for those living with HIV in the 1990s and early 2000s. Other side effects attributed to the early NRTIs are pancreatitis, neuropathy, lactic acidosis, hepatic steatosis and cardiomyopathy—all very unpleasant and some life-threatening.

Side effects result from damage to the mitochondria, energy-producing organelles that power all living cells. The number of mitochondria differs greatly depending on how much energy is needed, but on average there are between 100 and 1000 per cell. Mitochondrial DNA (mtDNA) and the enzyme that builds it (DNA polymerase γ) are affected by NRTIs. This inhibition of DNA polymerase γ and damage to mtDNA lead to cellular dysfunction, increasing levels of waste product and leading to eventual death. As mtDNA is ubiquitous in the body, the side effect profile of NRTIs is very diverse (Gerschenson & Brinkman, 2004).

Older NRTIs were particularly malign, with ddI (didanosine) and d4T (stavudine), two of the earliest NRTI, causing peripheral nerve damage in a third of patients exposed to these drugs (Simpson & Tagliati, 1995). The longer-term complications of nerve damage are unpleasant, painful and difficult to treat, often necessitating large doses of drugs to suppress nerve conduction (such as amitriptyline or gabapentin), which in turn can have their own fatigue-inducing side effects.

Another debilitating and sometimes life-limiting side effect of these early NRTI is liver disease. People who were exposed to ddI or d4T are, on average, 30–40% more likely to develop liver disease, and thus, these drugs have been discontinued in nearly all developed countries (Ryom et al., 2016).

One newer NRTI, abacavir, deserves special consideration here as its history is chequered, although it remains one of most commonly used

NRTI. Abacavir is one of the first drugs to have its side effect profile clarified in relation to the genetics of the person taking it. It is one of the first drugs personalised to one's genetic code. When abacavir was first used in 1998, it was found that between 5 and 8% of patients developed an unusual array of symptoms which mimicked a severe immune reaction (nausea, diarrhoea, rash, fatigue, fever, cough, shortness of breath) and when abacavir was restarted after a break, patients had severe anaphylactic reactions (Escaut, Liotier, Albengres, Cheminot, & Vittecoq, 1999; Walensky, Goldberg, & Daily, 1999). Initially it was unclear as to why only certain patients developed these side effects until 2002 when it was first linked to the gene HLA B*5701 (Mallal et al., 2002). Human leucocyte antigens (HLA) are a complex mechanism for recognising one's own proteins versus those from virus or bacteria, and they are expressed on most cells in the body. It was discovered that those with certain genetic codes (HLA B*5701 positive) recognised abacavir as a potential pathogen and inadvertently triggered and stimulated the immune system in an effort to destroy it. This gave rise to the abacavir hypersensitivity reaction manifesting as the symptoms described above (Illing, Purcell, & McCluskey, 2017).

Guidelines are now unanimous in relation to the testing of HLA B*5701 in all patients who would need to take abacavir. In certain instances, it can be given before the test is done if there is an urgent need, but with caution in higher-risk populations as the allele is much more likely in White patients (Cao et al., 2001; Hughes et al., 2004) than those with African heritage.

Non-nucleoside Reverse Transcriptase Inhibitors

Non-nucleoside reverse transcriptase inhibitors (NNRTI or 'non-nukes') have been the most popular third choice of drug since their development (with the other two drugs, or the 'backbone', usually being NRTIs). The most commonly used NNRTIs have been efavirenz and nevirapine, with efavirenz being one of the most commonly used agents globally to date.

NNRTIs still inhibit the reverse transcriptase enzyme but do not mimic the bases themselves. Instead, they directly interact with the reverse transcriptase enzyme to stop its activity. Three dimensionally, the enzyme looks like a hand, palm up; when it is active the thumb and index finger come together, a little like the universally recognised 'ok' sign with the genetic material being made in the space between thumb and index finger. NNRTI irreversibly binds to reverse transcriptase to induce a conformational change to the protein—it keeps the active sites apart (the thumb and index finger cannot touch) so the enzyme is unable to function.

Efavirenz has been a first-line treatment for HIV since 1998 and was used as a gold standard of treatment for over a decade. It has high potency against HIV, can be co-formulated easily, only needs to be taken once a day, is safe in pregnancy and has a more favourable safety profile than its main counterpart, nevirapine. It was also part of the first single-tablet regimen in the UK and US, Atripla.

The release of Atripla—the first ever one-tablet once-a-day regimen—in 2007 was a huge step forward not only for drug adherence but also for normalising HIV treatment. It proved popular among patients who may have previously struggled with taking up to 25 tablets a day and was a firm favourite for clinicians across the globe. Nowadays we have a wide array of single-tablet regimens for the treatment of HIV, but at the time this co-formulation was a pharmaceutical success with three separate drug companies (Gilead Sciences, Merck and Bristol-Myers Squibb) in an unusual but successful collaboration. To date, Atripla continues, in its generic formulation, to be one of the most popular single-tablet regimens to date globally.[1]

As with most medicines, however, it is not without its side effects. Up to a third of those taking efavirenz will experience dizziness and other neuropsychiatric effects such as anxiety, vivid dreams and poor sleep (Ford et al., 2015). These symptoms do eventually settle but can be persistent in many. Efavirenz use is avoided in those who work night shifts (it is taken before bed to reduce these side effects) and those with mental health issues.

Interestingly, it has been shown that these side effects may be related to the genetics of the person taking it. The CYP2B6 is a pathway in the liver which metabolises certain drugs. Those with certain mutations

---

[1] https://apps.who.int/iris/bitstream/handle/10665/179532/9789241509152_eng.pdf;jsessionid
=E0A1B30C508A16A7C461F87779762440?sequence=1.

metabolising efavirenz more slowly leading to higher concentrations and side effects (Gounden, van Niekerk, Snyman, & George, 2010). Another example of how genetics influences drug delivery and future dosing (many of those with the less efficient alleles can tolerate a dose reduction of efavirenz with fewer side effects and no loss in viral suppression).

A metabolite (8-hydroxyefavirenz) has been subject to much research as it has been shown that, in the central nervous system, the concentration can be high enough to cause direct neuronal damage possibly explaining why patients have such side effects from this drug (Tovar-y-Romo et al., 2012). To date, it is still used in developing countries but has largely been replaced by newer drugs with cleaner side effect profiles in resource-rich healthcare systems.

Protease Inhibitors

Protease inhibitors (PIs) remain an extremely useful and popular third-line agent for those who need HIV treatment. The HIV protease enzyme is used late in the HIV replication cycle when the immature HIV virion is being assembled within the CD4 cell. The protease helps to develop its outer shell and starts to mature into an infective virion ready to be released and infect other cells. If this enzyme is inhibited, HIV replication is halted.

The first PI to begin clinical trials in 1989 was saquinavir. It was shown to have potent anti-HIV activity making it very durable, especially if the HIV had been exposed to previous drugs and had developed resistance. This is the case with all PIs. This group of medicines was the final piece of the puzzle in highly active ART and heralded a new phase in sustained HIV suppression that came about in 1996 when effective ART was discovered.

PIs, however, are not without their drawbacks. Early PIs often had severe gastrointestinal side effects, mainly diarrhoea and nausea, with many patients stopping due to the unbearable side effects. This was in addition to marked changes in body fat distribution which gave patients hollow cheeks and had a significant psychological impact on those experiencing these side effects. Given the short half-life of the early PIs, they were often given three times a day with little forgiveness for poor adherence—virological failure was common. Ritonavir, a very early PI, was found to have potent inhibitory activity against the pathway that metabolises many medicines (cytochrome P450 [CYP] 3A4), thereby 'boosting' other PIs and is still used today.

This 'boosting' mechanism constituted an important development as it reduced doses of other toxic PIs and therefore side effects. However, a significant number of other drugs are affected leading to very complicated interactions if taken with other medicines. Often they are avoided as balancing these drug effects can be very difficult.

A common and sometimes serious interaction is with inhaled corticosteroids (such as those taken for asthma, especially fluticasone) which increase levels of the steroid when taken with ritonavir. The high levels of steroid from the inhalers, potentiated by ritonavir, can lead to Cushing syndrome, which is an endocrinological syndrome leading to swelling of the face and abnormal fat distribution. If the inhalers are stopped abruptly, this can result in an Addisonian crisis, an endocrinological emergency, which can be fatal if not treated early. Most HIV clinicians will have seen cases in their clinical practice which can be challenging to manage.

Patients who have poor adherence to ART are at risk of adverse health outcomes, and a careful history concerning concomitant medicines and attitudes towards HIV should be explored so that the clinician can challenge any myths or anxieties the patient may have. Often, reasons for not taking medicines may mask underlying acceptance issues in relation to the HIV diagnosis itself with the pills being a daily reminder of their status. Psychological support is key to overcoming this.

Integrase Strand Transfer Inhibitors

INSTIs (or integrases) were developed later than other classes of ARVs, with the first, raltegravir, being approved in 2007. It was given accelerated approval from the FDA due to its high effectiveness, especially in treatment-experienced patients who were resistant to other drugs. The enzyme, integrase, splices HIV DNA into the host cell's genome. Once this enzyme is inhibited, further replication of HIV is stopped.

Clinically, integrases have been an extremely useful addition to the HIV treatment armamentarium. Those who developed resistance to other classes of drugs exhibited a good response to this class of drugs providing a lifeline of effective treatment for those who would otherwise have struggled to remain virologically suppressed. Also, the rate of viral decline in those taking INSTIs is much quicker when compared to other agents (Messiaen et al., 2013; Rockstroh et al., 2013). It is therefore extremely effective for treating patients with very high viral loads, such as those who are seronconverting to reduce onward transmission.

INSTIs remain a popular choice for many patients due to a relatively clean side effect profile with only a minority of patients experiencing sleep disturbance and insomnia. They have few interactions with other medicines allowing effective viral suppression for those with other health conditions who may be taking a pharmacopeia of other medicines. In clinical practice, they have also proven to be very useful for those engaging in chemsex given the few interactions with recreational drugs with less inadvertent overdose—a lethal phenomenon seen in those taking enzyme inhibitors such as ritonavir.

The newer INSTI, dolutegravir, has proven very popular due to a high genetic barrier to resistance and excellent tolerability for patients. Two recent studies, TANGO (van Wyk et al., 2020) and GEMINI (Cahn et al., 2019), have both shown that dolutegravir plus either lamivudine (a NRTI) or rilpivarine (a NNRTI) as dual therapy is just as effective as taking the standard three-drug regimen, with few side effects and almost no viral resistance. This is an important step in challenging the dogma of three-drug regimens allows less drug exposure to NRTIs, the usual backbone for ART, and also significant cost savings (3TC is amongst the cheapest of ARVs due to it being off patent for a number of years). Dual therapy may be the future of modern ART as newer medicines have improved genetic barriers to resistance with favourable pharmacokinetic profiles.

CCR5 Receptor Inhibitors

Since the discovery of the CCR5 receptor on immune cells and its necessity for HIV entry into CD4 cells, it has long been a target for drug therapy. Maraviroc, currently the only licensed CCR5 receptor inhibitor for use in HIV, was developed at astonishing speed with only six years between identification in 2001 and approval in 2007.

Maraviroc is unique in that the target—the CCR5 receptor—is an external protein on the cell surface rather than an intracellular viral protein, the target of nearly all other HIV drugs. Maraviroc is a small molecule that causes a physical structural change to the CCR5 receptor which makes it impossible for HIV to enter the CD4 cell.

Maraviroc is used when a novel mechanism of HIV inhibition is needed, usually in the context of multi-drug-resistant HIV, and is an effective part of many salvage regimens for heavily treatment-experienced patients. Care must be taken to ensure the HIV is CCR5-tropic, that is, the HIV population uses CCR5 as its co-receptor, and not CXCR4, as this renders maraviroc useless.

HIV Treatment Failure and Resistance

Despite the huge advances in ART, treatment can still fail. Of those taking ART, 5–10% per year fail (Jose et al., 2016). The rate of failure differs by group, with gay men having the lowest rates of treatment failure when compared to heterosexual patients. Within the gay demographic, there are also variations in failure rates with those aged over 45 years having estimated failure rates of only 1% per year (O'Connor et al., 2017). Starting ART after 2008 is also a protective factor against treatment failure; this is likely due to the less toxic side effects and better adherence to the newer drugs.

Of those who do fail, some will go on to develop drug resistance rendering their current regimen inactive against their HIV. This is familiar territory for the HIV physician and testing for resistance should occur in this setting. The results of these resistance tests then allow a new and more effective regimen to be given to help re-suppress HIV replication.

HIV replicates quickly and efficiently once infection is established. Between 1 and 10 billion viruses are produced each day in an individual who is not on treatment. Reverse transcriptase, as with other enzymes, often makes random errors in the transcription of the genetic code. Therefore the daughter copy may differ from its parent which can result in HIV with new properties. Some mutations confer an advantage, most do not. These quasispecies, or sub-populations, which are related to the original but slightly different, may go on to become the dominant viral species.

Drug resistance arises when drugs exert pressure on those viruses whose mutation confers resistance to that particular drug. Commonly, these are the result of having sub-therapeutic drug levels within the body (i.e. the drug is present in the body, but not at high enough levels to fully suppress the virus). These low levels of drugs in the body can result from missing doses of ART or drug interactions with other medicines. Once this mutated family is resistant to a drug, it then becomes the main species of HIV and treatment failure occurs.

Generics

The annual budget in England for HIV care, provided by NHS England, is just over half a billion pounds per year, with the majority being spent on ART. The cost of these drugs is dictated by pharmaceutical companies and market forces. Often, new HIV drugs (especially single-tablet regimens containing two or more drugs) can cost over £500 per month.

Pharmaceutical companies spend vast sums of money on identifying and developing effective drugs that are safe, effective and tolerable. Companies have exclusivity of the drugs they develop for 20 years after approval. During this time, the pharmaceutical company can set whatever price it sees fit. Significant discounts can be given for large orders of drug, as seen in the HIV London Consortium who bulk buy all ARVs for those receiving care in London, saving millions of pounds in the process.

By 2033, nearly all of the HIV drugs we see on the market today will be beyond the patent period and can then be manufactured by any company at a fraction of the cost, often as low as 10% of the original price. For now, only some of the older HIV drugs are now available as generics, but the huge price reduction has led to a shift in prescribing the cheaper generic versions. A study led by Public Health England (Ong et al., 2019) showed that if clinicians switched all patients to generics as they are released, it could save the NHS up to £7 billion by 2033, allowing more funding to be directed towards HIV prevention and research into effective vaccines and a possible cure for HIV.

Choosing an Effective HIV Treatment Regimen

The HIV clinician has to choose an effective regimen for those newly diagnosed or who have failed on their previous treatment, for whatever reason. A number of factors must be taken into consideration before starting, giving different weight to each factor depending on the patient sitting in front of them. Often, patients are started on the accepted first- or second-line combinations (usually a Kivexa or Truvada backbone with the third agent as NNRTI, INSTI or PI) with the best virological efficacy and a side effect profile that is acceptable to both clinician and, more importantly, the patient. Some of the considerations associated with choosing an effective HIV treatment regimen are discussed below.

HIV Viral Load

The viral load at initiation of therapy can vary significantly and is dependent on the stage of infection, with those who are seroconverting or diagnosed very late often having very high viral loads which may need to be reduced quickly. Several factors must be considered, such as, if the person has an HIV-negative partner, if their occupation requires them to have undetectable virus (i.e. surgeon or dentist) or the need for urgent surgery. Also, some drugs may have unacceptable failure rates when the viral load is too high. Abacavir, for example, has been shown in some studies to have less efficacy for viral loads of over 100,000 copies/ml (Sax et al., 2009). This does not mean that patients cannot have this medicine, but that the HIV clinician will have to be very vigilant to ensure viral decay is progressing at the expected rate with a low threshold for intensifying or switching, if needed. There has been a recent shift to giving a standard three-drug regimen *plus* an INSTI to help bring the viral load down quickly. The INSTI can then be stopped once viral suppression is achieved.

Renal Function

Kidneys filter the blood and excrete waste products in the urine, including the majority of drugs, antiretrovirals included. Older age naturally leads to a decline in kidney function which may be worsened by other common conditions such as hypertension or diabetes. As one's ability to clear waste products and drugs decreases, there may be a risk of drug accumulation in the body, which may be toxic in extreme cases. Therefore, if renal function is impaired, some drug doses need to be reduced in order to avoid damaging toxicities. Also, some drugs may have a direct toxic effect on the kidneys, especially tenofovir disfumarate, which is avoided in patients with kidney impairment to slow the rate of further decline.

HLA B*5701

This genetic test is part of the baseline set of tests for all new diagnoses in the UK, with approximately 6% of Caucasian patients having the genes that make it dangerous to administer abacavir (Hughes et al., 2004). In certain settings (mainly emergencies and with no other options), abacavir can be given without the test results, but with extreme caution and a high level of suspicion for the abacavir sensitivity reaction if the patient becomes unwell.

Co-infections

In the UK, approximately 6.7% and 10.7% of people living with HIV are co-infected with hepatitis B (HBV) and C (HCV), respectively (Thornton, 2015). This is much higher than the general population (around 0.5–1.0% for each) and is reflective of high rates of sexually acquired infections (fisting, for example, has been shown to be a risk factor for HCV infection). Injecting drug use, as seen in some gay men who participate in chemsex, is also problematic despite robust needle exchange programmes available in the UK.

Treatment of HBV and HIV often overlap, particularly tenofovir and 3TC/FTC. Therefore, solutions of regimens containing both these drugs can simultaneously treat both infections with minimal drug exposure. For those diagnosed with HCV, the treatment now often includes oral therapy for 12 weeks but interactions between these and HIV drugs, especially PIs, can lead to unacceptable toxicities and modification of ART is required. TB is also much more common in those living with HIV, as HIV is in fact a risk factor for TB infection. The treatment for TB can often involve rifampicin, a potent anti-TB agent but an even more potent liver enzyme inducer which reduces the levels of many concomitant medications. Careful liaison with pharmacists and drug databases is required to ensure all drug levels are at an effective concentration.

Concomitant Medicines

A careful drug history from all patients is required at every visit for the HIV clinician—the frequency of drug interactions is high and almost every clinic requires a discussion with pharmacy colleagues to help decipher the often complicated interactions. This can even apply to over-the-counter medications, herbal remedies and recreational drugs.

HIV Resistance Test

All newly diagnosed patients in the UK should have baseline resistance patterns. The rates of transmitted drug resistance in the UK are between 6 and 10% of all new infections (Tostevin et al., 2017). However, this is decreasing with the advent of newer PI and INSTI. If drug mutations are found, this can influence the decision about which ART to prescribe as certain classes of drugs (or more than one in some cases) may not be effective in suppressing HIV. Discussion at team meetings at most HIV centres allows clinicians to reach an agreement about the best regimen for that patient.

Patient Acceptability

Most patients allow their HIV clinician to decide their most appropriate treatment regimen, although some will have expectations about what they will find acceptable or will have completed research (online or through friends who have HIV) before the consultation. This can significantly influence the decision-making process of the clinician, and conversations about the patient's expectations are helpful.

Some patients will not want to start ART immediately for a variety of reasons as they do not, for instance, feel ready to start medication for the rest of their life or they may be worried about the side effects or a household member finding their tablets. These decisions must be respected. However, it is also important to explore any possible factual errors and patients' fears and anxieties. Clinicians should be sensitive and responsive to patients' concerns in relation to their treatment—if patients are not fully invested in the process, adherence can be poor, resulting in treatment failure, a poor patient experience and opportunistic infections if treatment is not adhered to.

Social Background

All clinicians should be able to construct a fairly accurate idea of the social background for most patients (i.e. education level, occupation) as this may affect the treatment regimen given. For those who work nights, efavirenz should be avoided given the dosing at night and potential dizziness. Those who may have unstable social settings, such as those with substance use issues or who are homeless, HIV may not be their main priority and adherence can be poor. For these groups of patients, treatment with PIs or newer INSTI drugs are often preferred as they allow more doses to be missed without resultant treatment failure.

Future of HIV Treatment

Future treatment modalities for HIV seem promising, with the eventual goal of an HIV cure, either functional cure where viral suppression is achieved without ART, or a total cure where HIV is removed from all host cells.

The ultimate goal of future HIV treatment is the elusive cure. This has proved much more complicated than anyone first imagined. The challenge is that, once the HIV DNA is incorporated into the CD4 cells as part of its replication cycle, it is very difficult to 'splice' out the infected DNA portion. Indeed, the integration of viral DNA into our own is sometimes called the 'fatal step' as this then allows the creation of a *reservoir* of HIV that is difficult to treat even with the most effective ART (Wiegand et al., 2017). On treatment these latently infected cells escape immune recognition, and when ART is stopped, they begin producing HIV virus, and an HIV viral rebound ensues.

This reservoir is the cornerstone to HIV cure research. It is thought that the majority of the reservoir is created during the early stages of infection. Research has shown that those treated with effective ART during seroconversion, that is, very early on in the infection, have a reduced reservoir (and therefore have low levels of latently infected cells). Indeed, some patients who had treatment started during seroconversion and continued for a number of years, remained undetectable when treatment was stopped some years after starting—a so-called functional cure (Sáez-Cirión et al., 2013). This is in contrast to a sterilising cure, whereby all cells with HIV are eradicated, such as the two patients who were successfully 'cured' subsequent to being given new immune cells without CCR5 receptors, which inhibited the re-establishment of HIV, as part of a bone marrow transplant. For those who do subsequently develop haematological cancers, this approach may become standard practice in the future. This may have the advantage of a sterilising cure through the use of new cells that are immune to HIV (due to a lack of the CCR5 receptor).

Two of the most significant unanswered questions include how to precisely measure the size of the reservoir and how to activate the latent cells so they can be treated with ART, a therapeutic vaccine or broadly neutralising antibodies or a combination of all three—the 'kick and kill' theory. The standard of measurement is called a viral outgrowth assay (Bruner et al., 2016) where a concentration of T-cells is stimulated to produce HIV and measured quantitatively. However, this approach is costly, time-consuming and not all of the HIV produced is viable. Work continues on refining this process which has not yet been perfected to yield a cure (Bruner et al., 2019).

The activation of latent CD4 cells can be achieved with medications called histone deacetylation inhibitors. One of these drugs, vorinostat, was used with a therapeutic vaccine in the recent RIVER study (Fidler et al., 2020) but was shown to have no discernible effect on the HIV reservoir. Despite this disappointing result, the data produced will allow new avenues of research with a view to achieving a functional cure. Perhaps more effective histone deacetylation inhibitors with a combination of vaccines, ART and broadly neutralising antibodies may hold the key.

In the meantime, we are reliant on advances in drug technology. Recently, a successful combination of two long-acting medications has been used as an injection every two months negating the need for daily tablets. Patients find this therapeutic approach acceptable, but there remain questions about patient adherence and how the approach might fit into some patients' lifestyles. The ultimate goal would be for once or twice yearly treatments (either long-lasting injections or sub-dermal implants delivering sufficient drug to suppress HIV replication) which are now a very real possibility. This approach, coupled with advances in vaccine science or the addition of broadly neutralising antibodies, points to a future of much simpler and more effective treatment options.

The functional cure would revolutionise the lives of those living with HIV, with reduced clinic visits and potentially less HIV stigma. If this were coupled with a workable HIV vaccine received before sexual debut (not unlike the human papillomavirus vaccine administered to school children), HIV truly may well be consigned to the history books. When this becomes a reality—however distant this reality may be—equity of access and ensuring patient safety will be the primary concerns for the clinician.

Overview

It is safe to say that the development of effective ART has had the most profound impact on the course of HIV. A terrifying diagnosis, which often led to an undignified death for many gay men in the 1980s and 1990s, is now a manageable, long-term chronic condition. The drugs themselves have also evolved into extremely effective agents of viral suppression with relatively few serious side effects. The efficacy and tolerability of orally administered ART will continue to increase until we enter a world where an injection every three to six months, or a sub-dermal implant slowly releasing drug to suppress the virus for years at a time, will be the next standard of HIV care. The shape of HIV care will change dramatically over the next few decades as treatments improve, less monitoring from specialised HIV clinics is required, and HIV stigma is eradicated.

Another seminal moment in HIV treatment was the realisation that being on effective medication renders the patient uninfectious. Many patients living with HIV describe a torturous fear of passing the virus onto lovers, partners and children—a heavy burden for many. The U = U message (undetectable = transmittable) has been revolutionary for those who are HIV-positive and their partners, resulting in less anxiety, less stigma and a more enjoyable sex life.

Many patients in a clinical setting mention the hope for a cure and this is certainly possible in the future. A cure where all traces of HIV are eliminated from the body is the ultimate goal. However, treatment that can kill enough HIV to stop it replicating at high levels without ART is potentially the next logical step—a so-called functional cure. Cure research is the key to another stage in the fight against HIV, whereby gay men are slowly 'cured' and weaned off their medication. This will not be easy to achieve, and we must ensure equity of access to these services once they do become available.

A world without new HIV diagnoses and a functional cure for those who have been affected is the ideal future that is certainly attainable in the next phase of HIV treatments provided there is sufficient scientific innovation, political engagement and psychological readiness. Any milestones in drug development must be made available to all, and not just to those fortunate enough to live in developed nations. With the networks of treatment and care now more firmly established and the rapid rate of scientific development, there is a very real possibility of winning the battle against HIV.

References

Bruner, K. M., Murray, A. J., Pollack, R. A., Soliman, M. G., Laskey, S. B., Capoferri, A. A., … Siliciano, R. F. (2016). Defective proviruses rapidly accumulate during acute HIV-1 infection. *Nature Medicine, 22*(9), 1043–1049.

Bruner, K. M., Wang, Z., Simonetti, F. R., Bender, A. M., Kwon, K. J., Sengupta, S., … Siliciano, R. F. (2019). A quantitative approach for measuring the reservoir of latent HIV-1 proviruses. *Nature, 566*(7742), 120–125.

Cahn, P., Madero, J. S., Arribas, J. R., Antinori, A., Ortiz, R., Clarke, A. E., … Ustianowski, A. (2019). Dolutegravir plus lamivudine versus dolutegravir plus tenofovir disoproxil fumarate and emtricitabine in antiretroviral-naive adults with HIV-1 infection (GEMINI-1 and GEMINI-2): Week 48 results from two multicentre, double-blind, randomised, non-inferiority, phase 3 trials. *The Lancet, 393*(10167), 143–155.

Cao, K., Hollenbach, J., Shi, X., Shi, W., Chopek, M., & Fernández-Viña, M. A. (2001). Analysis of the frequencies of HLA-A, B, and C alleles and haplotypes in the five major ethnic groups of the United States reveals high levels of diversity in these loci and contrasting distribution patterns in these populations. *Human Immunology, 62*(9), 1009–1030.

Dillon, S. M., Lee, E. J., Kotter, C. V., Austin, G. L., Dong, Z., Hecht, D. K., … Wilson, C. C. (2014). An altered intestinal mucosal microbiome in HIV-1 infection is associated with mucosal and systemic immune activation and endotoxemia. *Mucosal Immunology, 7*(4), 983–994.

Dillon, S. M., Frank, D. N., & Wilson, C. C. (2016). The Gut microbiome and HIV-1 pathogenesis: A two way street. *AIDS, 30*(18), 2737–2751.

Escaut, L., Liotier, J. Y., Albengres, E., Cheminot, N., & Vittecoq, D. (1999). Abacavir rechallenge has to be avoided in case of hypersensitivity reaction. *AIDS, 13*(11), 1419–1420.

Fidler, S., Stöhr, W., Pace, M., Dorrell, L., Lever, A., Pett, S., … Murray, T. (2020). Antiretroviral therapy alone versus antiretroviral therapy with a kick and kill approach, on measures of the HIV reservoir in participants with recent HIV infection (the RIVER trial): A phase 2, randomised trial. *The Lancet, 395*(10227), 888–898.

Ford, N., Shubber, Z., Pozniak, A., Vitoria, M., Doherty, M., Kirby, C., & Calmy, A. (2015). Comparative safety and neuropsychiatric adverse events associated with efavirenz use in first-line antiretroviral therapy: A systematic review and meta-analysis of randomized trials. *Journal of Acquired Immune Deficiency Syndromes, 69*(4), 422–429.

Gerschenson, M., & Brinkman, K. (2004). Mitochondrial dysfunction in AIDS and its treatment. *Mitochondrion, 4*(5), 763–777.

Geskus, R. B., Prins, M., Hubert, J.-B., Miedema, F., Berkhout, B., Rouzioux, C., … Meyer, L. (2007). The HIV RNA setpoint theory revisited. *Retrovirology, 4*(1), 65. https://doi.org/10.1186/1742-4690-4-65

Gounden, V., van Niekerk, C., Snyman, T., & George, J. A. (2010). Presence of the CYP2B6 516G> T polymorphism, increased plasma Efavirenz concentrations and early neuropsychiatric side effects in South African HIV-infected patients. *AIDS Research and Therapy, 7*, 32. https://doi.org/10.1186/1742-6405-7-32

Hughes, A. R., Mosteller, M., Bansal, A. T., Davies, K., Haneline, S. A., Lai, E. H., … on behalf of the CNA30027 and CNA30032 study teams. (2004). Association of genetic variations in HLA-B region with hypersensitivity to abacavir in some, but not all, populations. *Pharmacogenomics, 5*(2), 203–211.

Illing, P. T., Purcell, A. W., & McCluskey, J. (2017). The role of HLA genes in pharmacogenomics: Unravelling HLA associated adverse drug reactions. *Immunogenetics, 69*(8–9), 617–630.

INSIGHT START Study Group, Lundgren, J. D., Babiker, A. G., Gordin, F., Emery, S., … Neaton, J. D. (2015). Initiation of antiretroviral therapy in early asymptomatic HIV infection. *The New England Journal of Medicine, 373*(9), 795–807.

Jayappa, K. D., Ao, Z., & Yao, X. (2012). The HIV-1 passage from cytoplasm to nucleus: The process involving a complex exchange between the components of HIV-1 and cellular machinery to access nucleus and successful integration. *International Journal of Biochemistry and Molecular Biology, 3*(1), 70–85.

Jose, S., Quinn, K., Dunn, D., Cox, A., Sabin, C., & Fidler, S. (2016). Virological failure and development of new resistance mutations according to CD4 count at combination antiretroviral therapy initiation. *HIV Medicine, 17*(5), 368–372.

Mallal, S., Nolan, D., Witt, C., Masel, G., Martin, A. M., Moore, C., … Christiansen, F. T. (2002). Association between presence of HLA-B*5701, HLA-DR7, and HLA-DQ3 and hypersensitivity to HIV-1 reverse-transcriptase inhibitor abacavir. *Lancet, 359*(9308), 727–732.

Messiaen, P., Wensing, A. M. J., Fun, A., Nijhuis, M., Brusselaers, N., & Vandekerckhove, L. (2013). Clinical use of HIV integrase inhibitors: A systematic review and meta-analysis. *PLoS ONE, 8*(1). https://doi.org/10.1371/journal.pone.0052562

Ni, J., Wang, D., & Wang, S. (2018). The CCR5-Delta32 genetic polymorphism and HIV-1 infection susceptibility: A meta-analysis. *Open Medicine, 13*, 467–474.

O'Connor, J., Smith, C., Lampe, F. C., Johnson, M. A., Chadwick, D. R., Nelson, M., … Delpech, V. (2017). Durability of viral suppression with first-line antiretroviral therapy in patients with HIV in the UK: An observational cohort study. *The Lancet HIV, 4*(7), e295–e302. https://doi.org/10.1016/S2352-3018(17)30053-X

Ong, K. J., van Hoek, A. J., Harris, R. J., Figueroa, J., Waters, L., Chau, C., … Delpech, V. (2019). HIV care cost in England: A cross-sectional analysis of antiretroviral treatment and the impact of generic introduction. *HIV Medicine, 20*(6), 377–391.

Rockstroh, J. K., DeJesus, E., Lennox, J. L., Yazdanpanah, Y., Saag, M. S., Wan, H., … STARTMRK Investigators. (2013). Durable efficacy and safety of raltegravir versus efavirenz when combined with tenofovir/emtricitabine in treatment-naive HIV-1-infected patients: Final 5-year results from STARTMRK. *Journal of Acquired Immune Deficiency Syndromes, 63*(1), 77–85.

Ryom, L., Lundgren, J. D., De Wit, S., Kovari, H., Reiss, P., Law, M., ... D:A:D Study Group. (2016). Use of antiretroviral therapy and risk of end-stage liver disease and hepatocellular carcinoma in HIV-positive persons. *AIDS, 30*(11), 1731–1743.

Sáez-Cirión, A., Bacchus, C., Hocqueloux, L., Avettand-Fenoel, V., Girault, I., Lecuroux, C., ... Rouzioux, C. (2013). Post-treatment HIV-1 controllers with a long-term virological remission after the interruption of early initiated antiretroviral therapy ANRS VISCONTI study. *PLoS Pathogens, 9*(3). https://doi.org/10.1371/journal.ppat.1003211

Sax, P. E., Tierney, C., Collier, A. C., Fischl, M. A., Mollan, K., Peeples, L., ... AIDS Clinical Trials Group Study A5202 Team. (2009). Abacavir-lamivudine versus tenofovir-emtricitabine for initial HIV-1 therapy. *The New England Journal of Medicine, 361*(23), 2230–2240.

Simpson, D. M., & Tagliati, M. (1995). Nucleoside analogue-associated peripheral neuropathy in human immunodeficiency virus infection. *Journal of Acquired Immune Deficiency Syndromes and Human Retrovirology: Official Publication of the International Retrovirology Association, 9*(2), 153–161.

Stein, D. S., Korvick, J. A., & Vermund, S. H. (1992). CD4+ lymphocyte cell enumeration for prediction of clinical course of human immunodeficiency virus disease: A review. *The Journal of Infectious Diseases, 165*(2), 352–363.

Strategies for Management of Antiretroviral Therapy (SMART) Study Group, El-Sadr, W. M., Lundgren, J. D., Neaton, J. D., Gordin, F., Abrams, D., ... Rappoport, C. (2006). CD4+ count-guided interruption of antiretroviral treatment. *The New England Journal of Medicine, 355*(22), 2283–2296.

Thornton, A. C. (2015). Viral hepatitis and HIV co-infection in the UK collaborative HIV cohort (UK CHIC) study [Doctoral, UCL (University College London)]. In Doctoral thesis, UCL (University College London). UCL. Retrieved from https://discovery.ucl.ac.uk/id/eprint/1473437/

Tostevin, A., White, E., Dunn, D., Croxford, S., Delpech, V., Williams, I., ... UK HIV Drug Resistance Database. (2017). Recent trends and patterns in HIV-1 transmitted drug resistance in the United Kingdom. *HIV Medicine, 18*(3), 204–213.

Tovar-y-Romo, L. B., Bumpus, N. N., Pomerantz, D., Avery, L. B., Sacktor, N., McArthur, J. C., & Haughey, N. J. (2012). Dendritic spine injury induced by the 8-hydroxy metabolite of efavirenz. *The Journal of Pharmacology and Experimental Therapeutics, 343*(3), 696–703.

van Wyk, J., Ajana, F., Bisshop, F., De Wit, S., Osiyemi, O., Portilla, J., … Smith, K. Y. (2020). Efficacy and safety of switching to dolutegravir/lamivudine fixed-dose two-drug regimen versus continuing a tenofovir alafenamide-based three- or four-drug regimen for maintenance of virologic suppression in adults with HIV-1: Phase 3, randomized, non-inferiority TANGO Study. *Clinical Infectious Diseases: An Official Publication of the Infectious Diseases Society of America.* https://doi.org/10.1093/cid/ciz1243

Verma, R. (2014). Decline in CD4 counts in HIV patients. *Medical Journal, Armed Forces India, 70*(3), 301. https://doi.org/10.1016/j.mjafi.2014.06.012

Walensky, R. P., Goldberg, J. H., & Daily, J. P. (1999). Anaphylaxis after rechallenge with abacavir. *AIDS, 13*(8), 999–1000.

Wiegand, A., Spindler, J., Hong, F. F., Shao, W., Cyktor, J. C., Cillo, A. R., … Kearney, M. F. (2017). Single-cell analysis of HIV-1 transcriptional activity reveals expression of proviruses in expanded clones during ART. *Proceedings of the National Academy of Sciences of the United States of America, 114*(18), E3659–E3668. https://doi.org/10.1073/pnas.1617961114

Wolbers, M., Babiker, A., Sabin, C., Young, J., Dorrucci, M., Chêne, G., … on behalf of the CASCADE Collaboration. (2010). Pretreatment CD4 cell slope and progression to AIDS or death in HIV-infected patients initiating antiretroviral therapy—The CASCADE collaboration: A collaboration of 23 cohort studies. *PLOS Medicine, 7*(2), e1000239. https://doi.org/10.1371/journal.pmed.1000239

Zicari, S., Sessa, L., Cotugno, N., Ruggiero, A., Morrocchi, E., Concato, C., … Palma, P. (2019). Immune activation, inflammation, and non-AIDS co-morbidities in HIV-infected patients under long-term ART. *Viruses, 11*(3). https://doi.org/10.3390/v11030200

6

HIV and Mental Health

What Is Mental Health?

Mental health is a complex construct. It consists of many distinct dimensions and poor mental health is characterised by a multitude of disorders. Mental health disorders often overlap in their antecedents, symptomatology and sequelae. Many co-occur. The World Health Organization (2001, p. 1) defines mental health as 'a state of well-being in which an individual realizes his or her own abilities, can cope with the normal stresses of life, can work productively, and is able to make a contribution to his or her community'.

This definition is useful for at least three reasons. First, it must be noted that the focus of this chapter is on the mental health disorders that are associated with HIV and how gay men attempt to cope with them. However, the definition rightly frames mental health in positive terms— mental health refers not only to the absence of disorder but also to the ability to be self-efficacious, productive and participatory. In Chap. 5, these factors were alluded to in relation to treatment success. This positive dimension of mental health must also be borne in mind, despite our focus on disorders in this chapter. Second, the definition implicitly

© The Author(s) 2020
R. Jaspal, J. Bayley, *HIV and Gay Men*, https://doi.org/10.1007/978-981-15-7226-5_6

acknowledges our inevitable exposure to events and situations which can cause psychological stress by referring to the 'normal stresses of life'. There are many events and situations that have the potential to disrupt our mental health, such as relationship breakdown, stress in the workplace and bereavement. However, these events and situations only succeed in undermining our mental health if we are unable to *cope* effectively. Our capacity to cope is thus an important dimension to mental health. Third, the definition captures the importance of both psychological factors (e.g. self-efficacy) and social factors (e.g. community belonging) in mental health. Mental health is indeed psychological in that it pertains to the mind of the individual. Yet, as social beings, we must belong and relate to other people effectively and productively, and we will be influenced by them.

Since the advent of antiretroviral therapy (ART), the prognosis of a person diagnosed with HIV is generally very good, even in most cases of late diagnosis. This has led to a decrease in cognitive impairment, including the overall incidence of depression in patients, although poor mental health does still remain the most significant comorbidity of HIV infection (Sherr, Clucas, Harding, Sibley, & Catalan, 2011). The interface of HIV and mental health among gay men is complex. As a stigmatised minority in a heteronormative world, gay men are more likely to experience poor mental health outcomes compared to heterosexual men, which can be attributed in part to greater levels of stigma, victimisation and bullying, and lower levels of self-disclosure, social support and institutional support in this population. There is now considerable evidence that HIV infection (as a significant psychosocial stressor) can further accentuate the mental health burden already faced by gay men worldwide. This can be regarded as a 'double jeopardy' for the mental health of gay men. There is a strong association between poor mental health and HIV infection—over 50% of HIV patients have a psychiatric comorbidity, such as depression and anxiety, and the prevalence of poor mental health is eight times higher than in the general population (Sherr et al., 2011).

In this chapter, we focus on some of the mental health disorders which commonly accompany HIV infection. Mental health disorders are multifarious and can include depression, anxiety and suicidal ideation. There is evidence of a higher prevalence of these specific psychopathological conditions in gay men than in the general population (e.g. Sandfort, Bakker, Schellevis, & Vanwesenbeeck, 2006), which is even higher in gay men living with HIV (e.g. Lyons, Pitts, & Grierson, 2012). This highlights the need to explore the social and psychological underpinnings of poor mental health among gay men living with HIV, and thus, we propose a social psychological model for doing so.

Explaining Mental Health in HIV

There are competing theories to explain the high prevalence of poor mental health in HIV patients, which can broadly be categorised into three paradigms: the biological paradigm, the social psychological paradigm and psychobiological paradigm. Researchers do not vastly disagree on the antecedents of poor mental health in HIV patients, but it is useful to explore the distinct *foci* of their explanations. Some argue that biology should be our starting point when considering mental health and HIV, while others claim that the social psychological context is key to understanding the onset of poor mental health. It is likely that a combination of these factors—biological and social psychological alike—affects the mental health of those living with HIV. In this section, each paradigm is considered briefly.

The Biological Paradigm

The biological model suggests that HIV infection can predispose the patient to various mental health disorders due to its physiological impact. Rivera-Rivera, Vázquez-Santiago, Albino, Sánchez, and Rivera-Amill (2016) show that HIV infection can cause depression through several interrelated mechanisms, namely, by inducing chronic elevation of cytokines through activation of microglia and astrocytes; decreasing monoaminergic function (essential for the maintenance of mood); inducing neurotoxicity, especially in dopaminergic neurons; and reducing brain-derived neurotrophic factor. It is thought that viral pathways inter-act with psychosocial triggers to create the depressive state.

Chronic inflammation associated with HIV infection, even when treated with ART, has been associated with the onset of depression in HIV patients. More specifically, chronic inflammation can induce the activation of the hypothalamic-pituitary-adrenal axis, which regulates the stress response in humans, thereby increasing the risk of depression and other mental health problems in response to stressors associated with HIV (Rivera-Rivera et al., 2016).

There may also be a pharmacological explanation for elevated mental health problems in some HIV patients (Treisman & Soudry, 2016). For instance, the non-nucleoside reverse transcriptase inhibitor efavirenz can induce mitochondrial dysfunction, which in turn is causally associated with the onset of depression and suicidal ideation (Treisman & Soudry, 2016).

The Social Psychological Paradigm

The social psychological paradigm focuses primarily on the impact of social factors (e.g. stigma and discrimination) and psychological factors (e.g. resilience and pessimism) on mental health outcomes. This para-digm takes the social and psychological 'triggers' for poor mental health as the starting point for understanding outcomes in patients.

While HIV is now a manageable chronic condition and those diag-nosed early generally have a good prognosis, diagnosis with HIV can induce significant social and psychological challenges (Jaspal, 2018). First, the individual will need to assimilate and accommodate a stigma-tised element (i.e. HIV-positive serostatus) into their identity and begin to view himself as HIV-positive. This can induce a threat to both their sense of continuity (i.e. that there is a thread between past, present and future) and self-esteem in view of the associated social stigma. Second, the individual will need to decide whether or not to disclose this new identity element to significant others, such as their sexual partner, family and friends, potentially risking stigma, rejection and abuse. Fear of rejec-tion can induce anxiety in the patient. Third, they will need to decide (in collaboration with healthcare professionals) whether or not to initiate ART, which constitutes a life-long commitment. This can represent a dilemma for the patient who may wish to forget about their infection rather than think about it on a daily basis as they take their medication. Fourth, people living with HIV do face significant social stigma—both enacted and real—which can undermine their psychological wellbeing. All these factors can plausibly decrease an individual's self-esteem and culminate in poor mental health, such as depression, anxiety and suicidal ideation.

Often, the decisions that people make—even those that are designed to protect their psychological wellbeing—can result in unintended consequences for their wellbeing and mental health. For instance, the newly diagnosed gay man may elect not to disclose his HIV status to others, not to initiate ART and to disengage from healthcare professionals, resulting in a *de facto* state of self-isolation. Though the individual will not be directly exposed to social stigma from other people, he may plausibly experience feelings of loneliness due to his self-isolation, which in turn may undermine his ability to derive social support. In this chapter, we draw on the Health Adversity Risk Model, inspired by identity process theory (Jaspal & Breakwell, 2014) from social psychology, to describe the ways in which these social psychological 'stressors' can culminate in poor mental health outcomes and, crucially, how we can intervene to enhance mental health in patients.

The Psychobiological Paradigm

The available evidence suggests that poor mental health is a combination of both biological and social psychological variables. As indicated in this chapter, HIV infection and ART can induce physiological changes in the patient that increase their risk of depression, anxiety and suicidal ideation. Moreover, a significant proportion of gay men diagnosed with HIV have pre-existing psychiatric disorders, which may be exacerbated by HIV disease and ART (Sherr et al., 2011).

Yet, there is much evidence that social context is a significant consideration in mental health. It is likely to mediate the relationship between

HIV and poor mental health. For instance, HIV diagnosis in a social context in which social representations (i.e. common understandings) of HIV are especially negative and stigmatising can increase the risk of decreased self-esteem and, thus, poor mental health outcomes among the newly diagnosed. Conversely, in a social context in which there is greater awareness and understanding of HIV and in which stigma is lower, the newly diagnosed individual may experience better mental health outcomes.

Furthermore, there is evidence that HIV patients who experience side effects associated with ART are more likely to report depressive symptomatology than those who do not (Chen, 2013). It could be predicted that those with less social support and decreased resilience would respond more negatively to side effects. Furthermore, gay men living with HIV are also likely to be exposed to psychologically adverse events, such as rejection and discrimination, which can lead them to derive a negative self-conception, potentially compromising their mental health. In view of the aforementioned physiological changes induced by HIV infection and some anti-HIV agents, patients exposed to social psychological stressors, such as rejection, may be at greater risk of poor mental health than the general population.

The psychobiological paradigm also acknowledges the role of individual psychological factors, such as personality. Personality traits can predispose an individual to poor mental health by determining their response to the adverse event (Jaspal, 2018). In other words, not everyone responds to the same 'adverse' event in quite the same way. For instance, gay men who are more optimistic and resilient might be more willing to reconstrue their HIV diagnosis in more positive terms and, thus, see a more positive future for themselves than those who are pessimistic and neurotic. The shy individual may have a proclivity to isolate himself, rather than to seek support and so on. It is easy to see how these distinct personality profiles can increase the risk of poor mental health.

In short, the psychobiological paradigm acknowledges the physiological reality of HIV and its impact on the biology of the individual, on the one hand, and the social context and psychological predisposition of the individual, on the other hand. The social psychological profile of the individual can predispose him to particular reactions to both the physiological reality of HIV and to the social 'triggers' that he experiences.

> **Clinical Snapshot 5: HIV Stigma and Relationships**
>
> *Decreased HIV knowledge and HIV stigma can lead some people to react negatively when a partner discloses HIV. This may increase anxiety and stress for the person living with HIV and adversely affect relationships. This is a common experience among gay men living with HIV. HIV stigma may also affect other parts of one's life, including relations with one's employer or family members who may also react negatively. HIV education consisting of positive media portrayals, dissemination of evidence-based health information and the challenging of myths concerning HIV is central to decreasing HIV stigma. The advent of U=U will undoubtedly also play a fundamental role in reducing HIV stigma, thereby enhancing relationship quality.*

Social Stigma

Three constructs are especially relevant to this chapter—mental health, HIV and homosexuality. All these constructs are stigmatised in society. Stigma is an overarching thread that underpins the lived experience of HIV-positive gay men.

Social stigma surrounds poor mental health, such as depression, suicidal ideation and self-harm, and the taboo of disclosing poor mental health leads some individuals to conceal symptoms, to delay seeking treatment and to adhere poorly to treatment. Furthermore, in collectivist cultures that value community, social stigma can also extend to the patient's family, which in turn could affect employment prospects, marriage prospects and, more generally, the family's standing in the community (Jaspal, 2020). Mental health remains a stigmatised topic in British society and that stigma appears to be more pronounced in ethnic minority communities (Memon et al., 2016).

One way in which people stigmatise mental health is by denying its significance or severity—they may believe that sufferers should 'pull themselves together', or pejoratively label poor mental health as 'madness' (Robinson, Turk, Jilka, & Cella, 2019). Because of the stigma underpinning poor mental health, self-disclosure and social networks might not provide the desired social support, but may inadvertently stigmatise the individual with poor mental health. Devoid of social support, the individual may resort to maladaptive strategies for coping with mental health problems, for example, self-medication, substance misuse, disengagement from mental health services. These strategies can in turn compromise HIV outcomes.

Social stigma on the basis of sexual orientation, which constitutes a fundamental, immutable aspect of the individual's identity, can take its toll on gay men's mental health. In a survey of 5375 lesbian, gay and bisexual people in the UK, it was found that 21% had experienced a hate crime; that 17% had faced discrimination in a café, restaurant or bar; and that 10% had experienced online abuse because of their sexual orientation (Stonewall, 2017). Exposure to stigma may lead some gay men to conceal or deny their sexual orientation, to feign heterosexuality under false pretences and to avoid seeking support with sexual identity issues. In a study of mental health in sexual minorities, it has been found that rejection from significant others, victimisation and discrimination are associated with the development of internalised homophobia and, in turn, with increased risk of psychological distress, depression, self-harm and suicidal ideation (Jaspal, Lopes, & Rehman, 2019; Rehman, Lopes, & Jaspal, 2020).

HIV stigma is a significant precursor of poor mental health. Since the first clinical observations of AIDS in 1981 and the subsequent discovery that gay men were disproportionately affected by HIV, the stigma of this 'gay disease' has become further entrenched in social representations, often reinforcing the stigma of homosexuality itself (Jaspal & Nerlich, 2020). There is little doubt that HIV is one of the most stigmatised health conditions and that people living with the condition generally report higher levels of stigma than patients living with other conditions, such as cancer or diabetes (e.g. Fife & Wright, 2000). HIV is stigmatised in part because of its association with taboo issues, such as sexual promiscuity, sex work, drug use and death. Given the stigma of HIV, many gay men prefer not to test for HIV, perceive themselves to be at low risk of infection and disengage from HIV care when diagnosed. Many anticipate negative reactions from others if they do disclose their HIV status and, thus, fail to do so.

Poor mental health may also increase the risk of HIV infection, often paving the way for engagement in high-risk behaviours. Yet, the stigma of HIV itself can adversely impact mental health among those who are diagnosed with the condition. Joffe (2007) sheds light on the mechanisms of stigma and how people engage with stigmatised phenomena—she has argued that people have a tendency to 'other' adversity, disease and markers of stigma from their own identity and, conversely, to associate them with others unlike themselves. In other words, individuals are inclined to view HIV as something that 'doesn't happen to people like us' but rather to others—especially those from other social groups. This in turn serves to increase the stigma of HIV.

Identity and Mental Health

Social stigma associated with some identity elements, such as one's sexuality and HIV status, can adversely impact mental health. Identity process theory (see Fig. 6.1) (Breakwell, 1986; Jaspal & Breakwell, 2014) provides a useful heuristic framework for understanding the interrelations between stigma, identity and mental health.

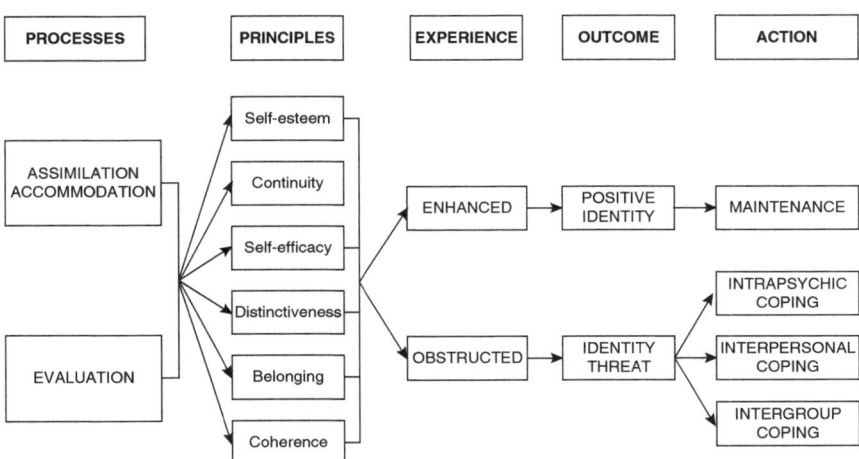

Fig. 6.1   Identity process theory (from Jaspal, 2018)

The theory postulates that individuals construct their identity through two processes:

- *Assimilation-accommodation* refers to the process of absorbing and creating space for new information in identity. For instance, upon diagnosis with HIV, one must absorb one's new HIV status in identity and potentially re-think other elements of identity.
- *Evaluation* refers to the process of attributing meaning/value to identity components. When diagnosed with HIV, one will contemplate what this really means, its implications for one's life and how others might react to it.

These processes are in turn guided by various motivational principles which essentially specify the desirable end-states for identity:

- *Self-esteem* refers to personal and social worth. For instance, in view of the stigma and the moralising social representations that surround HIV, the newly diagnosed may come to derive a negative self-conception due to their infection and believe that they are somehow 'flawed' as people (Jaspal & Williamson, 2017).
- *Self-efficacy* can be defined as the belief in one's competence and control. Even in the pre-ART era when HIV infection was a terminal illness, it was found that those gay men who perceived decreased control over their sexual behaviour were more likely to engage in sexual risk practices (Exner, Meyer-Bahlburg, & Ehrhardt, 1992).
- *Distinctiveness* refers to feelings of uniqueness and differentiation from others. Upon diagnosis with HIV, one may attempt to differentiate oneself from other people living with HIV in order to reduce exposure to stigma associated with the condition (Jaspal, 2018).
- *Continuity* is essentially the psychological thread between past, present and future. Diagnosis with a stigmatised chronic condition can disrupt the thread between past and present, and introduce an uncertain future, as this constitutes an example of undesirable change in one's life narrative.
- *Coherence* refers to the perception that relevant aspects of identity are coherent and compatible. It has been shown that gay men of religious

faith may perceive their sexual and religious identities to be incompatible, which can induce psychological stress (Jaspal & Cinnirella, 2010).

We construct our identities in ways that provide us with appropriate levels of these principles. We tend to see events, situations and identity elements that enhance the identity principles as being more important than those that do not. For instance, in societies in which homosexuality is deeply stigmatised, same-sex attracted men may downplay, or reject altogether, their gay identity because this may imperil the self-esteem and continuity principles of identity. In the era of ART, having an undetectable HIV viral load is socially represented as an achievement—in terms of both individual and public health promotion. It is easy to see how this can provide feelings of self-esteem, self-efficacy and continuity for the individual living with HIV. HIV undetectability now constitutes an identity element for those who have achieved it. It may be foregrounded both psychologically ('I am undetectable and I am proud of this') and socially ('I am undetectable and I like to tell others about this').

Conversely, when the principles are jeopardised, for instance, by changes in one's social context, *identity is threatened*. The experience of identity threat leads the individual to engage in strategies for coping. Coping in the face of psychological adversity associated with HIV is discussed later in this chapter. However, it must be noted at this stage that coping strategies are either adaptive or maladaptive. Some promote positive change in the long term because they resolve the source of the threat, while others fail to resolve the source of the threat in the long term although they may provide temporary respite from the threat. Identity process theory describes coping at three levels of human functioning:

- *Intrapsychic* strategies function at a psychological level. Some can be regarded as deflection strategies in that they enable the threatened individual to deny or reconceptualise the threat or the reasons for occupying the threatening position, while others are acceptance strategies that facilitate some form of cognitive re-structuring in anticipation of the threat. For instance, a gay man who engages in condomless sex with multiple partners may deny, rather than acknowledge, his risk of HIV because of the associated stigma.

- *Interpersonal* strategies focus on changing the nature of relationships with other individuals. Most are maladaptive given that the threatened individual may isolate himself from others or feign membership of a group or network of which he is not really a member, in order to avoid exposure to stigma, for instance. An example of an adaptive interpersonal strategy is that of self-disclosure, given that this can facilitate the acquisition of social support. Some gay men living with HIV disclose their HIV diagnosis to a trusted other, which can bring about respite from the initial threats associated with this experience. However, it must be noted that the success of this coping strategy is dependent in part on the reaction from one's interlocutor.

- *Intergroup* strategies are designed to change the nature of our relationships with groups. Most are adaptive. Individuals may join groups of like-minded others who share their predicament in order to access social support. They may create a new social group to derive support or a pressure group to influence social representations. Some gay men diagnosed with HIV report significant benefits of joining a support group in order to manage the psychosocial challenges of their diagnosis.

It is easy to see how the imposition of undesirable change as a result of being diagnosed with HIV could challenge continuity, self-esteem and self-efficacy and so on. In fact, there is much research that shows how these identity principles can be abrogated among those living with the condition (e.g. Jaspal, 2018). Unresolved, chronic threats to identity (like the chronic illness of HIV) can undermine psychological wellbeing and potentially lead to poor mental health, such as depression, anxiety and suicidal ideation (Breakwell, 1986; Jaspal et al., 2019).

In addition to the potential adverse impact of identity threat for mental health, some of the coping strategies intended to assuage identity threat may culminate in poor mental health. Intrapsychic strategies that are associated with deflection (such as denial, chemsex and substance misuse), rather than confrontation, of the threat to identity have limited effectiveness in the long term. Denial allows the threatened individual to ignore the threat, but the source of the threat continues to exist, though in a dormant state, and may in fact be reactivated or aggravated by inaction. Isolation can accentuate depression as it precludes group support for the threatened individual—a strategy, which, conversely, is associated with better mental health outcomes. Furthermore, some strategies themselves can become pathological—for instance, transient depersonalisation is a temporary state of psychological detachment from the self, which can buffer the negative effects of identity threat in the short term, but it may also be indicative of psychosis when it persists as a coping strategy. It is therefore essential that gay men who experience psychological adversity be guided towards adaptive and productive coping strategies (Jaspal, 2018). We return to this point later in this chapter.

Mental Health Disorders among Gay Men Living with HIV

In this chapter, there is a focus on depression, anxiety and suicidal ideation, which are known to be prevalent in gay men living with HIV, the possible reasons underpinning this increased prevalence and the potential ways in which individuals living with, or at risk of, poor mental health can be supported effectively.

> ### Clinical Snapshot 6: Depression and ART Adherence
>
> *Rates of depression and anxiety are higher in those living with HIV. This can in part be attributed to adjustment disorders and internalised stigma associated with one's HIV diagnosis. Furthermore, there are other possible triggers for depression, which are not associated with HIV, such as grief and relationship or work difficulties. It has been shown that low mood leads to a reduction in adherence to HIV treatment, leading to viral rebound, reductions in CD4 counts, endothelial dysfunction and potential AIDS-related conditions. This deterioration in physical health only serves to exacerbate the underlying mental health problems as patients can be admitted to hospital (an event that is often associated with deterioration in mood) or have to attend numerous medical appointments. This synergy between mental health, adherence and worsening physical health should be identified early, with all those who describe symptoms of depression (lack of energy, poor sleep, changes in appetite) being referred for talking therapy without delay. Patients who have complex depression (i.e. catatonic or elements of psychosis) should be referred to mental health services for assessment with close liaison about potential drug interactions, if applicable.*

Depression

Depression is associated with HIV in a variety of ways. On the one hand, it can precede HIV infection and lead to engagement in behaviours that increase one's risk of infection. This has been referred to as primary depression, which is often associated with a family history of affective disorders, personality traits that predispose one to depression such as neuroticism and adverse life experiences such as childhood sexual abuse. On the other hand, depression itself emerges as a consequence of HIV infection. This is referred to as secondary depression and may arise from exposure to social and psychological stressors, such as HIV stigma, but also from neurotropic effects of the virus on the subcortical neurological areas (Treisman, Fishman, Schwartz, Hutton, & Lyketsos, 1998).

Symptoms of depression include feelings of decreased self-worth, hopelessness, difficulties in showing an interest and in concentration, excessive pessimism, difficulties in sleeping, and loss of appetite. Depression appears to be very prevalent in patients living with HIV, with some studies suggesting that between 30 and 40% of HIV patients have clinical depression (e.g. Ferrando, 2009).

Several studies have focused on the possible antecedents of depression in gay men living with HIV. In an online survey with a convenience sample from the UK and Ireland, Murphy, Garrido-Hernansaiz, Mulcahy, and Hevey (2018) found that 57.9% of respondents reported symptoms of depression, which was predicted by internalised stigma, enacted stigma and decreased HIV health optimism. Internalised stigma emerged as the strongest predictor of depression, suggesting that the uncritical acceptance and internalisation of stigma encountered in social settings is particularly important in leading the individual to experience depressive symptoms.

Similarly, HIV-associated stigma and loneliness (possibly as a protective response in the face of stigma) has been found to be associated with depression among older HIV-positive adults (Grov et al., 2010). In their study of 357 Australian gay men living with HIV, Heywood and Lyons (2016) found that both depression and anxiety were related to HIV-related discrimination and internalised HIV stigma, suggesting that these social stressors may play a causal role in poor mental health outcomes. Furthermore, a Danish study revealed that stress, loneliness and constant rumination about HIV were predictive of depression in HIV patients and that those patients at risk of major depression were six times more likely to have missed doses of ART, shedding light on the potential consequences of depression (Rodkjaer, Laursen, Balle, & Sodemann, 2010).

Type of coping strategy also appears to play an important role in the onset of depression—in their study of 200 people living with HIV, Varni, Miller, McCuin, and Solomon (2012) found that participants who reported 'felt' stigma but who engaged in disengagement coping strategies were more likely to exhibit depression and anxiety than those who reported low levels of disengagement coping. As highlighted in Chap. 1, body image concerns are another significant predictor of depression (Blashill, Gordon, & Safren, 2012)—one study revealed a 31% prevalence of body dissatisfaction in a cohort of HIV-positive gay men (Sharma et al., 2007).

There does appear to be a reciprocal relationship between depression and other maladaptive practices and poor psychosocial outcomes, such as low self-efficacy and substance misuse, suggesting that these factors may reinforce depressive symptomatology in the patient. Indeed, Bhatia, Hartman, Kallen, Graham, and Giordano (2011) found that depressed HIV patients were between two and four times more likely to use substances than non-depressed patients and that the depressed cohort was twice as likely to have low levels of self-efficacy and decreased access to social support.

The sequelae of depression include decreased cognitive functioning and reduced levels of energy among older people living with HIV (Grov et al., 2010). Indeed, in their study of 130 HIV patients with CD4 >200 cells/mm^3, Bragança and Palha (2011) found a 34% prevalence of depression in their sample, and within this cohort, depression had an effect on the following components of cognitive function: speed of information processing, attention/working memory, learning and psychomotor functions. Depression can adversely impact self-efficacy, that is, the person's sense of control and competence and belief in their abilities, and thus lead them to believe that they cannot cope with their diagnosis (Kavanagh & Bower, 1985). As indicated in the clinical snapshot above, it is easy to see how this can in turn decrease adherence to ART and engagement with HIV care—the individual may simply believe that he is unable to do so (Uthman, Magidson, Safren, & Nachega, 2014).

In a meta-analysis of studies of 95 independent samples (Gonzalez, Batchelder, Psaros & Safren, 2011), it was found that depression was significantly related to non-adherence to ART. This was both a consistent finding and non-adherence was associated not only with clinical depression but also with mild and moderate forms of depression. Studies using more sophisticated statistical techniques such as structural equation modelling suggest that depressive symptoms mediate the relationship between HIV stigma and poor adherence to ART (e.g. Uthman et al., 2014). It is likely that individuals who are depressed are less self-efficacious in the face of HIV stigma and, thus, cope less effectively with it, which in turn results in the adoption of maladaptive coping responses, such as suboptimal adherence to ART. It is also possible that HIV stigma which succeeds in inducing depression in the individual results in more insidious effects, such as poor adherence to ART. In addition to the empirical observations that HIV patients with clinical depression are less likely to engage with HIV care or initiate ART, it has been found that, even when controlling for ART, depression is associated with an increase in viral load and with a decline in CD4 counts (Ironson et al., 2005). In their review of the literature on the impact of depression, Schuster, Bornovalova, and Hunt (2012) show that severe depression among HIV patients can lead to accelerated progression to AIDS.

When body dissatisfaction causes depression, as it appears to do in some cases, it is more likely to lead to decreased engagement with ART (Blashill & Vander Wal, 2010), which can undermine both HIV disease prognosis and prevention efforts. Indeed, it has been found that depressive symptomatology is associated with earlier mortality and elevated HIV-specific morbidity in patients, often due to poor adherence to ART (Lima et al., 2007).

In addition to poor adherence to ART, engagement in sexual behaviours that increase the risk of onward HIV transmission is related to depression. Babowitch, Mitzel, Vanable, and Sweeney (2018) have found that moderate levels of depression predict engagement in condomless anal sex with a casual sexual partner, which in turn can increase the risk of both the acquisition of bacterial STIs and onward HIV transmission. This could be attributed to low sexual self-efficacy (e.g. the inability to negotiate condom use), low self-esteem and, thus, decreased self-care. In their study, individuals with low and high levels of depression were less likely to engage in sexual risk. This may be attributed to the possibility that individuals with moderate (as opposed to severe) depression are less likely to seek treatment and to come to the attention of medical or psychological practitioners. This in turn can enable depression to escalate and culminate in maladaptive coping strategies, such as substance misuse and engagement in sexual risk behaviour, such as chemsex. On the other hand, individuals with severe depression may not necessarily exhibit the same level of sexual risk given that it is associated with complete loss of interest in sex. Indeed, O'Cleirigh et al. (2013) found only a modest decline in sexual transmission behaviour in HIV-positive gay men with moderate depression who participated in a risk reduction behavioural intervention, compared to those with low or severe levels of depression.

In view of the insidious effects of depression on both the health and wellbeing of the HIV patient and public health more generally, researchers have understandably focused on strategies for decreasing depression. In a study of 210 South Africans living with HIV, Breet, Kagee, and Seedat (2014) found that social support mediated the relationship between HIV-related stigma and symptoms of post-traumatic stress disorder, suggesting that the derivation of social support may break the link between this social stressor and adverse social psychological outcomes. However, they also found that social support did not buffer the effects of HIV-related stigma on depression, suggesting that there are other factors that undermine the ability of social support to buffer the effects of HIV-related stigma on specific mental health outcomes.

In a study of 450 people living with HIV, it was found that spiritual peace was inversely associated with depression (Yi et al., 2006). Sherr et al. (2011) conducted a systematic review of the literature on interventions for decreasing depressive symptomatology in HIV patients and found that psychological interventions were most effective—especially those incorporating principles of the cognitive behavioural approach. A randomised control trial of a mindfulness-based intervention to improve psychological wellbeing in Canadian gay men living with HIV revealed an improvement in symptoms of depression in patients in the treatment arm of the study (Gayner et al., 2012). There is evidence that cognitive behavioural group therapy using art as a medium can have a favourable effect on depressive symptomatology in HIV-infected gay men, as demonstrated in a Thai quasi-experimental study (Sahassanon, Pisitsungkagarn, & Taephant, 2019).

Yet, there remains much to be done in the fight against depression in HIV patients. Pence, O'Donnell, and Gaynes (2012) estimate that up to 82% of HIV patients with depression are not currently in receipt of any treatment, that 93% are not receiving adequate treatment and that 95% are not in remission from depression. This demonstrates the severe epidemic of depression in the HIV population.

Anxiety

Anxiety shares many common features with depression, such as feeling distressed, experiencing low mood and restlessness, but it does have many distinctive elements and should therefore be regarded as a separate disorder. Anxiety can be thought of as an umbrella category which encompasses a series of distinct but related disorders. These include but are not limited to phobias, social anxiety disorder, panic disorder, agoraphobia and generalised anxiety disorder. These disorders share at least three characteristics: they are characterised by excessive fear in response to a perceived threat; they reflect an irrational anticipation of future threat; and they entail the enactment of one or more 'anxiety states' which may be physiological, cognitive or behavioural. Anxiety symptoms vary in severity and sometimes wane over time. Often, anxiety is attributed to the personality of the individual, with some traits (e.g. neuroticism) evidently predisposing individuals to this condition. However, as with depression, there are clearly also social psychological antecedents to anxiety, including adverse life experiences, such as childhood sexual abuse, intimate partner violence, assault and others.

Like depression, anxiety is more prevalent in HIV patients than in the general population, with a meta-analysis suggesting that 22.8% of patients experience at least one anxiety disorder (Brandt et al., 2017). O'Cleirigh et al. (2013) found that almost half of their sample of gay men living with HIV met the clinical criteria for one of the three anxiety disorders they measured in their study, namely, post-traumatic stress disorder, social anxiety and panic disorder. Anxiety also appears to be more prevalent in HIV patients than in patients suffering from other chronic conditions.

While death anxiety was prevalent in HIV patients (Hintze, Templer, Cappelletty, & Frederick, 1993), in part because of the lack of effective HIV treatment prior to 1996, the continued incidence of anxiety can now be attributed to a more diverse and complex myriad of factors—ranging from the biology of HIV to its social psychological dimension. In their 2-year longitudinal study of 173 gay men living with HIV, Sewell et al. (2000) found an association between anxiety and HIV-related symptoms, fatigue and physical limitations. This suggests that HIV symptomatology induces anxiety in the patient, potentially because of concerns about the impact of HIV on their health. In addition to HIV symptomatology, social factors such as homelessness and lifetime sexual abuse have also been found to be associated with anxiety symptoms in HIV patients—most likely as antecedents (Semple, Strathdee, Zians, McQuaid, & Patterson, 2011).

Understandably, much research into mental health in the pre-ART era focused on death anxiety, because in the absence of effective treatment there was a high mortality rate in HIV-infected patients and a dominant social representation was that HIV would lead to a slow, painful and horrific death (Miller, Lee, & Henderson, 2012). Yet, among older HIV patients who may have other comorbidities and who personally witnessed the pre-ART era and newly diagnosed patients with lower levels of HIV knowledge, death anxiety persists as a significant psychological concern. There is also evidence of 'survivor guilt' among some gay men who survived through the epidemic while many of their loved ones did not (Broun, 1998).

There is evidence that HIV patients who hold irrational beliefs (in general—not necessarily about HIV) are more susceptible to death anxiety (Braunstein, 2004). Moreover, there is a correlation between death anxiety and the severity of post-traumatic stress disorder symptoms, which suggests that unresolved trauma may increase death anxiety in patients (Safren, Gershuny, & Hendriksen, 2003). In a study of 635 HIV patients (Shacham, Morgan, Önen, Taniguchi, & Overton, 2012), it was found that individuals who had not initiated ART were 1.61 times more likely to exhibit symptoms of anxiety, while those patients on ART who had high levels of anxiety were less likely to adhere to their medication, to have higher viral loads and to have lower CD4 counts.

Panic disorder is more prevalent in HIV patients than in the general population. It has been found that those patients with resolved grief in relation to their HIV infection are less likely to suffer from panic disorder than those with unresolved grief (Summers et al., 1995). This demonstrates the importance of effective coping with psychological adversity (in this case, grief) in the mitigation of panic disorder in patients.

Anxiety can have insidious effects on the health and wellbeing of people living with HIV. It can have significant physiological effects. It has been found that anxiety can impair stress hormones, norepinephrine and cortisol; cause dysregulation of the immune system by increasing viral replication or causing viral rebound; and impair the patient's response to HIV therapy (e.g. Lampe et al., 2010).

There appears to be an empirical relationship between anxiety and emotional dysregulation, which refers to difficulties in regulating affective experiences and in controlling behaviours that are associated with these affective experiences (Brandt et al., 2017). In their study of HIV patients, Brandt, Gonzalez, Grover, and Zvolensky (2013) found that emotional dysregulation was associated with both general anxiety and pain-related anxiety. In view of the many social, psychological and physiological 'triggers' for psychological distress among HIV patients, patients with emotional dysregulation may be more susceptible to anxiety, which itself has many sequelae.

Emotional dysregulation can actually limit the range of adaptive coping strategies to which individuals have access, thereby reducing their capacity to cope effectively with the stressors associated with HIV infection. For instance, individuals with emotional dysregulation may find it difficult to interact with other people in order to derive social support from them or they may react adversely to innocuous remarks from other people, leading to a proclivity to isolate themselves from care providers and others in their social network. Consequently, it is recommended that HIV patients be assessed for emotional dysregulation and that this mutable condition be treated proactively before the onset of more severe psychological conditions, such as anxiety.

Brandt et al. (2017) describe several sequelae of HIV-related anxiety. First, there is evidence that anxiety can increase HIV disease severity and accelerate progression to AIDS. Second, having an anxiety disorder is negatively associated with adherence to ART. Third, HIV patients with anxiety disorder are more likely to misuse substances, possibly as a maladaptive coping strategy, which in turn can have negative health and HIV outcomes. Fourth, people living with both HIV and anxiety are more likely to contemplate and attempt suicide than HIV patients who do not have anxiety. Fifth, cognitive impairment, such as accelerated cognitive ageing and memory loss, is prevalent in HIV patients with anxiety disorders. Sixth, quality of life is observably lower in HIV patients with anxiety, affecting key principles such as self-esteem, life satisfaction, sense of meaning and purpose, and other psychosocial components. Seventh, there is increased prevalence of HIV transmission behaviours in HIV patients with anxiety—this includes sex with multiple partners, sexual compulsivity, condomless sex and sex while under the influence of alcohol and substances.

Sexual risk-taking is a significant public health concern associated with HIV patients with anxiety. In their study of HIV-positive gay men, O'Cleirigh et al. (2013) found a significant relationship between post-traumatic stress disorder and HIV transmission risk behaviour, which was moderated by age, with younger gay men being more likely to engage in transmission risk behaviour. Younger people (including those who are gay) do tend to take more sexual risks and also did not grow up in the pre-ART era when an AIDS diagnosis was associated with death.

Therefore, there tend to be lower levels of fear and death anxiety in this group.

In particular, *social* anxiety (i.e. the irrational fear of judgement and negative evaluation by other people in social situations) is strongly associated with sexual risk-taking behaviour in gay men. In their study of 100 young gay men, Hart and Heimberg (2005) found that social anxiety (operationalised in terms of social interaction anxiety and observation anxiety) predicted engagement in condomless insertive sexual intercourse. It can therefore be argued that gay men who are anxious about social interaction will be less self-efficacious in communicating their desires to others, including sexual partners. They may not feel empowered to negotiate condom use. Moreover, those who are anxious about being observed by others will be more attentive to their sexual performance because they will be focused on how they are perceived and evaluated by others. Erectile dysfunction (or fear thereof) may be a significant factor. Therefore, their sexual performance may constitute their focus, rather than engagement in protective behaviour, such as condom use.

Anxiety appears to function as a mediator of the relationship between psychological adversity and sexual risk-taking behaviour. In their study of 456 HIV-positive gay men in the US, O'Leary, Purcell, Remien, and Gomez (2003) found that the relationship between childhood sexual abuse and sexual risk-taking behaviour was mediated by anxiety. This suggests that when childhood sexual abuse induces anxiety, it is more likely to lead to engagement in HIV transmission behaviours. Semple et al. (2011) found that anxiety was associated with injection drug use, engagement in sexual risk behaviour and the pursuit of sexual partners when 'high' on methamphetamine, which could plausibly be conceptualised as maladaptive coping behaviours, that is, as possible consequences of anxiety.

A systematic review of 39 studies of interventions for treating anxiety in HIV patients, most of which focused on male patients in Western countries, revealed that psychological interventions, such as cognitive behavioural therapy, were more effective than pharmacological interventions (Clucas et al., 2011). This review and others have generally indicated that cognitive behavioural interventions are especially effective in the treatment of anxiety (e.g. Spies, Asmal, & Seedat, 2013).

Suicidal Ideation

Suicidal ideation refers to the contemplation of taking one's own life and may include an actual plan to do so. Like other mental health conditions, suicidal ideation is especially high among gay men, regardless of HIV status (Michaels, Parent, & Torrey, 2016).

In the early days of the HIV epidemic, suicidal ideation was common in HIV patients given the poor prognosis associated with the condition prior to the advent of ART. Despite the enormous advances made in HIV medicine, suicide rates in HIV patients do remain higher than in the general population (Schlebusch & Govender, 2015). Moreover, suicidal ideation is higher in those gay men living with HIV than in the general population (Ferlatte, Salway, Oliffe, & Trussler, 2017). Indeed, a French study of 2973 HIV patients revealed a 6.3% prevalence of suicidal ideation in the sample, with gay and bisexual men exhibiting the highest scores on this variable (Carrieri et al., 2017).

In their US study, Carrico, Neilands, and Johnson (2010) found that 28% of their gay and bisexual participants had contemplated suicide in the last two weeks. In a US study of 2694 people who died by suicide between 2000 and 2013 (Ahmedani et al., 2017), HIV/AIDS was identified as one of the three conditions (out of a total of 19) which were most strongly associated with suicide risk. In a systematic review of 66 studies 27% of individuals living with HIV reported suicidal ideation (Catalan et al., 2011). A study of five HIV clinics in England revealed a 31% prevalence of suicidal thoughts in the last week among HIV patients and noted that suicide is a significant cause of death in this cohort (Sherr et al., 2008). A sense of hopelessness and futility may accompany HIV infection in those who are uninformed about HIV.

The early post-diagnosis phase can be construed as a 'high-risk' period for suicidal ideation in HIV patients particularly if the individual is not well informed about HIV and holds stigmatising beliefs about the condition. With the passage of time, however, the infected individual may develop personal and social resources for coping more effectively with their HIV diagnosis and its associated stressors. As outlined elsewhere in this chapter, these stressors include stigma, discrimination and rejection, as well as financial worries, homelessness, and challenging personal relationships. These stressors do appear to be more prevalent in HIV-positive gay men than in those who are HIV-negative.

HIV disease progression and low CD4 cell count are associated with increased risk of suicide (Ruffieux et al., 2019), suggesting that poor HIV outcomes may have the psychological effect of decreasing hope in the patient, thereby rendering suicide a more attractive option than life. The most powerful predictor is an existing diagnosis with another psychiatric illness, such as depression, anxiety or psychosis. Indeed, suicidal ideation often co-occurs with these other conditions. In a study of 211 Brazilian patients (Passos, Souza, & Spessato, 2014), 34.1% of the sample was at risk of suicide, and it was found that depression and anxiety independently predicted suicidal ideation.

Carrico et al. (2010) have described a stress and coping model of suicide risk in relation to HIV patients, which postulates that HIV-specific vulnerability factors, such as stigma and HIV biological processes, can lead to disengagement (as a coping response) and negative emotions such as hopelessness and pessimism, heightening the risk of suicidal ideation.

There is evidence that adverse life experiences may predispose gay men living with HIV to poor mental health, including suicidal ideation. For instance, it has been shown that childhood sexual abuse, which is prevalent among HIV patients, is associated with both depression and anxiety (Gibb, Chelminski, & Zimmerman, 2007). These conditions in turn increase the risk of suicide in gay men newly diagnosed with HIV. In his study of 149 HIV patients in New Jersey, Roy (2003) found that almost half of the sample participants had attempted suicide and that individuals in this cohort were more likely to have suffered childhood abuse, to exhibit higher levels of neuroticism and to have a comorbidity of depression. This demonstrates the multi-faceted risk profile of HIV patients who attempt suicide—they may have a complex profile with particular personality traits, a history of adverse life events and other psychopathologies, thereby creating the ideal conditions for suicidal ideation to occur.

Preau et al. (2008) surveyed 2932 people living with HIV in France and found that almost a quarter of them had attempted suicide. In addition to HIV discrimination, having been infected with HIV through gay sex was a significant predictor of attempted suicide, suggesting that there is a compounded sense of stigma in relation to both HIV and sexual orientation. Furthermore, in their study of French HIV patients, Carrieri et al. (2017) found that HIV-related discrimination, homelessness and loneliness predicted increased suicide risk in patients. In a study of 673 HIV-positive men, Ferlatte et al. (2017) found that social exclusion, sexual rejection, verbal and physical abuse were positively associated with suicidal ideation and that experiencing more of these adverse events increased suicidal ideation.

Using the Interpersonal-Psychological Theory of Suicidal Behavior (Joiner, 2005), Manetta and Cox (2014) found that HIV patients with suicidal ideation experienced more feelings of perceived burdensomeness and of thwarted belongingness than those with no suicidal ideation. In other words, people living with HIV and contemplating suicide may hold the belief that they are a burden to others around them, for instance, because their condition may cause their family members distress or expose them to HIV stigma. Moreover, they may experience disconnection or alienation from others, believing themselves to be outsiders, which itself may be self-imposed isolation as a means of self-protection from anticipated stigma.

Carrico et al. (2010) studied 232 gay and bisexual men living with HIV and found that 28% of participants reported suicidal ideation in the past fortnight and that suicidal ideation was associated with a threefold increase in engagement in HIV risk behaviour (as the receptive partner, which is the most risky acquisition mode). Moreover, suicidal ideation was associated with a threefold increase in stimulant use, which itself may increase behavioural disinhibition and, thus, engagement in HIV risk behaviours.

Coping

In this chapter, it has been shown that gay men living with HIV may face significant situational stressors, that they may develop negative self-schemata and that they are disproportionately affected by poor mental health. Consistent with identity process theory, they use a variety of strategies—some maladaptive—to cope.

In a study of 502 HIV patients in Norway, Taiwan and the US, Kemppainen et al. (2006) found that there were cross-cultural differences in choice of coping strategy in response to HIV-related anxiety. In the US, praying was by far the most preferable strategy, while in Norway respondents preferred exercising and walking and in Taiwan they prioritised talking to others and attending support groups. In their cross-sectional survey of 465 people living with HIV, Chaudoir et al. (2012) found that the relationship between HIV stigma and depression was moderated by spiritual peace, that is, the extent to which spiritual beliefs provide the individual with a sense of peace. Spiritual peace may buffer the insidious effects of HIV stigma, which continues to be pervasive in society, on mental health outcomes, such as depression. Intrinsic religiosity has been shown to be a protective factor against death anxiety although the role of extrinsic religiosity is inconclusive—in some contexts, it can attenuate symptoms of death anxiety, while in others, it could accentuate them (Miller et al., 2012). These studies suggest that social and cultural norms will influence the choice, and indeed effectiveness, of particular coping strategies.

Like the choice of coping strategy, its effectiveness in resolving threat is likely to vary by context. Kraaij et al. (2008) studied cognitive and behavioural coping strategies in response to HIV and found that only use of the cognitive strategies (e.g. positive reappraisal, positive refocusing, putting things into perspective) was associated with decreased symptoms of depression and anxiety. Conversely, behavioural coping strategies (e.g. use of emotional support, substance use) did not successfully decrease symptoms of anxiety or depression. There is nothing maladaptive or unsustainable about the strategy of deriving emotional support for instance, but for a specific population in any given context this may fail to resolve threat.

Although there is much evidence that social support is an effective strategy for coping with psychological adversity, some research shows that social support alone may not be sufficient. In a study of 320 individuals living with HIV, Liu et al. (2013) found that the relationship between social support and depressive symptoms was mediated by psychological capital, that is, hope and optimism, and by self-efficacy. This suggests that, in order to benefit from social support, one must have access to, or develop, particular skills, such as being more hopeful, optimistic and self-efficacious.

The derivation of social support is known to be an effective coping strategy, but this is dependent on its availability in one's social context. In a study of older people living with HIV, Kalichman, Heckman, Kochman, Sikkema, and Bergholte (2000) found that over a quarter of respondents had contemplated suicide and that they reported higher levels of emotional distress, poorer health-related quality of life and were more likely to use avoidance strategies for coping. Crucially, individuals with suicidal ideation were also more likely to have disclosed their HIV status to people close to them, suggesting that this strategy had not always resulted in the acquisition of social support but had sometimes driven them towards avoidant, isolationist strategies for coping.

Heywood and Lyons (2016) found that social support was protective against anxiety and depression among gay men living with HIV. However, their findings suggested that the source of social support (e.g. family, a friend, a partner) was less decisive in buffering the effects of psychological adversity on mental health than the *type* of social support. More specifically, emotional support was more effective than other types of support as a buffer against poor mental health outcomes in their sample of gay men living with HIV. It is possible that for particular individuals, cultures and situations, specific types of support will be more effective than others. The challenge is to identify the factors that predict the effectiveness of any given type of support for particular individuals, groups and situations.

Some strategies employed by gay men are clearly maladaptive and may perpetuate threats to identity and intensify poor mental health. In their study of 95 HIV patients, Garey et al. (2015) found that hazardous alcohol consumption was associated with depressive and anxious symptoms, which might suggest that individuals are using alcohol as a strategy to cope with their poor mental health. There are now several studies which show that substance misuse is more prevalent in gay men living with HIV than in those who are uninfected and that this practice is associated with poor mental health outcomes. This suggests that substance misuse is a coping response.

Crucially, the practice of chemsex, discussed throughout this volume, is more common in gay men living with HIV than in HIV-negative gay men. This has been attributed to the status of chemsex as an 'escapist' strategy for coping with adversity—gay men who practice chemsex are able to escape transiently from their social and psychological difficulties and, thus, to shield themselves from threats to identity. For instance, it has been reported that individuals face less HIV prejudice, stigma and rejection on the chemsex scene and that it is uncommon for gay men in this context to enquire about HIV status despite non-use of condoms in chemsex parties (Bourne, Reid, Hickson, Torres Rueda, & Weatherburn, 2014). Another maladaptive strategy, which itself is related to alcohol and substance misuse, is sexual compulsivity, that is, a preoccupation with sexual fantasy or behaviour which is characterised by a loss of self-control and with unhealthy outcomes for the individual. Gay men living with HIV are more likely to report sexual compulsivity, which may represent an attempt to derive transient feelings of intimacy from sexual partners in the face of prejudice, stigma and rejection. Furthermore, sexual compulsivity can bolster feelings of self-esteem when this principle of identity is chronically threatened by other social stressors—not least HIV stigma itself.

Predicting Poor Mental and Sexual Health Outcomes

The capacity to cope effectively with these situational stressors is key to both psychological and physical wellbeing. Those who cope are less likely to develop a negative self-schema, such as internalised homophobia, which is known to yield negative mental health outcomes. Jaspal (2018) has proposed what is now referred to as the Health Adversity Risk Model, a multi-level model that can enable us to predict poor mental health and sexual health outcomes in gay men (see Fig. 6.2).

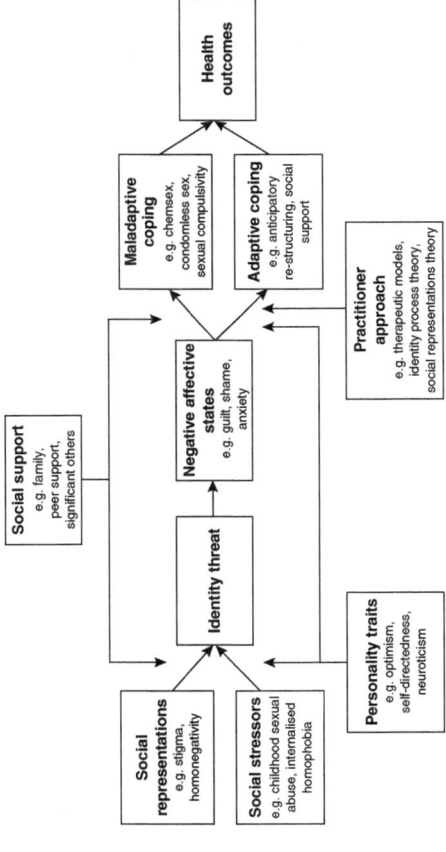

Fig. 6.2   The Health Adversity Risk Model (from Jaspal, 2018)

Situational Stressors and Negative Psychological Self-Schemata

In this chapter, possible antecedents of poor mental health are discussed. The Health Adversity Risk Model for understanding self-identity, well-being and sexual health among gay men attempts to articulate the pathways between situational stressors and poor mental and sexual health outcomes.

Gay men living with HIV are at risk of situational stressors, that is, social representations, events and situations which can induce psychological stress. As demonstrated throughout this volume, gay men are, to varying extents, exposed to negative social representations of their sexual orientation due to both heteronormativity and homophobia in society. Some gay men internalise the homophobia that they encounter, which is transformed into a psychological self-schema. They may do so when there is no recourse perhaps because the stigmatising social representations are so coercive and consensually accepted in their social context that there is no scope for challenging them. In addition to these stigmatising social representations to which gay men are exposed, there is a higher prevalence of adverse life events in this population, such as childhood sexual abuse and homophobic bullying.

Both these negative social representations and the situational stressors could undermine the principles of self-esteem, continuity, self-efficacy and so on, leading to identity threat. Yet, it is clear that not everyone exposed to negative social representations or situational stressors will necessarily experience identity threat. The relationship between the adverse event and identity threat is mediated by at least two variables: personality traits and the availability of social support. Some personality traits, such as conservatism, can increase the likelihood of identity threat when continuity is challenged, for instance (e.g. Bardi, Jaspal, Polek, & Schwartz, 2014). Moreover, social support is simply not available to some people who require it, which increases the likelihood of threat (Jaspal, 2015).

If the adverse event does lead to identity threat, the individual will experience a negative affective state, such as guilt, shame or anxiety. It is plausible to hypothesise that an event or situation that abrogates more than one identity principle will intensify negative affect. As demonstrated in this chapter, HIV infection does have the capacity to threaten several, if not all, identity principles. Negative affect amounts to poor mental health—in its most chronic and severe form, it can cause depressive psychopathology, such as depression, anxiety and suicidal ideation.

Coping with Threats to Identity

A central tenet of identity process theory is that the threatened individual will react to threat by engaging in coping strategies. Methods of coping can also be meaningfully categorised into adaptive and maladaptive strategies. Adaptive coping strategies include *inter alia* making pre-emptive changes to identity in anticipation of a threat (anticipatory re-structuring), re-thinking the meanings of a threatening event (re-conceptualisation) and the derivation of social support, while those that are maladaptive include *inter alia* denial of one's reality, engagement in chemsex and sexual compulsivity. At least three variables will determine the choice of coping strategy: personality, the availability of social support and the practitioner.

First, personality traits do appear to predispose people to cope in particular ways. For instance, gay men who value conservation may be less inclined to engage in anticipatory re-structuring due to their desire to maintain a sense of continuity between past, present and future. Gay men who value conservation may find it difficult to imagine and implement significant changes to their patterns of thought and behaviour because they are more inclined to hold onto the past and maintain the status quo. Thus, the hypothetical gay man who values conservation and who is diagnosed with HIV may respond to this potential threat to identity in a way that enables him to minimise the need for change—this may necessitate a maladaptive coping strategy like denial, rather than anticipatory re-structuring.

Second, the availability of social support is a significant determinant of coping strategy. Only those gay men who actually possess a social support network can make use of it. Not all gay men are themselves comfortable with their sexual orientation; some have not come out as gay or bisexual;

and some avoid involvement in the gay community. It must also be noted that in some social contexts social support for gay men and indeed those living with HIV is simply not available. This may be especially acute in socially conservative contexts in which being gay or bisexual is highly stigmatised and in which HIV is never acknowledged.

Conversely, gay men with access to social support are more likely to engage in other effective coping strategies, such as self-disclosure, and to make use of the support offered by others than those without access to a social support network. For instance, in their study of 371 highly sexually active gay men, Salfas, Rendina, and Parsons (2019) reported that involvement in the gay community was significantly associated with better mental health outcomes and that it buffered the adverse impact of internalised homophobia (a negative self-schema) on mental health outcomes. In short, some gay men may actively disengage from social support, while others simply have no access to it because social support is not available in their context. They are likely to engage in more individualised and, unfortunately, maladaptive strategies for coping in the absence of social support.

Third, practitioners working with gay men living with, or at risk of, HIV may be able to intervene to channel their clients and patients towards more effective and sustainable coping strategies. They may be able to intervene to prevent engagement in maladaptive coping strategies if they succeed in predicting this by identifying the associated risk factors. Undoubtedly, this will require some knowledge of social representations theory, which outlines how knowledge of HIV and risk are popularised, and identity process theory, which focuses on the pathways between psychological adversity and behaviour (Jaspal, 2018). For instance, an HIV patient with low self-esteem who has not disclosed his HIV status to others may not have access to social support and may be at risk of engaging in chemsex, which, in their view, may be the only strategy available to them. The practitioner may be able to facilitate access to HIV peer support before chemsex becomes a first-line coping response. In short, the practitioner can often predict and mitigate the risk of maladaptive coping behaviours in gay men living with HIV.

Overview

There is an important relationship between HIV and mental health. Poor mental health can increase the risk of infection, on the one hand, and HIV infection can induce or exacerbate poor mental health, on the other hand. It is argued that the psychobiological paradigm of mental health is important as it can capture both the social psychological and biological aspects, and indeed drivers, of poor mental health. By identifying the potential drivers, we will be better positioned to address them at a clinical level. Social stigma is a key determinant of poor mental health in those at risk of, and living with, HIV. The social stigma appended to both sexual orientation and to HIV must be challenged at various levels. This will enable gay men to reduce their likelihood of engagement in risk behaviours and to access the multitude of HIV prevention tools available to them. In this chapter, we describe the Health Adversity Risk Model, which allows us to predict how adverse events and experiences (e.g. stigma) might impact on identity processes, potentially leading to engagement in maladaptive risk behaviours and, thus, poor clinical outcomes. Mental health is at the heart of the model, as it is postulated that gay men react to adversity in the way that they do in order to protect their mental health. The challenge for clinicians and practitioners will be to ensure that mental health remains central to effective HIV care.

References

Ahmedani, B. K., Peterson, E. L., Hu, Y., Rossom, R. C., Lynch, F., Lu, C. Y., … Simon, G. E. (2017). Major physical health conditions and risk of suicide. *American Journal of Preventive Medicine, 53*(3), 308–315.

Babowitch, J. D., Mitzel, L. D., Vanable, P. A., & Sweeney, S. M. (2018). Depressive symptoms and condomless sex among men who have sex with men living with HIV: A curvilinear association. *Archives of Sexual Behavior, 47*(7), 2035–2040.

Bardi, A., Jaspal, R., Polek, E., & Schwartz, S. (2014). Values and IPT: Theoretical integration and empirical interactions. In R. Jaspal &

G. M. Breakwell (Eds.), *Identity process theory: Identity, social action and social change* (pp. 175–200). Cambridge: Cambridge University Press.

Bhatia, R., Hartman, C., Kallen, M. A., Graham, J., & Giordano, T. P. (2011). Persons newly diagnosed with HIV infection are at high risk for depression and poor linkage to care: Results from the Steps Study. *AIDS and Behavior, 15*(6), 1161–1170.

Blashill, A. J., & Vander Wal, J. S. (2010). Gender role conflict as a mediator between social sensitivity and depression in a sample of gay men. *International Journal of Men's Health, 9*(1), 26–39.

Blashill, A. J., Gordon, J. R., & Safren, S. A. (2012). Appearance concerns and psychological distress among HIV-infected individuals with injection drug use histories: prospective analyses. *AIDS Patient Care and STDs, 26*(9), 557–561. https://doi.org/10.1089/apc.2012.0122

Bourne, A., Reid, D., Hickson, F., Torres Rueda, S., & Weatherburn, P. (2014). *The Chemsex study: Drug use in sexual settings among gay & bisexual men in Lambeth, Southwark & Lewisham*. London: Sigma Research, London School of Hygiene & Tropical Medicine. Retrieved June 2, 2020, from https://www.lambeth.gov.uk/sites/default/files/ssh-chemsex-study-final-main-report.pdf.

Bragança, M., & Palha, A. (2011). Depression and neurocognitive performance in Portuguese patients infected with HIV. *AIDS and Behavior, 15*(8), 1879–1887.

Brandt, C., Zvolensky, M. J., Woods, S. P., Gonzalez, A., Safren, S. A., & O'Cleirigh, C. M. (2017). Anxiety symptoms and disorders among adults living with HIV and AIDS: A critical review and integrative synthesis of the empirical literature. *Clinical Psychology Review, 51*, 164–184.

Brandt, C. P., Gonzalez, A., Grover, K. W., & Zvolensky, M. J. (2013). The relation between emotional dysregulation and anxiety and depressive symptoms, pain-related anxiety, and HIV-symptom distress among adults with HIV/AIDS. *Journal of Psychopathology and Behavioral Assessment, 35*(2), 197–204.

Braunstein, J. W. (2004). An investigation of irrational beliefs and death anxiety as a function of HIV status. *Journal of Rational-Emotive & Cognitive-Behavior Therapy, 22*(1), 21–38.

Breakwell, G. M. (1986). *Coping with threatened identities*. London: Methuen.

Breet, E., Kagee, A., & Seedat, S. (2014). HIV-related stigma and symptoms of post-traumatic stress disorder and depression in HIV-infected individuals: Does social support play a mediating or moderating role? *AIDS Care, 26*(8), 947–951.

Broun, S. N. (1998). Understanding "post-AIDS survivor syndrome": A record of personal experiences. *AIDS Patient Care and STDs, 12*(6), 481–488.

Carrico, A. W., Neilands, T. B., & Johnson, M. O. (2010). Suicidal ideation is associated with HIV transmission risk in men who have sex with men. *Journal of Acquired Immune Deficiency Syndromes, 54*(4), e3–e4. https://doi.org/10.1097/QAI.0b013e3181da1270

Carrieri, M. P., Marcellin, F., Fressard, L., Préau, M., Sagaon-Teyssier, L., Suzan-Monti, M., … ANRS-VESPA2 Study Group. (2017). Suicide risk in a representative sample of people receiving HIV care: Time to target most-at-risk populations (ANRS VESPA2 French national survey). *PloS One, 12*(2), e0171645. https://doi.org/10.1371/journal.pone.0171645

Catalan, J., Harding, R., Sibley, E., Clucas, C., Croome, N., & Sherr, L. (2011). HIV infection and mental health: Suicidal behaviour—systematic review. *Psychology, Health & Medicine, 16*(5), 588–611.

Chaudoir, S. R., Norton, W. E., Earnshaw, V. A., Moneyham, L., Mugavero, M. J., & Hiers, K. M. (2012). Coping with HIV stigma: Do proactive coping and spiritual peace buffer the effect of stigma on depression? *AIDS and Behavior, 16*, 2382–2391.

Chen, W.-T. (2013). Side effects of antiretroviral therapy (ART) are associated with depression in Chinese individuals with HIV: A mixed methods study. *Journal of Midwifery & Women's Health, 58*, 585–585.

Clucas, C., Sibley, E., Harding, R., Liu, L., Catalan, J., & Sherr, L. (2011). A systematic review of interventions for anxiety in people with HIV. *Psychology, Health & Medicine, 16*(5), 528–547.

Exner, T. M., Meyer-Bahlburg, H. F., & Ehrhardt, A. A. (1992). Sexual self control as a mediator of high risk sexual behavior in a New York City cohort of HIV+ and HIV- gay men. *Journal of Sex Research, 29*(3), 389–406.

Ferlatte, O., Salway, T., Oliffe, J. L., & Trussler, T. (2017). Stigma and suicide among gay and bisexual men living with HIV. *AIDS Care, 29*(11), 1346–1350.

Ferrando, S. J. (2009). Psychopharmacologic treatment of patients with HIV/AIDS. *Current Psychiatry Reports, 11*(3), 235–242.

Fife, B. L., & Wright, E. R. (2000). The dimensionality of stigma: A comparison of its impact on the self of persons with HIV/AIDS and cancer. *Journal of Health and Social Behavior, 41*(1), 50–67.

Garey, L., Bakhshaie, J., Sharp, C., Neighbors, C., Zvolensky, M. J., & Gonzalez, A. (2015). Anxiety, depression, and HIV symptoms among persons living with HIV/AIDS: The role of hazardous drinking. *AIDS Care, 27*(1), 80–85.

Gayner, B., Esplen, M. J., DeRoche, P., Wong, J., Bishop, S., Kavanagh, L., & Butler, K. (2012). A randomized controlled trial of mindfulness-based stress reduction to manage affective symptoms and improve quality of life in gay men living with HIV. *Journal of Behavioral Medicine, 35*(3), 272–285.

Gibb, B. E., Chelminski, I., & Zimmerman, M. (2007). Childhood emotional, physical, and sexual abuse, and diagnoses of depressive and anxiety disorders in adult psychiatric outpatients. *Depression and Anxiety, 24*(4), 256–263.

Gonzalez, J. S., Batchelder, A. W., Psaros, C., & Safren, S. A. (2011). Depression and HIV/AIDS treatment nonadherence: A review and meta-analysis. *Journal of Acquired Immune Deficiency Syndromes, 58*(2), 181–187. https://doi.org/10.1097/QAI.0b013e31822d490a

Grov, C., Golub, S. A., Parsons, J. T., Brennan, M., & Karpiak, S. E. (2010). Loneliness and HIV-related stigma explain depression among older HIV-positive adults. *AIDS Care, 22*(5), 630–639. https://doi.org/10.1080/09540120903280901

Hart, T. A., & Heimberg, R. G. (2005). Social anxiety as a risk factor for unprotected intercourse among gay and bisexual male youth. *AIDS and Behavior, 9*(4), 505–512.

Heywood, W., & Lyons, A. (2016). HIV and elevated mental health problems: Diagnostic, treatment, and risk patterns for symptoms of depression, anxiety, and stress in a national community-based cohort of gay men living with HIV. *AIDS and Behavior, 20*(8), 1632–1645.

Hintze, J., Templer, D., Cappelletty, G. G., & Frederick, W. (1993). Death depression and death anxiety in HIV-infected males. *Death Studies, 17*(4), 333–341.

Ironson, G., O'Cleirigh, C., Fletcher, M. A., Laurenceau, J. P., Balbin, E., Klimas, N., … Solomon, G. (2005). Psychosocial factors predict CD4 and viral load change in men and women with human immunodeficiency virus in the era of highly active antiretroviral treatment. *Psychosomatic Medicine, 67*(6), 1013–1021.

Jaspal, R. (2015). The experience of relationship dissolution among British Asian gay men: Identity threat and protection. *Sexuality Research & Social Policy, 12*(1), 34–46.

Jaspal, R. (2018). *Enhancing sexual health, self-identity and wellbeing among men who have sex with men: A guide for practitioners.* London: Jessica Kingsley Publishers.

Jaspal, R. (2020). Honour beliefs and identity among British South Asian gay men. In M. M. Idriss (Ed.), *Men, masculinities and honour-based abuse* (pp. 114–127). London: Routledge.

Jaspal, R., & Breakwell, G. M. (Eds.). (2014). *Identity process theory: Identity, social action and social change.* Cambridge: Cambridge University Press.

Jaspal, R., & Cinnirella, M. (2010). Coping with potentially incompatible identities: Accounts of religious, ethnic and sexual identities from British Pakistani men who identify as Muslim and gay. *British Journal of Social Psychology, 49*(4), 849–870.

Jaspal, R., & Nerlich, B. (2020). HIV stigma in UK press reporting of a case of intentional HIV transmission. *Health: An Interdisciplinary Journal for the Social Study of Health, Illness & Medicine.* https://doi.org/10.1177/1363459320949901

Jaspal, R., Lopes, B., & Rehman, Z. (2019). A structural equation model for predicting depressive symptomatology in Black, Asian and Minority Ethnic lesbian, gay and bisexual people in the UK. *Psychology and Sexuality.* https://doi.org/10.1080/19419899.2019.1690560

Jaspal, R., & Williamson, I. (2017). Identity management strategies among HIV-positive Colombian gay men in London. *Culture, Health and Sexuality: An International Journal for Research, Intervention and Care, 19*(2), 1374–1388.

Joffe, H. (2007). Identity, self-control, and risk. In G. Moloney & I. Walker (Eds.), *Social representations and identity* (pp. 197–213). London: Palgrave Macmillan.

Joiner, T. E. (2005). *Why people die by suicide.* Cambridge, MA: Harvard University Press.

Kalichman, S. C., Heckman, T., Kochman, A., Sikkema, K., & Bergholte, J. (2000). Depression and thoughts of suicide among middle-aged and older persons living with HIV-AIDS. *Psychiatric Services* (Washington, D.C.), *51*(7), 903–907.

Kavanagh, D. J., & Bower, G. H. (1985). Mood and self-efficacy: Impact of joy and sadness on perceived capabilities. *Cognitive Therapy and Research, 9*(5), 507–525.

Kemppainen, J. K., Eller, L. S., Bunch, E., Hamilton, M. J., Dole, P., Holzemer, W., … Tsai, Y. F. (2006). Strategies for self-management of HIV-related anxiety. *AIDS Care, 18*(6), 597–607.

Kraaij, V., van der Veek, S. M., Garnefski, N., Schroevers, M., Witlox, R., & Maes, S. (2008). Coping, goal adjustment, and psychological well-being in HIV-infected men who have sex with men. *AIDS Patient Care and STDs, 22*(5), 395–402.

Lampe, F. C., Harding, R., Smith, C. J., Phillips, A. N., Johnson, M., & Sherr, L. (2010). Physical and psychological symptoms and risk of virologic rebound among patients with virologic suppression on antiretroviral therapy. *Journal of Acquired Immune Deficiency Syndromes (1999), 54*(5), 500–505.

Lima, V. D., Geller, J., Bangsberg, D. R., Patterson, T. L., Daniel, M., Kerr, T., … Hogg, R. S. (2007). The effect of adherence on the association between depressive symptoms and mortality among HIV-infected individuals first initiating HAART. *AIDS, 21*(9), 1175–1183.

Liu, L., Pang, R., Sun, W., Wu, M., Qu, P., Lu, C., & Wang, L. (2013). Functional social support, psychological capital, and depressive and anxiety symptoms among people living with HIV/AIDS employed full-time. *BMC Psychiatry, 13*, 324. https://doi.org/10.1186/1471-244X-13-324

Lyons, A., Pitts, M., & Grierson, J. (2012). Exploring the psychological impact of HIV: Health comparisons of older Australian HIV-positive and HIV-negative gay men. *AIDS and Behavior, 16*(8), 2340–2349.

Manetta, A. M., & Cox, L. E. (2014). Suicidal behavior and HIV/AIDS: A partial test of Joiner's Theory of why people die by suicide. *Social Work in Mental Health, 12*(1), 20–35. https://doi.org/10.1080/15332985.2013.832717

Memon, A., Taylor, K., Mohebati, L. M., Sundin, J., Cooper, M., Scanlon, T., & de Visser, R. (2016). Perceived barriers to accessing mental health services among black and minority ethnic (BME) communities: A qualitative study in Southeast England. *BMJ Open, 6*(11), e012337. https://doi.org/10.1136/bmjopen-2016-012337

Michaels, M. S., Parent, M. C., & Torrey, C. L. (2016). A minority stress model for suicidal ideation in gay men. *Suicide and Life-Threatening Behavior, 46*(1), 23–34.

Miller, A. K., Lee, B. L., & Henderson, C. E. (2012). Death anxiety in persons with HIV/AIDS: A systematic review and meta-analysis. *Death Studies, 36*(7), 640–663.

Murphy, P. J., Garrido-Hernansaiz, H., Mulcahy, F., & Hevey, D. (2018). HIV-related stigma and optimism as predictors of anxiety and depression among HIV-positive men who have sex with men in the United Kingdom and Ireland. *AIDS Care, 30*(9), 1173–1179.

O'Cleirigh, C., Newcomb, M. E., Mayer, K. H., Skeer, M., Traeger, L., & Safren, S. A. (2013). Moderate levels of depression predict sexual transmission risk in HIV-infected MSM: A longitudinal analysis of data from six sites involved in a "prevention for positives" study. *AIDS and Behavior, 17*(5), 1764–1769.

O'Leary, A., Purcell, D., Remien, R. H., & Gomez, C. (2003). Childhood sexual abuse and sexual transmission risk behaviour among HIV-positive men who have sex with men. *AIDS Care, 15*(1), 17–26.

Passos, S. M., Souza, L. D., & Spessato, B. C. (2014). High prevalence of suicide risk in people living with HIV: Who is at higher risk? *AIDS Care, 26*(11), 1379–1382.

Pence, B. W., O'Donnell, J. K., & Gaynes, B. N. (2012). Falling through the cracks: The gaps between depression prevalence, diagnosis, treatment, and response in HIV care. *AIDS (London, England), 26*(5), 656–658.

Préau, M., Bouhnik, A. D., Peretti-Watel, P., Obadia, Y., Spire, B., & ANRS-EN12-VESPA Group. (2008). Suicide attempts among people living with HIV in France. *AIDS Care, 20*(8), 917–924.

Rehman, Z., Lopes, B., & Jaspal, R. (2020). Predicting self-harm in an ethnically diverse sample of lesbian, gay and bisexual people in the United Kingdom. *International Journal of Social Psychiatry, 66*(4), 349–360.

Rivera-Rivera, Y., Vázquez-Santiago, F. J., Albino, E., Sánchez, M. D., & Rivera-Amill, V. (2016). Impact of depression and inflammation on the progression of HIV disease. *Journal of Clinical & Cellular Immunology, 7*(3), 423. https://doi.org/10.4172/2155-9899.1000423

Robinson, P., Turk, D., Jilka, S., & Cella, M. (2019). Measuring attitudes towards mental health using social media: Investigating stigma and trivialisation. *Social Psychiatry and Psychiatric Epidemiology, 54*(1), 51–58.

Rodkjaer, L., Laursen, T., Balle, N., & Sodemann, M. (2010). Depression in patients with HIV is under-diagnosed: A cross-sectional study in Denmark. *HIV Medicine, 11*(1), 46–53.

Roy, A. (2003). Characteristics of HIV patients who attempt suicide. *Acta Psychiatrica Scandinavica, 107*(1), 41–44.

Ruffieux, Y., Lemsalu, L., Aebi-Popp, K., Calmy, A., Cavassini, M., Fux, C. A., … Swiss HIV Cohort Study and the Swiss National Cohort. (2019). Mortality from suicide among people living with HIV and the general Swiss population: 1988–2017. *Journal of the International AIDS Society, 22*(8), e25339. https://doi.org/10.1002/jia2.25339

Safren, S. A., Gershuny, B. S., & Hendriksen, E. (2003). Symptoms of post-traumatic stress and death anxiety in persons with HIV and medication adherence difficulties. *AIDS Patient Care and STDs, 17*(12), 657–664. https://doi.org/10.1089/108729103771928717

Sahassanon, P., Pisitsungkagarn, K., & Taephant, N. (2019). The effect of cognitive-behavioral group therapy using art as a medium on depressive symptoms and HIV antiretroviral medication adherence. *International Journal for the Advancement of Counselling, 41*, 530–543.

Salfas, B., Rendina, H. J., & Parsons, J. T. (2019). What is the role of the community? Examining minority stress processes among gay and bisexual men. *Stigma and Health, 4*(3), 300–309.

Sandfort, T. G., Bakker, F., Schellevis, F. G., & Vanwesenbeeck, I. (2006). Sexual orientation and mental and physical health status: Findings from a Dutch population survey. *American Journal of Public Health, 96*(6), 1119–1125.

Schlebusch, L., & Govender, R. D. (2015). Elevated risk of suicidal ideation in HIV-positive persons. *Depression Research and Treatment*, 609172. https://doi.org/10.1155/2015/609172

Schuster, R., Bornovalova, M., & Hunt, E. (2012). The influence of depression on the progression of HIV: Direct and indirect effects. *Behavior Modification, 36*(2), 123–145.

Semple, S. J., Strathdee, S. A., Zians, J., McQuaid, J., & Patterson, T. L. (2011). Psychosocial and behavioral correlates of anxiety symptoms in a sample of HIV-positive, methamphetamine-using men who have sex with men. *AIDS Care, 23*(5), 628–637.

Sewell, M. C., Goggin, K. J., Rabkin, J. G., Ferrando, S. J., McElhiney, M. C., & Evans, S. (2000). Anxiety syndromes and symptoms among men with AIDS: A longitudinal controlled study. *Psychosomatics, 41*(4), 294–300.

Shacham, E., Morgan, J. C., Önen, N. F., Taniguchi, T., & Overton, E. T. (2012). Screening anxiety in the HIV clinic. *AIDS and Behavior, 16*(8), 2407–2413.

Sharma, A., Howard, A. A., Klein, R. S., Schoenbaum, E. E., Buono, D., & Webber, M. P. (2007). Body image in older men with or at-risk for HIV infection. *AIDS Care, 19*(2), 235–241.

Sherr, L., Clucas, C., Harding, R., Sibley, E., & Catalan, J. (2011). HIV and depression—a systematic review of interventions. *Psychology, Health & Medicine, 16*(5), 493–527.

Sherr, L., Lampe, F., Fisher, M., Arthur, G., Anderson, J., Zetler, S., ... Harding, R. (2008). Suicidal ideation in UK HIV clinic attenders. *AIDS, 22*(13), 1651–1658.

Spies, G., Asmal, L., & Seedat, S. (2013). Cognitive-behavioural interventions for mood and anxiety disorders in HIV: A systematic review. *Journal of Affective Disorders, 150*(2), 171–180.

Stonewall. (2017). *LGBT in Britain: Hate crime and discrimination*. London: Stonewall. Retrieved June 3, 2020, from https://www.stonewall.org.uk/system/files/lgbt_in_britain_hate_crime.pdf.

Summers, J., Zisook, S., Atkinson, J. H., Sciolla, A., Whitehall, W., Brown, S., ... Grant, I. (1995). Psychiatric morbidity associated with acquired immune deficiency syndrome-related grief resolution. *The Journal of Nervous and Mental Disease, 183*(6), 384–389.

Treisman, G., Fishman, M., Schwartz, J., Hutton, H., & Lyketsos, C. (1998). Mood disorders in HIV infection. *Depression and Anxiety, 7*(4), 178–187.

Treisman, G. J., & Soudry, O. (2016). Neuropsychiatric effects of HIV antiviral medications. *Drug Safety, 39*(10), 945–957.

Uthman, O. A., Magidson, J. F., Safren, S. A., & Nachega, J. B. (2014). Depression and adherence to antiretroviral therapy in low-, middle- and high-income countries: A systematic review and meta-analysis. *Current HIV/ AIDS Reports, 11*(3), 291–307.

Varni, S. E., Miller, C. T., McCuin, T., & Solomon, S. E. (2012). Disengagement and engagement coping with HIV/AIDS stigma and psychological well-being of people with HIV/AIDS. *Journal of Social and Clinical Psychology, 31*(2), 123–150.

World Health Organization. (2001). *Strengthening mental health promotion (Fact sheet No. 220)*. Geneva: World Health Organization.

Yi, M. S., Mrus, J. M., Wade, T. J., Ho, M. L., Hornung, R. W., Cotton, S., ... Tsevat, J. (2006). Religion, spirituality, and depressive symptoms in patients with HIV/AIDS. *Journal of General Internal Medicine, 21*(Suppl 5), S21–S27. https://doi.org/10.1111/j.1525-1497.2006.00643.x

7

Intersecting Identities

Introduction

Our identities are multi-faceted. Throughout the life course, we join and leave social groups. Some group memberships are transient, such as having a particular job role. Others are perceived to be 'essential' to the self, such as ethnicity and, for many people of religious faith, their religion. Some elements of our identities can become 'interconnected' over time often because other people in our social context highlight the connections between them. For instance, sexuality and religion are not *intrinsically* connected, but when religious authorities criticise same-sex relationships and attribute them to 'sin', these identity elements can become interconnected in people's minds. Consequently, we begin to think about how these two identity elements fit together, that is, their compatibility and coherence.

This is a book about HIV and gay men. Gay men are by no means a homogeneous group, and perhaps for that reason, the notion of 'community' has frequently been problematised (e.g. Holt, 2011). Gay men have multiple identities—many identify as gay/bisexual but also as members of a particular ethnicity, religion, social class and so on. Throughout

© The Author(s) 2020
R. Jaspal, J. Bayley, *HIV and Gay Men*, https://doi.org/10.1007/978-981-15-7226-5_7

this volume, it is argued that identity is a key determinant of cognition and behaviour in relation to HIV risk. It can plausibly be hypothesised that the multiple identities of gay men will produce distinct HIV outcomes. This question is the focus of the present chapter. Although recent epidemiological data suggest that there has been an overall decline in new HIV diagnoses among gay men, there has been no such decline in those of Black, Asian and minority ethnic (BAME) backgrounds (Bayley, Williams, & Singh, 2017).

Definitions

Ethnicity

Ethnicity refers to a *belief* in common descent which is shared across an entire group. It can also include institutionalised religion, especially when one's religion is perceived to be a key tenet of one's ethnicity. Although ethnicity is often perceived to be objective, primordial and stable, there is significant evidence to the contrary. Ethnicity is not a reflection of genealogical facts but rather a reflection of beliefs about these 'facts', which may or may not be true—its very existence is dependent on belief (Abizadeh, 2001). Thus, ethnicity is what we might describe as 'socially constructed' although ethnic demarcation lines 'are real in the sense that they form an important part of people's *psychological* realities' (Zagefka, 2009, p. 231).

In medical science and public health, we often refer to ethnic differences, which can sometimes give the impression that any given ethnic group is *inherently* predisposed to a particular medical condition or that it *inherently* displays a particular symptomatology. There is often nothing inherent about vulnerability to disease and illness. For instance, in the context of HIV, we correctly note that Black Africans are at higher risk of HIV infection than other groups. Yet, the reasons underlying this increased risk are actually social, rather than inherent to the ethnicity of Black Africans. It is because of social, cultural, historical, epidemiological, rather than physiological, factors that individuals of Black African ethnicities have been disproportionately affected by HIV.

It is also important to point out that the ethnic labels that are ascribed to individuals, such as 'Asian', 'BAME', may not necessarily align with the *self-identification* of those individuals to whom they are ascribed (Jaspal, Lopes & Breakwell, 2020). This can be problematic on several levels, not least because our attempts to engage individuals from these 'communities' (which may or may not exist in the eyes of individuals themselves) are seen as irrelevant to them and, thus, fail. For instance, the inclusion of people of Latin American descent in the UK in the category 'White Other' may not resonate among individuals of Latin American descent and, thus, fail to capture them adequately or obscure them within a broad and rather meaningless category.

Sexual Orientation and Identity

Sexual orientation can be defined as a trait that predisposes an individual to experience sexual attraction to people of the same sex (gay), to people of the opposite sex (heterosexual) or to people of both sexes (bisexual). Sexual orientation is often assessed using self-report methods, focusing on a combination of self-reported sexual attraction, emotional attraction and sexual behaviour, but it may also be assessed using physiological methods for detecting sexual arousal in response to stimuli (Jaspal, 2019). Over the years, many sexual orientation categories and terms have been used to describe sexual attraction among men, such as homosexual, gay, bisexual, heterosexual, straight and others. Each of these categories and future ones can also be thought of as social representations, evoking distinct meanings, images and values. However, whether or not these categories represent sexual orientation or sexual identity is another matter.

Sexual identity can be defined in terms of the individual's subjective perception, appraisal and categorisation of his sexual orientation. More specifically, the individual derives a sexual identity from the recognition, evaluation and labelling of his sexual orientation. Sexual identity interacts with other components of identity when determined by the social context. It is important to reiterate that sexual orientation and sexual identity are not interchangeable, despite the fact that some people appear to use the terms synonymously. For instance, it is quite possible for a man with a homosexual orientation to have sex with other men, but not to self-identify as gay, as has been observed in Middle Eastern societies, for instance (Maatouk & Jaspal, 2019). The individual may continue to perceive himself to be heterosexual, or perhaps bisexual, although, to the outside observer, this identity appears to be inconsistent with his behaviour. In this chapter, we discuss potential sexual identity issues that can arise among BAME gay men, such as internalised homophobia and the motivation to conceal one's sexual identity.

BAME Communities in the UK

Demography and Sociology

The UK has a long-standing history of ethnic diversity. BAME people are generally defined in the UK according to the following six specific ethnic group categories: Black Caribbean, Black African, Black Other, South Asian (Indian, Bangladeshi, Pakistani), South East Asian (described as Oriental) and dual heritage (described as mixed). However, in our research (e.g. Jaspal, Fish, Williamson, & Papaloukas, 2016; Jaspal & Williamson, 2017), we have also included recent minority groups in the UK, such as Spanish-/Portuguese-speaking Latin American men. Although the term 'BAME' is often used to refer to visible ethnic minority (i.e. those who are not White), it seems appropriate to include in this category some groups traditionally referred to as 'White Other', such as those of Eastern European descent. Like other BAME groups, they too face significant social and health inequalities vis-à-vis the White British population (Fish, Papaloukas, Jaspal, & Williamson, 2016).

The BAME population in the UK grew from 6.6 million in 2001 to 9.1 million in 2009 (7.9% and 14.1% of the UK population, respectively) (UK Census, 2011). In the 2011 census, 19.5% of respondents in England and Wales indicated that they were of BAME backgrounds.[1] Although there are no recent census data on ethnicity, it is likely that there has been an increase in the BAME population. According to

---

[1] https://www.ethnicity-facts-figures.service.gov.uk/uk-population-by-ethnicity.

Stonewall (2012), there are approximately 400,000 BAME LGB people in the UK.

Today, individuals of South Asian descent make up 7.5% of the population in England and Wales, making them the largest ethnic minority category in Britain.[2] Much of the research summarised in this chapter focuses on this population. The term 'British South Asian' is a superordinate ethno-cultural category, used typically to refer to individuals of Indian, Pakistani, Bangladeshi or Sri Lankan descent.

The majority of first-generation British South Asians arrived in the UK in the 1960s and 1970s in order to fill a labour shortage in the largely industrial towns and cities of Northern England and the Midlands. Many had originally intended to return but instead settled in the UK—there are now second, third and even fourth generations of British South Asians. Individuals from this population tend to live in relatively close-knit communities, retaining both a connection with their respective heritage countries and with the norms, values and cultural orientation associated with them. As Jaspal and Cinnirella (2013) outline, national identification among British South Asians is a complex issue—many feel that they are not accepted by their White British co-nationals and, therefore, cannot be British. On the whole, they share a collectivist cultural orientation, which appends importance to notions of kinship ('biraderi'), honour ('izzat') and shame ('sharam'). Jaspal (2020) has explored the significance of kinship, honour and shame, which can impact on identity construction, interpersonal relations and psychological wellbeing among BAME gay men. As shown in this chapter, these factors can in turn impinge on HIV risk and epidemiology.

HIV Epidemiology

Both gay men and BAME groups experience significant inequalities in relation to sexual health in general and HIV, in particular. BAME gay men face a double jeopardy vis-à-vis sexual health. There is a relationship

---

[2] Office for National Statistics 2011, http://www.ons.gov.uk/ons/rel/census/2011-census/key-statistics-for-local-authorities-in-england-and-wales/rpt-ethnicity.html#tab-Ethnicity-in-England-and-Wales.

between HIV risk awareness and risk behaviour—people who have adequate risk awareness may take steps to reduce their risk. However, in their survey of 538 BAME gay and bisexual men in the UK, Jaspal, Lopes, Jamal, Paccoud, and Sekhon (2017) found that participants scored an average of 3.7 (out of a possible score of 10) on HIV knowledge and that South Asians possessed the least knowledge of all BAME groups. Crucially, those who perceived their sexual risk behaviour to be safe possessed the least HIV knowledge, suggesting that their risk appraisals might be inaccurate.

HIV incidence in BAME communities is high—in 2015, two thirds of all new HIV diagnoses among heterosexuals in the UK were in people of BAME background, and BAME people are more likely to be diagnosed at an advanced stage of infection (Public Health England, 2016). Black gay and bisexual men are more likely to be diagnosed with a bacterial STI than other ethnic groups and six times more likely to live with undiagnosed HIV than other gay and bisexual men (Fish et al., 2016). According to Public Health England, there has been a greater than 82% increase in new HIV diagnoses among gay and bisexual men of 'other' and mixed heritage. In their analysis of STI surveillance data in England, Mohammed, Furegato, and Hughes (2016) report that just 5.6% of the 326,820 attendances by gay and bisexual men at sexual health clinics were among those of BAME background. However, BAME gay and bisexual men were more likely to be diagnosed with bacterial STIs and HIV than White gay and bisexual men, with higher incidence of chlamydia in Black Caribbean gay and bisexual men and higher incidence of HIV in those of mixed heritage. The authors suggest that more culturally appropriate prevention messages might help reduce the incidence of bacterial STIs and HIV in BAME gay and bisexual men.

In their analysis of new HIV diagnoses in their London clinic from 2016 to 2018, Stegmann, Scott, Jones, and Rayment (2019) found that 88% of new diagnoses were among gay and bisexual men, of whom just over a quarter were from Poland. As noted earlier, it may be appropriate to consider Eastern Europeans as BAME. Moreover, 59% of those under the age of 25 were of BAME background, with most self-identifying as Black British. In their analysis of testing rates at their London clinic between 2015 and 2016, Bayley, Williams and Singh (2017) observed a

42% decline in new HIV diagnoses among gay and bisexual men but noted that no such decline was observable in those of South Asian ethnicity. They attributed this continued incidence in South Asian gay and bisexual men to low engagement with sexual health services.

In a case notes review of 203 BAME gay and bisexual men attending a London sexual health clinic (Soni, Bond, Fox, Grieve, & Sethi, 2008), it was found that they were more likely to report unprotected anal sex with casual male partners in the past three months, indicating a high risk of HIV acquisition. BAME gay men are more likely to have a history of substance abuse and less likely to have heard of biomedical HIV prevention approaches, namely, post-exposure prophylaxis (PEP) and pre-exposure prophylaxis (PrEP), than other gay and bisexual men (Millett et al., 2012). Furthermore, the same study reported that BAME gay and bisexual men were three times more likely to test positive for HIV than White gay and bisexual men. In an analysis of the GUM clinical activity dataset in England (Mohammed et al., 2016), it was found that, among all gay and bisexual men attending sexual health services, those of BAME background were more likely to be diagnosed with an STI than other gay and bisexual men and that those of White mixed and Black African backgrounds were more likely to be diagnosed with HIV than other groups.

In a study of uptake of and retention in HIV care among gay and bisexual men by ethnic group, the United Kingdom Collaborative HIV Cohort Study Group (2012) found that BAME gay and bisexual men are more likely to be lost to follow-up after HIV diagnosis than White men and that permanent loss to follow-up is especially prevalent in those of South Asian heritage. Moreover, BAME gay and bisexual men are 18% less likely than White men to initiate ART following diagnosis, although once they do their clinical outcomes appear to be the same as those of White ethnicity. Thus, treatment outcomes appear to be good in BAME gay and bisexual men, but retaining them in HIV care following HIV diagnosis remains a challenge. Moreover, BAME gay and bisexual men were 18% less likely to initiate ART than White gay and bisexual men with a similar CD4 cell count. These studies highlight not only a higher prevalence of HIV in BAME gay men but also a higher risk of infection and onward transmission in this population.

The epidemiological data present clear evidence that BAME gay men are disproportionately affected by poor sexual health, including HIV. Theories from social psychology can enable us to understand the possible risk factors.

Theories of Social Knowledge and Intersecting Identities

There is now a body of research into identity processes among gay men from BAME backgrounds (Coyle & Rafalin, 2000; Jaspal & Cinnirella, 2010, 2012a), which shows that contemplating the relationship between sexuality, ethnicity and religion can be a source of psychological distress. Moreover, BAME gay men may face multiple forms of stigma, including homophobia, racism and HIV stigma. There is of course nothing inherently problematic about being BAME and gay—rather, the 'messages' disseminated in these groups, and to group members, may *construct* this identity configuration (i.e. being both BAME and gay) as problematic. In this section, theories of social knowledge and intersecting identities are briefly outlined.

Social Representations Theory

Social representations theory (Moscovici, 1988) from social psychology postulates that social knowledge arises from social representations. A social representation can be defined as a collective 'elaboration' of a given social object which enables individuals to think and talk about it. This elaboration includes emerging beliefs, values, ideas, images and metaphors that are used to conceptualise the social object. For instance, in attempting to make sense of one's same-sex attraction, BAME gay men will draw on those social representations of homosexuality that are most readily available to them.

If one appends importance to one's ethnic group, it is likely that this group will become the main source of social representations. Furthermore, it is true that some groups have more to say about particular issues—religious institutions are often concerned with issues of morality and ethics; some represent homosexuality as immoral and unethical and provide elaborate explanations for this stance; and sometimes religious institutions impose these social representations on their followers. This is of course not to deny that people of religious faith are exposed only to negative social representations, but it is unlikely that the positive social representations of homosexuality (e.g. being gay is fine) will be as readily available to those gay men whose principal group memberships espouse only negative representations (e.g. being gay is immoral).

Social representations theory describes two social psychological processes which are said to converge in the creation of social representations:

- *Anchoring* refers to the process whereby a novel, unfamiliar phenomenon is integrated into existing ways of thinking. For instance, in research with gay Muslims (Jaspal & Cinnirella, 2010), it has been found that homosexuality is sometimes linked to 'liberal Western culture'. It is easy to see how this could encourage the social representation that homosexuality is the product of one's social environment and upbringing and, thus, that it can be changed.
- *Objectification* refers to the process whereby an abstract phenomenon is rendered concrete and tangible. The use of metaphors is a prime example of objectification. For example, homosexuality has been described in terms of an illness, which implies that it can be treated or cured, but also in terms of sin, suggesting that one can repent and change.

Anchoring and objectification are the key components of a social representation, that is, they give rise to that collective 'elaboration' that facilitates thought and action.

Breakwell (2014) has described the social and psychological processes that govern the individual's relationship with a social representation. After all, the social representation is social and needs to be personalised at the individual level.

The individual takes a stance on the social representation, that is, they differ in their awareness, understanding and acceptance of it. For instance, although a BAME gay or bisexual man of religious faith is aware of, and understands, the social representation in his religious group that homosexuality is immoral, he might not accept it. Yet, this is possible only if the individual has access to competing social representations and possesses the personal and social resources to reject the representation. How an individual personalises a social representation will have significant implications for their own identity, wellbeing and indeed health. If one accepts the social representation that homosexuality is immoral, one is at risk of developing internalised homophobia, which in turn could undermine self-esteem. Moreover, as outlined in Chap. 3, this can increase engagement in HIV risk behaviour.

It is also important to point out that our group memberships determine the extent of our exposure to particular social representations, which in turn can shape HIV awareness. If HIV is particularly stigmatised in one's ethnic group and one's ethnic group is important and salient, it is likely that one will have only limited exposure to social representations of HIV from this group membership. Furthermore, those social representations which are available will be negative and stigmatising, rather than constructive and geared towards awareness-raising. This may explain the finding that HIV awareness is very low in BAME gay men and especially in those of South Asian background (Jaspal et al., 2017).

Psychological Coherence

The psychological coherence principle captures how the individual feels subjectively about the different elements that define who they are as a person. Psychological coherence refers to the individual's need to perceive compatibility and coherence between *interconnected* self-aspects or elements of the identity structure (Jaspal & Cinnirella, 2010). In view of the multiplicity of identity, the individual is typically presented with a vast amount of information, some of which may be contradictory and incompatible.

Drawing upon identity process theory (see Chap. 6), it is hypothesised that people are psychologically motivated to enhance feelings of compatibility and coherence between these elements of themselves, especially in contexts of multiple identification with interconnected identity elements (Jaspal & Cinnirella, 2010; Jaspal & Siraj, 2011). If the need for psychological coherence is not fulfilled, identity becomes susceptible to threat, leading the threatened individual to engage in strategies to counteract the threat. In this sense, psychological coherence can be seen as an important principle of identity. Yet, the perceived coherence between identity elements is fluid, context-dependent, and subjective—it resides 'in the eye of the perceiver and [is] not some objective quality of the identities under scrutiny' (Jaspal & Cinnirella, 2010, p. 866).

Social psychologists have employed the concept of psychological coherence in order to understand how individuals subjectively manage potentially competing or contradictory social representations, which are associated with distinct identity elements. For instance, gay Muslims may simultaneously be exposed to the religious representation that marriage is a union between a man or a woman and the competing social representation (associated with the sexual ingroup) that gay marriage is important and worth fighting for. The construct of psychological coherence acknowledges the influence of prevailing social representations concerning identities, their qualitative nature and their compatibility. For instance, British Muslim gay men may fear 'coming out', that is, publicly disclosing membership in the categories 'Muslim' and 'gay', due to their awareness of negative social representations of homosexuality within religious circles (Jaspal & Siraj, 2011). In the next section, we explore the psychological impact of intersecting identities, focusing on the social representations that they can generate and the implications for psychological coherence.

The Psychological Impact of Intersecting Identities

Drawing mainly, but not exclusively, on empirical research into the identities and experiences of British South Asian gay men as a case study, this section of the chapter focuses on how individuals make sense of homosexuality, the threats to psychological coherence that can arise as they take a stance on the connections between their ethnicity and sexual orientation, and the ways in which they attempt to maintain a sense of belonging in the social groups which matter to them.

Deriving a Sexual Identity from Sexual Orientation

As noted earlier in this chapter, there is often alignment between sexual orientation and sexual identity, but this is not always the case—some individuals do not identify in a way that seems consistent with their sexual orientation. This is especially observable among gay men from BAME backgrounds who may perceive barriers to the assimilation and accommodation of a gay or bisexual identity.

Some gay men report very early awareness of their sexual orientation (e.g. 'I have always known'), while others identify a particular temporal point at which they became aware of it (e.g. 'I realised I was gay when I was twenty'). Although the individual may become aware of their same-sex attractions at a particular point in time, these attractions may be dismissed as a 'phase', reconceptualised as platonic or denied because this information is too difficult to assimilate and accommodate in identity. These actions amount to strategies for coping with the psychological distress that some gay men experience when thinking about their (stigmatised) sexual orientation. By engaging in what can loosely be described as 'deflection' strategies, such as those described above, the individual is able to maintain their previous self-image and to avoid a situation where the psychological coherence principle is jeopardised.

BAME gay men may experience difficulties in making sense of their sexual orientation and the feelings, emotions and desires associated with it, largely because of the stigmatising social representations of homosexuality which are associated with their ethnic communities (e.g. Jaspal & Cinnirella, 2010). Gay men attempt to define and append meaning to their sexual orientation, which in turn will determine the way in which they decide to 'categorise' themselves. Possible self-categories include inter alia gay, homosexual, bisexual and heterosexual. Several scholars have noted that the category 'gay' is a Western construct, which BAME people with same-sex desires may therefore reject as an inaccurate category of self-identification (e.g. Carlson, 1997; Jaspal, 2019). In Western cultures, being gay is often understood as a group-level identity element, which implies a sense of commonality and solidarity with other members of this group. According to this perspective, the individual perceives a sense of affiliation to the group and shares some key norms, values and practices with other group members (Tajfel & Turner, 1986).

Some BAME gay men construe homosexuality in terms of an individual characteristic, rather than as a social group membership. In other words, they may perceive their sexual orientation as an entirely personal characteristic and eschew any sense of social identification with other gay men. Some may even stigmatise and denigrate other gay in order to retain a psychological distance from them and indeed from a gay or bisexual identity (Jaspal & Cinnirella, 2014). This may be symptomatic of the individual's internalised homophobia in that they uncritically accept negative social representations of homosexuality. Yet, this strategy for coping with internalised homophobia reduces the likelihood of developing friendships with other gay men, which in turn may deprive them of social support networks that might offer more effective respite from psychological distress.

In view of the importance appended to religion in many BAME communities, individuals may come to view their sexual orientation through the lens of their religious identity and draw upon theological representations of it. In attempting to make sense of their sexual orientation, BAME gay men of religious faith may make theologically informed attributions, which in turn can have implications for the ways in which they evaluate their sexual orientation, that is, the meanings that they append to it.

Some British Muslim gay men, for instance, attribute their sexual orientation to God, and given the social representation in Islam that God is perfect, this attributional tendency can enable them to deduce that God's creation (viz. their sexual orientation) cannot possibly be imperfect or wrong (Jaspal & Cinnirella, 2010). This amounts to a form of anchoring—a link is established between homosexuality and divinity. Moreover, homosexuality is metaphorically represented as God's 'creation', which constitutes an example of objectification. In view of the importance appended to their religious identity, this can enable gay Muslims to evaluate their sexual orientation positively, that is, to derive positive social representations of it. Accordingly, some individuals distance the notion of sex from their homosexual relationships and instead emphasise the importance of companionship, security and intimacy in these relationships.

In previous research (e.g. Jaspal & Cinnirella, 2010), gay Muslims have rejected the focus on sexual behaviour in social representations of homosexuality and claimed that it was promiscuity, not homosexuality, which invited disapproval from God in the Story of Lot in Islam (see also Kugle, 2010). Unsurprisingly, this positive evaluation of homosexuality can facilitate the assimilation and accommodation of sexual orientation in identity. Given that this identity element can contribute favourably to self-esteem (and possibly to other principles of identity), gay Muslims may more readily assimilate and accommodate it in their self-concept.

Conversely, some gay Muslims attribute their sexual orientation to malevolent forces, such as Satan, and deduce from this the notion that homosexuality is imperfect and perhaps even evil. In previous work (Jaspal & Cinnirella, 2010), interviewees have expressed the social representation that homosexuality is a Satanic corruption, which they, as followers of God, must attempt to resist, rather than embrace. In short, homosexuality is anchored to images of evil and sin. When perceived in terms of 'Satanic corruption', the reality of one's homosexuality may undermine one's self-esteem. This attributional style can therefore preclude the assimilation and accommodation of homosexuality in the self-concept. People wish to distance from their self-concept those identity elements that challenge the integrity of identity. As a means of coping with the ensuing psychological distress, some gay Muslims hope to change their sexual orientation (Jaspal, 2014a). The principal aim is to align their sexual orientation with the perceived norms, values and expectations associated with their religious identity. Yet, by anchoring homosexuality to sin and evil, individuals may face an additional threat to psychological coherence. Indeed, some BAME gay men of religious faith question the feasibility of religious self-identification and engagement in homosexual behaviour.

In making sense of their sexual orientation, individuals consider the extent to which they wish to disclose it to other people. In Western societies, there is a strong positive social representation of 'coming out' as gay. When celebrities come out as gay, this is often presented as a positive personal and societal action. There is also much social sciences research that highlights the social and psychological benefits of 'coming out' (Lasala, 2000; Rosario, Hunter, Maguen, Gwadz, & Smith, 2001). Yet, this is not necessarily the case for all BAME gay men, whose ethnic communities may construe 'coming out' as negative, leading to social, legal and indeed psychological challenges.

Some BAME gay men are fearful of 'bringing shame on the family' by disclosing their sexual identity and of the negative social consequences that this could entail (Jaspal, 2020). Some believe that it is impossible to be gay and a member of their ethnic group. This may render the prospect of 'coming out' challenging or even impossible. The more feasible alternative may be for BAME gay men to develop ways of constructing and manifesting their sexual identities in ways that do not threaten their physical and psychological wellbeing (see Jaspal, 2014b). Yet, the challenges to psychological perception can nevertheless remain.

Challenges to Psychological Coherence

BAME gay men may regard their sexual orientation through the lens of their ethnic identity and therefore make attributions associated with their ethnic identity to make sense of their sexual orientation. For instance, those of religious faith may believe that their sexual orientation is a sin. This renders the two identities—ethnicity and sexuality—interconnected and gives rise to the need to take a stance on their compatibility. It is clear that some BAME gay men do struggle to derive a sense of coherence between these identities (Jaspal & Cinnirella, 2010). For instance, British Pakistani Muslim gay men may feel that homosexuality is 'wrong' or 'sinful' from the perspective of their Muslim identity and that homosexuality prevents them from being 'good Muslims'. In the process of attempting to establish coherence between their ethnic and sexual identities, some BAME gay men may come to question the authenticity of other identity elements, such as their religion.

Although some BAME gay men of religious faith are unaware of the theological stance on homosexuality, they may continue to believe that same-sex behaviour is incompatible with their religious identity. What they come to believe is often based on dominant social representations in their ethnic group, rather than any 'objective' theological pronouncement on their sexual orientation. In other words, although individuals may not necessarily possess first-hand knowledge of holy scripture, they draw upon negative social representations of homosexuality. For instance, some gay Muslims describe the Prophet Mohammed's alleged disgust towards homosexuality, as well as God's intolerance of it, which resonates with the Story of Lot from the Koran. Individuals may draw upon an important identity—their religion—in substantiating their views about homosexuality. Many BAME gay men do value their religious identity, which may lead them to accept uncritically and to internalise the social representations that they perceive to be associated with this identity. Internalised homophobia, coupled with consciousness of one's own homosexual behaviour, can accentuate the perception of incompatibility between ethnic and sexual identities and induce psychological distress.

BAME gay men in previous studies (e.g. Jaspal, 2012a) have described threats to psychological coherence by making metaphorical statements, such as 'my worlds were clashing' and 'I was fighting with myself'. These statements suggest that their distinct identities represent separate 'worlds' in their minds and that their combination entails a degree of internal conflict. However, as BAME gay men struggle to reconcile their sexual orientation and their ethnicity, they may attenuate the significance of, or deny altogether, the identity aspect of lesser importance. In many cases, their sexual orientation is relegated to an inferior position in the identity structure. Accordingly, individuals may view themselves as heterosexuals while acknowledging occasional engagement in homosexual behaviour (Maatouk & Jaspal, 2020). The perception of homosexuality in terms of a behaviour, rather than a characteristic of identity, essentially obviates the need to acknowledge the threat to psychological coherence. Behaviours can seem more mutable than identity elements, which people conversely tend to view as essential to their sense of self and thus immutable.

In explicating their engagement in homosexual 'behaviours', some BAME gay men engage in the psychological process of external attribution whereby they identify an external source (external to the self) which can be held responsible/accountable for their homosexuality (see Kelley,

1967). Indeed, as noted above, some gay Muslims may attribute their sexual orientation externally—to either God or Satan. Additionally, previous studies have described a tendency for some BAME gay men who live in the UK to attribute their sexual orientation to 'Western culture' (Jaspal & Cinnirella, 2010). According to this attribution, individuals were able to distance their sexual orientation from their valued ethnicity and, thus, the self and instead argued that, due to Western cultural influences (and particularly the 'normalisation' of homosexuality in Western societies), they had 'adopted' homosexual practices.

Some BAME gay men believe that, if they had grown up in their heritage countries (associated with their ethnicities), they would not have engaged in homosexual behaviours. Similarly, some of the Iranian Muslim gay men who participated in our interview studies attributed their homosexual behaviour to their migration to Britain where it was reportedly 'easier' to meet other men for sex (e.g. Jaspal, 2014b). This attributional style enables individuals to objectify their sexual orientation as a 'sinful behaviour' and to distance it from the self, which in turn protects identity from threat. In previous research (e.g. Jaspal & Cinnirella, 2010), Muslim gay men have sometimes constructed their homosexuality as a behaviour, rather than as an identity aspect, possibly as a means of minimising threats to the psychological coherence principle.

However, those BAME gay men who, for whatever reason, cannot deny their sexual orientation and who acknowledge the difficulties in 'resisting' it, may come to question the authenticity of their ethnic identity. It is important to note that ethnicity constitutes an important identity for many BAME gay men and one that they wish to maintain. Doubts surrounding the authenticity of their ethnic identity can essentially represent a rupture between past, present and future (Jaspal & Cinnirella, 2012b). Loss of ethnic identity may amount to a perceived loss of community, which may plausibly affect other dimensions of life, such as family identity.

People employ various strategies for aligning their sexual orientation and ethnic identity in a way that might enhance the psychological coherence principle of identity. These include self-distancing from the gay community, contemplating an arranged heterosexual marriage and seeking religious guidance to 'convert' to heterosexuality (e.g. Jaspal, 2014a).

Yet, the recognition that it is impossible to change their sexual orientation in real terms may lead some individuals to perceive decreased self-efficacy, that is, some may feel helpless and resign themselves to the psychologically undesirable reality of their homosexual orientation. In short, the strategies deployed to enhance the psychological coherence principle of identity can be ineffective in the long term and undermine other psychological needs, such as belongingness in valued groups.

Maintaining Belongingness in Valued Ingroups

In view of the negative social representation of homosexuality associated with their ethnic identity, BAME gay men may fear exclusion from their ethnic ingroup. British South Asian gay men have reported fears that they will no longer be accepted by fellow members of their ethnic group in view of the negative social representations which prevail in their ethnic groups (Jaspal, 2012b). The prospect of ostracism may represent a threat to their sense of belongingness within their respective communities.

Furthermore, recent research suggests that ethnic and religious minority groups face racism and other forms of exclusion on the gay scene, which can inhibit access to social support in this context (Jaspal, 2017). They may face 'sexual racism' whereby they are rejected by White gay men under the pretext that they are not sexually attractive or sexually objectified, that is, perceived to be sexually desirable solely on the basis of the physical characteristics associated with race and ethnicity. There is evidence that this is psychologically distressing for BAME gay men (Jaspal, 2017). In the face of exclusion, BAME individuals may become more immersed in their ethnic ingroup as this group membership can come to constitute a strong and reliable source of belongingness, that is, individuals derive a sense of acceptance and inclusion from it. This can make some BAME gay men even more reliant on their ethnic ingroup as they fear exclusion from it, which would leave them with few alternative social support options. In previous research (Jaspal, 2012a), one interviewee described his fear of being 'kicked out of the community' and of 'being alone in the world', while another noted that he was 'not networked or well connected' outside of his ethnic and family networks. This highlights the need for belongingness within the ethnic ingroup.

BAME gay men may employ a variety of strategies for attempting to maintain a sense of connection with their ethnic identity in the face of threats to belongingness. For instance, in their focus group and interview study of 85 gay men of ethnic minority backgrounds in the US, Choi, Han, Paul, and Ayala (2011) found that individuals tended to conceal their sexual orientation from members of their ethnic communities to avoid homophobia and to avoid frequenting contexts in which they anticipated racism from other gay men. In short, a combination of passing and self-isolation is employed in order to evade these forms of stigma. Furthermore, psychologists have described the strategy of 'compartmentalisation', which refers to the psychological process of keeping elements of identity separate in the mind as a means of reducing perceived incompatibilities between them (Breakwell, 1986). Indeed, use of this strategy is also observable in work on sexual and religious identification among BAME gay men of Muslim background (e.g. Jaspal, 2014a). However, compartmentalisation may not be a sustainable as a long-term strategy in this group. Although some individuals do report initially compartmentalising their identity elements, there are some contexts in which compartmentalisation ceases to function effectively.

In an interview for a previous study (Jaspal, 2012a), a gay Muslim described his experience of sitting in a mosque during Friday prayers and suddenly becoming aware of his sexual orientation and the implications that this had for his Muslim identity. The interviewee described the onset of his feelings of insecurity and inauthenticity (in relation to his Muslim identity) and realised that compartmentalisation was no longer viable as a coping strategy. Furthermore, there are some social and interpersonal issues that can undermine the efficacy of compartmentalisation. Given the cultural expectation for a heterosexual (often arranged) marriage in some BAME communities, gay men from these communities may be pressured into considering marital offers (Jaspal, 2014a). This can undermine the compartmentalisation strategy as social cues of this nature essentially compel the individual to take a stance on the compatibility of their sexual orientation and ethnicity.

BAME gay men may engage in the strategy of hyper-affiliation to the ethnic ingroup. Hyper-affiliation can be defined as 'accentuated social and psychological identification with a social group in response to threatened group membership' (Jaspal & Cinnirella, 2014, p. 266). This essentially means that the individual may actively attempt to reconnect with their ethnic group to 'prove' the legitimacy of their membership. When BAME gay men deploy this strategy, they become immersed in the ethnic group, adopting all its norms, values and social representations and, conversely, distance themselves from other groups, including the sexual ingroup. This can serve to fortify ethnic identification but does not resolve the threats to psychological coherence or to self-esteem when norms, values and social representations explicitly denigrate the sexual ingroup, for instance. In short, hyper-affiliation can transiently make individuals feel more connected to their ethnic community, although the threat to belongingness may resurface and continue to challenge psychological wellbeing.

Furthermore, there are socially oriented methods of safeguarding ethnic authenticity and belongingness. In seeking to demonstrate the authenticity of one's ethnic identity in public settings, individuals may reproduce social representations, which they perceive to be central to their ethnic identity. For instance, some express homophobic social representations despite having same-sex attractions themselves, which itself may be associated with internalised homophobia. However, it may also constitute a means of 'convincing' other people within one's ethnic ingroup that one is an authentic group member, thereby safeguarding belongingness in that group. This means of authenticating one's ethnic identity may be problematic because the perceived ingroup position on any given issue (i.e. homosexuality) may not necessarily be consistent with the individual's own personal identity (i.e. as a gay or bisexual man). In other words, one may publicly express the social representation that homosexuality is a sin but not actually believe it oneself.

Intersecting identities—in this case, ethnicity and sexual orientation among BAME gay men—can present significant social and psychological challenges, including threats to psychological coherence and belongingness in valued groups. This in turn can lead to a precarious sense of identity and internalised homophobia as individuals attempt to reduce threats to psychological coherence and belongingness. In the next section, we consider the potential impact of intersecting identities and the associated stressors on HIV risk and outcomes.

Clinical Snapshot 7: Religion and Gay Men

In general, homosexuality has not been accepted as normal or 'healthy' in many religious communities. There is a slow shift in some religions, but there remains a level of prejudice and stigma within them. Men who have sex with men (note, not gay men as many do not identify as such) from a Muslim background very often find it hard to disclose their sexual behaviour and struggle to reconcile their Muslim identity with their sexual identity—often leading to psychological conflict, substance use issues or mood disorders. This is exacerbated by a lack of discussion about sexual health or function, potential ostracisation from friends and family or repression of their sexual identity. In clinic, these men can also have low levels of knowledge concerning HIV transmission which can lead to increased risk-taking. It is important to increase HIV awareness and understanding and to improve access to prevention and care in these communities.

Intersecting Identities, Social Stressors and HIV

Sexual identity issues can have important direct and indirect effects on sexual health outcomes. Threats to identity, as outlined in identity process theory (see Chap. 6), may lead to engagement in sexual risk-taking behaviours, while the desire to protect identity can sometimes lead to disengagement from sexual health services. This may mean that opportunities are missed to prevent HIV among BAME gay men, to test and diagnose them and to retain those who are living with HIV in clinical care. In view of the social stigma appended to homosexuality in their respective communities, BAME gay men may be concerned about the possible negative consequences of disclosing their sexual orientation to significant others, such as rejection, which can lead them to conceal it from others (Jaspal & Siraj, 2011; Jaspal & Williamson, 2017).

There is evidence that prejudice faced by BAME gay men can also have negative outcomes for their sexual health. For instance, in their study of the correlates of sexual risk-taking among 2235 Latino and Black gay men in the US, Ayala, Bingham, Kim, Wheeler, and Millett (2012) found that experiences of racism and homophobia were associated with a lack of social support, potentially suggesting that these experiences make individuals feel that support (e.g. from their ethnic communities and other gay men) is not readily available to them and, thus, do not seek it. Furthermore, in their study, the relationship between discrimination and engagement in unprotected anal intercourse was mediated by participation in risky sexual situations (i.e. being in a situation which makes the use of condoms difficult). Thus, exposure to discrimination may lead individuals to put themselves in risky sexual situations, which in turn heightens the risk of actual engagement in sexual risk behaviours.

Bogart et al. (2011) conducted a survey of 181 Black gay and bisexual living with HIV in the US to assess levels of perceived discrimination due to ethnicity, sexual orientation and HIV status. They found that all three forms of discrimination were associated with depressive symptomatology, which in turn has been linked to poor clinical outcomes in HIV patients (see Chap. 7). It is noteworthy that Black gay men may be at greater risk of discrimination on the basis of their sexual orientation due to dominant social representations within their ethnic communities and are certainly at greater risk of racial discrimination due to their stigmatised ethnic minority status. Both racism and homophobia are significant stressors experienced by BAME gay men.

Racism

In Jaspal's (2017) study of racism on the gay scene, British South Asian gay men described experiences of rejection from White British gay men as well as overt stigma due to Islamophobia, which inhibited feelings of belongingness and, thus, impeded the formation of enduring interpersonal relationships in these contexts. Some interviewees also described the low self-confidence and vulnerability that arose from exposure to such stigma. Racism is associated with decreased self-esteem, and that decreased self-esteem may in turn give rise to engagement in sexual risk-taking behaviours. In Jaspal's (2017) study, some individuals felt unable to negotiate condom use with their sexual partners, fearing that this could lead to further rejection and, thus, resorted to sexual behaviours that increased their risk of HIV and other STIs.

Some attempts have been made to understand the relationship between prejudice and engagement in sexual risk behaviours. In an important sociological study of sexual risk-taking among gay and bisexual men of Asian and Pacific Islander descent in the US, Han (2008) focused on the structural conditions and social norms underpinning sexual behaviour among men from this population. Individuals in this study reported both subtle and blatant forms of racism, including 'fetishisation' of their ethnicity from White people. The author argued that, in view of the racism experienced by these men, they come to express a preference for White men who are deemed to be 'hard to get'. Given that partnering with White men is viewed as a challenge, self-esteem might be enhanced when one does succeed in securing a White man as one's (sexual) partner.

Yet, this does come with potential costs—participants in Han's (2008) study reported putting themselves at risk of HIV in the quest to win the favour of White men. They reported acquiescing to the sexual desires and demands of their White sexual partners, with whom relations were precarious—some believed, and were led to believe, that their primary function was to satisfy their White sexual partner through passivity and submissiveness and, in some cases, by agreeing to condomless sex. The author argues that this pattern of behaviour is sustained by the dominant social representation of gay men of Asian and Pacific Islander descent as sexually passive and submissive, which in turn leads to the expectation that they adopt the sexually receptive role—itself associated with greater HIV risk.

Furthermore, Raymond and McFarland (2009) focus on the broader ramifications of racism for HIV incidence in Black gay men in the US. In their cross-sectional survey of 1142 gay and bisexual men, they found that Black participants were more likely to engage in same race sexual partnering and that, among respondents of other ethnicities, Black individuals were the least preferred sexual partners and they were believed to be at higher risk of HIV. Similarly, Phillips, Birkett, Hammond, and Mustanski (2016) found that Black, Hispanic and Asian gay and bisexual men in their study were more likely to express a partner preference for ethnic ingroup members, further demonstrating the sexual 'interconnectedness', that is, sexual activity concentrated within a relatively small subsection of the population, of ethnic minority gay communities. It is possible that negative attitudes towards ethnic minority gay men may be the causal factor in the 'interconnectedness' of these groups, which in turn can lead to a more rapid and sustained spread of HIV among ethnic minority gay men.

In their survey of 1196 Black, Latino and Asian/Pacific Islander gay and bisexual men in the US, Han et al. (2015) found that 65% of participants reported feeling stressed as a result of racism in the gay community and that both racism-related stress and avoidance coping were associated with increased odds of unprotected anal intercourse. This suggests that, because individuals express a preference for avoidance, they are less likely to engage in adaptive strategies for coping such as the derivation of social support, which conversely can buffer the effects of racism on sexual risk (Jaspal, 2018a).

While these studies all focus on HIV prevention, their findings may also be transferable to gay men living with HIV who may transmit the virus to others. Bogart, Landrine, Galvan, Wagner, and Klein (2013) studied HIV outcomes among 181 Black and 167 Latino gay and bisexual men living with HIV in the US and showed that perceived discrimination was associated with poor HIV outcomes. More specifically, Black respondents who perceived greater racial discrimination were less likely to have a high CD4 cell count and an undetectable viral load and were more likely to have visited an emergency department in the last six months. Among both Black and Latino participants, high levels of perceived discrimination due to ethnicity, sexual orientation and HIV status were associated with AIDS symptomatology. In view of the evidence showing that discrimination is associated with condomless sex, it is possible that these stressors could lead to increased HIV transmission risk.

Homophobia

Like racism, the experience of homophobia from within both one's ethno-religious group and from the general population is also associated with decreased self-esteem, which in turn is related to sexual risk-taking (Thomas, Mience, Masson, & Bernoussi, 2014).

Fear of involuntary disclosure of their sexual identity, which could in turn induce threats to belongingess, self-esteem and continuity, may lead some BAME gay men to focus principally on concealing their sexual identity from significant others. In the process, BAME gay men may be more concerned with protecting their identity than their sexual health (e.g. Jaspal & Williamson, 2017). For some individuals, the aim is to have sex covertly and, thus, condoms and other precautionary measures are frequently overlooked in the process. Furthermore, as outlined above, long-term exposure to multiple forms of discrimination may take its toll on self-esteem, leading some BAME gay men to develop both internalised homophobia and a long-standing self-deprecation due to their sexual orientation.

In their study of the correlates of sexual risk-taking among US-born and foreign-born Latino gay men in the US, Mizuno, Borkowf, Ayala, Carballo-Diéguez, and Millett (2015) found that neither homophobia nor racism was independently associated with sexual risk-taking behaviour. However, when they co-occurred among foreign-born gay men only, this was positively associated with risk-taking behaviour in this population. Although the authors did not clarify the possible reasons for the association of discrimination and sexual risk in foreign-born men specifically, it could be speculated that foreign-born gay men possess fewer social and psychological resources, such as access to social support, for coping effectively with discrimination. This may lead to less effective and potentially maladaptive coping strategies, such as engagement in sexual risk behaviours.

In their study of 1154 Black gay men in the US, Jeffries, Marks, Lauby, Murrill, and Millett (2013) found that verbal homophobia (i.e. being called names) was associated with increased odds of sexual risk behaviour in undiagnosed gay men, while all forms of homophobia were related to increased odds of HIV transmission behaviour in HIV-diagnosed individuals. They argue that possible exposure to HIV stigma may disempower Black gay men who face homophobia and lead to the adoption of maladaptive coping strategies, such as sexual risk/transmission behaviour. The authors also found that social integration failed to buffer the effects of homophobia, which they attributed to the *nature* of homophobia faced by individuals in this population. More specifically, homophobia often originates from family members, close relatives and members of the church, who have formally been construed as a reliable source of social support in relation to other issues. It may be more psychologically threatening than homophobia from less significant others, such as the general population, and lead to internalised homophobia.

Internalised homophobia, that is, the individual's acceptance and internalisation of stigma in relation to their sexual orientation (Herek, Gillis, & Cogan, 2009), and the ensuing threat to self-esteem that acknowledgement of one's sexual orientation can induce may also lead to barriers to engagement with sexual health services. As a consequence, some BAME gay men will not receive an early HIV diagnosis, potentially undermining disease prognosis. Internalised homophobia may inhibit the assimilation and accommodation of a gay identity, and consequently some BAME gay men may continue to view themselves as exclusively heterosexual and, thus, as ineligible for sexual health screening. It has been observed that individuals tend to 'other' risk, that is, they attribute it to people 'unlike themselves' (Joffe, 2007). Accordingly, sexual health screening may be viewed as relevant to 'others' and irrelevant to oneself.

Furthermore, given the association of sexual health screening with homosexuality and the fluidity of sexual identity among some BAME gay men—some transiently self-identify as 'straight'—engagement with sexual health services may represent a threat to their sense of continuity. This may represent a 'rupture' in the self-narrative that has been constructed over time. It may compel the individual to acknowledge an aspect of their identity and behaviour that they wish to deny. Moreover, some BAME gay men have expressed fear of being seen (especially by other ethno-religious ingroup members) in a sexual health clinic (Jaspal, 2018b; McKeown et al., 2012). This could represent a threat not only to individual continuity, given the acknowledgement of sexual identity, but also to the continuity of their 'public' identity as heterosexual, that is, the self-image that they wish to display to others. Consequently, they may disengage from sexual health services.

In order to conceal their sexual identities, some BAME gay men report seeking sexual partners on mobile social networking applications, such as

Grindr, where they can remain anonymous. Similarly, they may express a preference for using gay saunas for the same purpose, given that there is less risk of non-voluntary disclosure of their sexual orientation to others (Jaspal, 2020). Some BAME gay men avoid gay bars and nightclubs because of perceived racism in these venues. This can essentially deprive them of access to social representations that can facilitate awareness and understanding of HIV and prevention methods.

Overview

In this chapter, the notion of intersecting identities and its impact on HIV have been explored through the case study of BAME gay men. For many in this population, their ethnic and religious identities are important but can be construed as incompatible with their sexual identity. This in turn can produce psychological distress as they struggle to reconcile these identities. Moreover, they may be motivated to engage in behaviours that put them at risk of HIV. The Health Adversity Risk Model, which was described in the previous chapter, provides some insight into the psychological mechanisms of this process. Focusing on BAME gay men, who are at high risk of HIV, it has been shown that the stressors of homophobia, racism and decreased belongingness can lead them to engage in risk behaviours and, potentially, to disengage from sexual health services. It is important to understand the total identity of the individual in order to optimise their prevention and care outcomes. Finally, it is noteworthy that, although this chapter focuses on BAME gay men as a case study, many of the observations may be transferable to other identity configurations, that is, other identities in combination. Future research should examine how these other identity configurations may impact on HIV risk. For instance, the intersection of social class and sexual orientation is an important and fruitful area to consider, especially as those of lower socio-economic status appear to be disproportionately impacted by poor sexual health. Gay men constitute an extremely diverse group—this diversity must be studied, and both the challenges and opportunities for HIV, which are associated with this diversity, must be understood.

References

Abizadeh, A. (2001). Ethnicity, race, and a possible humanity. *World Order, 33*(1), 23–34.

Ayala, G., Bingham, T., Kim, J., Wheeler, D. P., & Millett, G. A. (2012). Modeling the impact of social discrimination and financial hardship on the sexual risk of HIV among Latino and Black men who have sex with men. *American Journal of Public Health, 102*(Suppl 2), S242–S249. https://doi.org/10.2105/AJPH.2011.300641

Bayley, J., Williams, A., & Singh, S. (2017). Dramatic reductions in new HIV diagnoses for MSM in England are not uniform for all ethnicities in a large London clinic. *Sexually Transmitted Infections, 93*(S1), A43. 10.1136/sextrans-2017-053232.125.

Bogart, L. M., Landrine, H., Galvan, F. H., Wagner, G. J., & Klein, D. J. (2013). Perceived discrimination and physical health among HIV-positive Black and Latino men who have sex with men. *AIDS and Behavior, 17*(4), 1431–1441.

Bogart, L. M., Wagner, G. J., Galvan, F. H., Landrine, H., Klein, D. J., & Sticklor, L. A. (2011). Perceived discrimination and mental health symptoms among Black men with HIV. *Cultural Diversity & Ethnic Minority Psychology, 17*(3), 295–302.

Breakwell, G. M. (1986). *Coping with threatened identities*. London: Methuen.

Breakwell, G. M. (2014). Identity and social representations. In R. Jaspal & G. M. Breakwell (Eds.), *Identity process theory: Identity, social action and social change* (pp. 118–134). Cambridge: Cambridge University Press.

Carlson, D. (1997). Gayness, multicultural education and community. In M. S. Seller & L. Weis (Eds.), *Beyond black and white* (pp. 233–256). Albany, NY: State University of New York Press.

Choi, K. H., Han, C. S., Paul, J., & Ayala, G. (2011). Strategies for managing racism and homophobia among U.S. ethnic and racial minority men who have sex with men. *AIDS Education and Prevention: Official Publication of the International Society for AIDS Education, 23*(2), 145–158.

Coyle, A., & Rafalin, D. (2000). Jewish gay men's accounts of negotiating cultural, religious and sexual identity: A qualitative study. *Journal of Psychology and Human Sexuality, 12*, 21–48.

Fish, J., Papaloukas, P., Jaspal, R., & Williamson, I. (2016). Equality in sexual health promotion: A systematic review of effective interventions for black and minority ethnic men who have sex with men. *BMC Public Health, 16*, 810.

Han, C. S. (2008). A qualitative exploration of the relationship between racism and unsafe sex among Asian Pacific Islander gay men. *Archives of Sexual Behavior, 37*(5), 827–837.

Han, C. S., Ayala, G., Paul, J. P., Boylan, R., Gregorich, S. E., & Choi, K. H. (2015). Stress and coping with racism and their role in sexual risk for HIV among African American, Asian/Pacific Islander, and Latino men who have sex with men. *Archives of Sexual Behavior, 44*(2), 411–420.

Herek, G. M. J., Gillis, R., & Cogan, J. C. (2009). Internalized stigma among sexual minority adults: Insights from a social psychological perspective. *Journal of Counseling Psychology, 56*, 32–43.

Holt, M. (2011). Gay men and ambivalence about 'gay community': From gay community attachment to personal communities. *Culture, Health & Sexuality, 13*(8), 857–871.

Jaspal, R. (2012a). "I never faced up to being gay": Sexual, religious and ethnic identities among British South Asian gay men. *Culture, Health and Sexuality: An International Journal for Research, Intervention and Care, 14*(7), 767–780.

Jaspal, R. (2012b). Coping with religious and cultural homophobia: Emotion and narratives of identity threat from British Muslim gay men. In P. Nynäs & A. K. T. Yip (Eds.), *Religion, gender and sexuality in everyday life* (pp. 71–90). Farnham: Ashgate.

Jaspal, R. (2014a). Arranged marriage, identity and psychological wellbeing among British Asian gay men. *Journal of GLBT Family Studies, 10*(5), 425–448.

Jaspal, R. (2014b). Sexuality, migration and identity among gay Iranian migrants to the UK. In Y. Taylor & R. Snowdon (Eds.), *Queering religion, religious queers* (pp. 44–60). London: Routledge.

Jaspal, R. (2017). Coping with ethnic prejudice on the gay scene: British South Asian gay men. *Journal of LGBT Youth, 14*(2), 172–190.

Jaspal, R. (2018a). *Enhancing sexual health, self-identity and wellbeing among men who have sex with men: A guide for practitioners*. London: Jessica Kingsley Publishers.

Jaspal, R. (2018b). Perceptions of HIV testing venues among men who have sex with men in London and the Midlands, United Kingdom. *Journal of Gay & Lesbian Social Services, 30*(4), 336–355.

Jaspal, R. (2019). *The social psychology of gay men*. London: Palgrave Macmillan.

Jaspal, R. (2020). Honour beliefs and identity among British South Asian gay men. In M. M. Idriss (Ed.), *Men, masculinities and honour-based abuse* (pp. 114–127). London: Routledge.

Jaspal, R., Lopes, B., & Breakwell, G. M. (2020). British national identity and life satisfaction in ethnic minority groups in the United Kingdom. *National Identities*. https://doi.org/10.1080/14608944.2020.1822793.

Jaspal, R., & Cinnirella, M. (2010). Coping with potentially incompatible identities: Accounts of religious, ethnic and sexual identities from British Pakistani men who identify as Muslim and gay. *British Journal of Social Psychology, 49*(4), 849–870.

Jaspal, R., & Cinnirella, M. (2012a). Identity processes, threat and interpersonal relations: Accounts from British Muslim gay men. *Journal of Homosexuality, 59*(2), 215–240.

Jaspal, R., & Cinnirella, M. (2012b). The construction of ethnic identity: Insights from identity process theory. *Ethnicities, 12*(5), 503–530.

Jaspal, R., & Cinnirella, M. (2013). The construction of British national identity among British South Asians. *National Identities, 15*(2), 157–175.

Jaspal, R., & Cinnirella, M. (2014). Hyper-affiliation to the religious ingroup among British Pakistani Muslim gay men. *Journal of Community and Applied Social Psychology, 24*(4), 265–277.

Jaspal, R., Fish, J., Williamson, I., & Papaloukas, P. (2016). *Public Health England black and minority ethnic men who have sex with men project evaluation report*. London: Public Health England.

Jaspal, R., Lopes, B., Jamal, Z., Paccoud, I., & Sekhon, P. (2017). Sexual abuse and HIV risk behaviour among black and minority ethnic men who have sex with men in the UK. *Mental Health, Religion & Culture, 20*(8), 841–853.

Jaspal, R., & Siraj, A. (2011). Perceptions of 'coming out' among British Muslim gay men. *Psychology and Sexuality, 2*(3), 183–197.

Jaspal, R., & Williamson, I. (2017). Identity management strategies among HIV-positive Colombian gay men in London. *Culture, Health and Sexuality: An International Journal for Research, Intervention and Care, 19*(2), 1374–1388.

Jeffries, W. L., Marks, G., Lauby, J., Murrill, C. S., & Millett, G. A. (2013). Homophobia is associated with sexual behavior that increases risk of acquiring and transmitting HIV infection among black men who have sex with men. *AIDS and Behavior, 17*(4), 1442–1453.

Joffe, H. (2007). Identity, self-control, and risk. In G. Moloney & I. Walker (Eds.), *Social representations and identity* (pp. 197–213). London: Palgrave Macmillan.

Kelley, H. H. (1967). Attribution theory in social psychology. In D. Levine (Ed.), *Nebraska Symposium on motivation* (Vol. 15, pp. 192–238). Lincoln: University of Nebraska Press.

Kugle, S. S. H. (2010). *Homosexuality in Islam: Critical reflection on gay, lesbian, and transgender muslims.* Oxford: Oneworld Publications.

Lasala, M. C. (2000). Gay male couples: The importance of coming out and being out to parents. *Journal of Homosexuality, 39*(2), 47–71.

Maatouk, I., & Jaspal, R. (2019). HIV in men who have sex with men in Lebanon: Clinical & psychosocial aspects. *BMJ Journal of Sexual & Reproductive Health, 45*(3), 175–176.

Maatouk, I., & Jaspal, R. (2020). Religion, male bisexuality and sexual health in Lebanon. In A.K.T. Yip & A. Toft (eds.), *Bisexuality, Spirituality and Identity: Critical Perspectives* (pp. 137–155). London: Routledge.

McKeown, E., Doerner, R., Nelson, S., Low, N., Robinson, A., Anderson, J., … Elford, J. (2012). The experiences of ethnic minority MSM using NHS sexual health clinics in Britain. *Sexually Transmitted Infections, 88*(8), 595–600.

Millett, G. A., Peterson, J. L., Flores, S. A., Hart, T. A., Jeffries, W. L., Wilson, P. A., … Remis, R. S. (2012). Comparisons of disparities and risks of HIV infection in black and other men who have sex with men in Canada, UK, and USA: A meta-analysis. *Lancet, 380*(9839), 341–348.

Mizuno, Y., Borkowf, C. B., Ayala, G., Carballo-Diéguez, A., & Millett, G. A. (2015). Correlates of sexual risk for HIV among US-born and foreign-born Latino men who have sex with men (MSM): An analysis from the Brothers y Hermanos study. *Journal of Immigrant and Minority Health, 17*(1), 47–55.

Mohammed, H., Furegato, M., & Hughes, G. (2016). P068 Inequalities in sexually transmitted infection risk among black and minority ethnic men who have sex with men in England. *Sexually Transmitted Infections, 92*, A42.

Moscovici, S. (1988). Notes towards a description of social representations. *European Journal of Social Psychology, 18*, 211–250.

Phillips, G., Birkett, M., Hammond, S., & Mustanski, B. (2016). Partner preference among men who have sex with men: Potential contribution to spread of HIV within minority populations. *LGBT Health, 3*(3), 225–232.

Public Health England. (2016). *HIV in the UK: 2016 report.* London: Public Health England. Retrieved June 2, 2020, from https://assets.publishing.service.gov.uk/government/uploads/system/uploads/attachment_data/file/602942/HIV_in_the_UK_report.pdf.

Raymond, H. F., & McFarland, W. (2009). Racial mixing and HIV risk among men who have sex with men. *AIDS and Behavior, 13*(4), 630–637.

Rosario, M., Hunter, J., Maguen, S., Gwadz, M., & Smith, R. (2001). The coming-out process and its adaptational and health-related associations among gay, lesbian, and bisexual youths: Stipulation and exploration of a model. *American Journal of Community Psychology, 29*(1), 133–160.

Soni, S., Bond, K., Fox, E., Grieve, A. P., & Sethi, G. (2008). Black and minority ethnic men who have sex with men: A London genitourinary medicine clinic experience. *International Journal of STD & AIDS, 19*(9), 617–619.

Stegmann, K., Scott, C., Jones, R., & Rayment, M. (2019). P97 Mind the gap: New diagnoses of HIV in a London clinic (2016–2018). In *Poster presented at the 25th Annual Conference of the British HIV Association (BHIVA),* Bournemouth, UK, 2–5 April 2019. Retrieved from https://onlinelibrary.wiley.com/doi/full/10.1111/hiv.12739

Stonewall. (2012). *One minority at a time: Being black and gay.* London: Stonewall. Retrieved June 2, 2020, from https://www.stonewall.org.uk/system/files/One_Minority_At_A_Time__2012_.pdf.

Tajfel, H., & Turner, J. C. (1986). The social identity theory of intergroup behaviour. In S. Worchel & W. G. Austin (Eds.), *Psychology of intergroup relations* (pp. 7–24). Chicago, IL: Nelson-Hall.

Thomas, F., Mience, M. C., Masson, J., & Bernoussi, A. (2014). Unprotected sex and internalized homophobia. *The Journal of Men's Studies, 22*(2), 155–162.

UK Census. (2011). UK population by ethnicity. Retrieved May 10, 2020, from https://www.ethnicity-facts-figures.service.gov.uk/uk-population-by-ethnicity.

United Kingdom Collaborative HIV Cohort Study Group. (2012). Uptake and outcome of combination antiretroviral therapy in men who have sex with men according to ethnic group: The UK CHIC Study. *Journal of Acquired Immune Deficiency Syndromes, 59*(5), 523–529.

Zagefka, H. (2009). The concept of ethnicity in socio-psychological research: Definitional issues. *International Journal of Intercultural Relations, 33*, 228–241.

8

Looking to the Future: Eradication by 2030?

Introduction

The primary objective of this volume was to provide insights into the clinical, social and psychological aspects of HIV—both its prevention and care—among gay men. Given that HIV is a clinical issue with significant social, psychological and behavioural underpinnings, it is clear that all of these aspects will need to be closely examined if we are to achieve the zero-infections target by 2030. It is also clear that, in order to prevent HIV, we must focus on optimising HIV care and ensuring that all people living with HIV are able to access it.

In this volume, we have discussed many distinct facets of the HIV epidemic in the UK, including its history, science and epidemiology; its biological and social and psychological risk factors; HIV diagnosis and treatment options; the mental health burden of HIV; and the role of identity in relation to HIV-related cognition and behaviour. The multitude of topics covered in this book are testimony to the complexity of HIV—both its prevention and treatment. The impact of gay history on the sexual behaviour of gay men may not seem immediately obvious to the outside observer. Yet, our analysis demonstrates that a history

© The Author(s) 2020
R. Jaspal, J. Bayley, *HIV and Gay Men*, https://doi.org/10.1007/978-981-15-7226-5_8

characterised by prejudice, rejection and identity concealment has clear implications for how gay men think about their identity and express it in the heteronormative contexts that they inhabit. Furthermore, the short-sighted attempt to manage HIV by silencing the voices of young gay adolescents, with the damaging Section 28 legislation, probably had counter-productive effects on the epidemic in the UK.

It is essential to learn from these historical lessons and to ensure that the potential future implications of today's policy remain at the forefront of our thinking and serve to reduce health inequalities. Only a serious consideration of all these issues will enable us to achieve the ambitious zero-infections target by 2030.

A key aim of this volume was to address three specific questions which were posed in the introduction:

- What are the major clinical and social psychological challenges associated with HIV risk, prevention and treatment among gay men?
- How can theoretical, empirical and methodological tools from the clinical and social psychological sciences be bridged in order to address some of these challenges?
- What are the next steps for HIV research, theory and practice among gay men?

This is not the type of book in which neat conclusions can be drawn in relation to these questions. However, the discussion that has unfolded in this volume does highlight the key debates that we should be having in order to realise the zero-infections target by 2030. It elucidates the gaps in our knowledge, in policy and in practice, which may curtail our ability to prevent HIV in the future. As the epidemic progresses, identifying new cases does remain a challenge—1 in 10 gay men is unaware of his diagnosis despite the best efforts of public health campaigns. More research is needed in order for us to close this gap in diagnoses. In order for this to be a well-informed debate, there are some key components that must not be overlooked by researchers, clinicians and policymakers.

The Key Components of HIV Prevention and Treatment

Our discussion of HIV in the preceding chapters suggests that the following seven factors, which are the key theoretical building blocks for understanding social psychological issues (Breakwell, 2007; Jaspal, 2019), must be considered in order to provide reliable responses to these questions.

- The *physical/biological context* includes the physiological aspects of HIV. Some sexual behaviours are riskier than others. Substance use can create both physiological and psychological conditions for HIV transmission to occur. One may fail an ART regimen requiring more intensive support. At the most basic level, one may not physically be able to access HIV prevention services. The list is not exhaustive, and there are of course many other examples of how the physical and biological context is important.
- The *socio-historical context* determines the individual and social attitudes that exist today. Gay men have acquired a sense of self on the basis of previous experiences, that is, their socio-historical context. Similarly, heterosexual people base their perceptions and understandings of HIV on the socio-historical context of the epidemic. This context must therefore be understood.
- The *'macro' level* includes societal and institutional structures, such as ideology, legislation and policy. Gay men are more likely to engage with healthcare if the institutional approach to gay men's health is characterised by acceptance and inclusion. A good example of this is the recent initiative for NHS staff to wear rainbow badges to signal that LGBT people are welcome. Furthermore, individuals can access PEP, PrEP and TasP only if health policy provides access to them. State ideology determines whether HIV should be a health priority and how it should be dealt with. All of these 'macro' level issues have significant implications for both HIV prevention and treatment.
- *Social representations* are key. As outlined in Chap. 7, these collective understandings inform how gay men think, feel and act in relation to

HIV and its prevention methods. Their level of access to particular social representations will develop in social context.

- The *intrapsychic level* must be acknowledged. This refers to the psychological aspects of HIV, such as how gay men think about themselves in relation to the epidemic, their perceived risk of infection, stigma and so on. Identity, cognition and emotion are three examples of the intrapsychic level.
- Gay men's *interpersonal relationships* matter, since relationships with other individuals and groups provide access and exposure to particular social representations and constitute a source of social support. However, particular interpersonal relationships may also expose an individual to stigma or to situations of risk. All these factors shape HIV prevention.
- Gay men's *behaviour* is at the heart of HIV prevention. Ultimately, it is behaviour that determines one's level of risk. Moreover, effective behaviour change can result in reduced risk. It is likely that all of the aforementioned factors shape behaviour, which remains a central focus of HIV research and subsequent public health campaigns.

The Importance of Combination HIV Prevention

It is evident that we now possess sophisticated clinical tools for the effective prevention of HIV, which include condom use, PEP, PrEP, TasP and other emerging methods, such as a potential vaccine against HIV. These approaches have varying degrees of efficacy and are characterised by some pitfalls, and each will be acceptable to only some gay men. For instance, while condom use is one of the most effective prevention options and has been promoted since the very beginning of the epidemic in the UK, it has not been consistently observed by all gay men. Moreover, although PrEP performs even more efficaciously than a condom, not all gay men personally endorse this method for themselves due to stigma and other issues. There are many reasons why an individual may reject one method over another and these reasons must be explored and understood. This is especially important in a clinical setting where these factors must be examined in order to ensure the best outcome for the patient. Assumptions about the acceptability of certain methods may prove to be erroneous.

Potential barriers to these prevention methods must be removed. In the meantime, it is important to refrain from favouring any single approach at the expense of another. It is short-sighted to focus only on the pitfalls of any particular method and to discard it altogether. As highlighted in this volume, this has been a recurrent theme in discussions about PrEP since it is sometimes feared that PrEP use will lead to the abandonment of condoms by all gay men. It appears that all possible prevention options must all be included within a broad and inclusive 'toolbox' of HIV prevention approaches so that the clinician (and indeed patient) can draw upon a particular method or set of methods at any given time.

Another important point is that sexual risk-taking can be in flux—some who go through periods of risk behaviour (e.g. chemsex as a consequence of recent psychological trauma) may find PrEP acceptable. If they were to settle with one partner, their acceptability of PrEP may subsequently reduce. This is why it is vital to engage with gay men in clinic (and in fact in all healthcare appointments). Their HIV prevention package should be modified accordingly. The effective engagement with communities (led by culturally competent healthcare workers) lies at the very heart of our ability to deliver excellent care to those who are at risk of HIV.

In this volume, the fundamental importance of patient-centred care has been emphasised in the battle against HIV. An adequate understanding of the patient's identity, social context and cultural norms is crucial to ensuring that patients from all backgrounds are engaged in prevention and treatment. The inextricable relationship between sexual health and HIV has been illustrated. Psychological services must complement sexual health services, and vice versa. These are just some reasons why it is essential for the adequate funding of sexual health and HIV services in the UK. Although the UK has made enormous strides in preventing HIV, resulting in a recent continued decline in new infections, there remains much work to be done, especially in some groups, such as ethnic minority gay men and those of lower socio-economic status. It would be counter-productive to deprive sexual health services of the funding required to perform adequately in order to realise the zero-infections target. The target can be achieved only if combination prevention remains a reality, not an aspiration.

Yet, at the time of writing, the UK is in the grip of a significant global challenge. The outbreak of COVID-19 precipitated a nationwide lockdown and the enforcement of social distancing (Jaspal & Nerlich, 2020). Giving the rising number of infections, hospitalisation and deaths associated with the disease, the main focus of the NHS has understandably been on the treatment of COVID-19. Clinicians from all specialties, including sexual health and HIV, have been redeployed to join the fight against COVID-19. This in turn has meant that many other services, including sexual health and HIV services, have been curtailed and that the roll-out of PrEP to those at risk of HIV has been delayed. We must ensure that sexual health and HIV does not fall off the policy agenda across the world as we deal with the aftermath of COVID-19. In fact, the COVID-19 outbreak may well provide the ideal conditions for detecting more early infections than ever before. In short, it will be vital to continue to work collaboratively with HIV charities and activists in order to promote sustainable change in relation to HIV prevention.

Consistent with the social distancing measures, gay men have been strongly advised to avoid meeting casual partners for sex—advice that has been reiterated on gay mobile social networking applications, such as Grindr. However, the extent to which gay men adhere to this policy is unclear. Therefore, it is possible, but not yet known with certainty, that the unprecedented public health emergency of COVID-19 may translate into poorer HIV and sexual health outcomes in gay men. There may also be an accentuation of poor mental health, especially in vulnerable groups, as a result of the outbreak (Lopes & Jaspal, 2020). The closure of 'non-essential' sexual health services may have a deleterious effect on health and wellbeing, and will need to be closely monitored. Furthermore, there are broader questions about the future of HIV prevention and care in the UK. There is of course much uncertainty about the economic, social and political landscape that awaits us after the COVID-19 pandemic. Will the economic challenges ahead lead to decreased funding for sexual health services? Will funding for all communicable diseases be increased in the future? How will any possible austerity measures impact on HIV incidence among gay men? What will this mean for the zero-infections target?

The Future of HIV Prevention

Notwithstanding the unsettling challenges posed by COVID-19, each chapter in this volume highlights the tremendous advances made in HIV prevention and care over the last four decades. Collectively, these steps have resulted in a significant reduction in HIV incidence in gay men which continues to fall each year. The UN 90-90-90 target has of course already been achieved in the UK. Yet, the assessment of performance in relation to HIV depends on the measure that it used. Psychological wellbeing is a recurrent theme in this volume. The available evidence suggests that gay men face challenges to psychological wellbeing, which can lead to increased risk-taking, and that those living with HIV also face poor psychological health outcomes. Yet, psychological wellbeing and living free of side effects of ART and of HIV stigma are not currently one of the measures in the 90-90-90 target. They should be.

The goal of HIV medicine has traditionally focused on the physical health of those at risk of, or living with, HIV. In the case of HIV prevention, the focus has been on keeping people HIV-negative, and in the context of HIV care, the principal aim has been to get people undetectable and to keep them physically well. Psychological health is inextricably entwined with both risk and wellness—those who are not psychologically well are more likely to take risks and to experience poorer physical health outcomes. Although over 90% of people living with HIV have received a diagnosis, are on ART and are undetectable, it is unlikely that the same proportion of individuals experience a high level of psychological wellbeing. Indeed, much of the existing evidence on psychological wellbeing among gay men living with HIV suggests a very high prevalence of anxiety, depression and other forms of psychological adversity. Although a 'fourth 90' focusing on quality of life has been discussed, a specific emphasis on psychological wellbeing (which does indeed encompass quality of life) would be fruitful for future research, policy and practice.

This should also be formally included in the UNAIDS targets (see also Jaspal & Lopes, 2020).

Both effective HIV care and HIV prevention are important in their own right. They are also are inextricably entwined. If a person living with HIV is not engaging with care, they will not be able to achieve viral suppression through the use of ART and may therefore transmit HIV to others. If a person is experiencing poor quality of care, they are more likely to disengage or to interrupt ART, yielding the same risks for onward transmission. In this volume, a series of clinical and social psychological barriers to effective care and prevention have been described. These include lack of HIV knowledge, inaccurate risk appraisal, actual and anticipated side effects, stigma and many others. Moreover, it is clear that not all of these barriers affect all groups in society in quite the same way. In Chap. 7, the impact of ethnicity and culture on both HIV prevention and care were explored. Individuals from ethnic and religious minority groups also appear to be at disproportionately high risk of poor outcomes than the general population. Thus, it is necessary to ensure that our approach to prevention and care is underpinned by cultural competence, identity awareness and robust evidence.

It is evident that a variety of disciplines have contributed to HIV research evidence. While clinical scientists focus on the physiological aspects of HIV, its treatment and prevention, social scientists are grappling with empirical questions concerning human behaviour. Both are essential for the zero-infections target. The future of prevention and treatments for HIV is an exhilarating story that is now turning to the prospect of two- or three-monthly injectable medication and sub-dermal implants negating the use of daily pills and dramatically improving adherence to medication. These methods should also be just as effective for prevention with the tantalising prospect of protection lasting months with ART administered in this fashion. A 'functional cure' whereby people remain undetectable without the use of drugs is also an exciting chapter in the story of HIV—researchers are eagerly trying to unlock this puzzle which would have life-changing results for millions of people.

The research outlined in this volume has been driven by many theoretical approaches—some focusing on the individual, others on societal and institutional structures. The research studies have been underpinned by a multitude of methodological approaches, including randomised control trials, phylogenetics, behavioural experiments, surveys, qualitative interviews, media analyses and others. Moreover, the data generated by this research have been analysed using a similarly diverse range of methods, including structural equation modelling, multi-level modelling, interpretative phenomenological analysis and discourse analysis. In order to provide nuanced analyses of the seven aforementioned dimensions of HIV, it will be necessary to use the full plethora of methods of data generation and analysis at our disposal (see Breakwell, Wright, & Barnett, 2020). Our repertoire of theories and methods grows as we bridge disciplinary approaches, as we have attempted to do in this volume. It is hoped that future research into HIV will be theoretically, methodologically and analytically eclectic.

At the beginning of this volume, two case studies were illustrated, which explored various social psychological issues peripherally related to HIV risk. Throughout the chapters of this volume, it has been shown how these issues—body image, sense of community, friendship, the digital world of gay dating, identity and culture—may impinge on HIV risk. Clearly, more social psychological opportunities and challenges will emerge in the future. In order to achieve the zero-infections target, these must be continually monitored and addressed in the research questions we pose in the future.

Future research into HIV among gay men must focus on those groups in society in which there remain significant barriers to effective HIV prevention and care. There are significant lacunae in our knowledge about the HIV prevention and care needs of some subgroups of gay men, such as those who do not consistently self-identify as gay but have sex with men, gay men from ethnic and religious minority communities, and those with poor mental health. Although individuals in these subgroups are often deemed to be 'hard-to-reach', it is necessary to use the full plethora of tools available to us to attempt to reach and to engage them in research. It has unfortunately been shown that their rates of participation in research appear to be lower than other groups, which means that their specific needs may not be captured in the data that this research generates.

Final Thoughts

There is much to be gained from bridging clinical medicine and social psychology in the context of HIV prevention. This volume is an attempt to do just that. There must be a reciprocal relationship between these fields of study but also between key communities in the area of HIV prevention among gay men—researchers, practitioners, policymakers and, of course, gay men themselves. By working in partnership, using clinical practice to establish research questions and drawing on that research to inform clinical practice, we will be better positioned to achieve the ambitious goal of ending all HIV transmissions by 2030. We will need to use the lessons learned from history to shape our future. We will need to think creatively and to take some risks to reduce risk. This is a goal worth pursuing since the end of HIV is clearly in sight.

References

Breakwell, G. M. (2007). *The psychology of risk*. Cambridge: Cambridge University Press.

Breakwell, G. M., Wright, D., & Barnett, J. (2020). *Research methods in psychology* (5th ed.). London: SAGE.

Jaspal, R. (2019). *The social psychology of gay men*. London: Palgrave Macmillan.

Jaspal, R., & Lopes, B. (2020). Psychological wellbeing facilitates accurate HIV risk appraisal in gay and bisexual men. *Sexual Health, 17*(3), 288–295.

Jaspal, R., & Nerlich, B. (2020). Social representations, identity threat and coping amid COVID-19. *Psychological Trauma: Theory, Research, Practice and Policy, 2*(S1), S249–S251.

Lopes, B., & Jaspal, R. (2020). Understanding the mental health burden of COVID-19 in the United Kingdom. *Psychological Trauma: Theory, Research, Practice and Policy, 12*(5), 465–467.

Acronyms

AIDS	acquired immune deficiency syndrome
ART	antiretroviral therapy
ARV	antiretroviral
AZT	zidovudine
BAME	Black, Asian and Minority Ethnic
BBC	British Broadcasting Corporation
BHIVA	British HIV Association
CDC	Center for Disease Control and Prevention
CMV	cytomegalovirus
COVID-19	coronavirus disease 2019
d4T	stavudine
ddI	didanosine
DNA	deoxyribonucleic acid
FDA	Food and Drug Administration
FLV	feline leukaemia virus
GBL	gamma butyrolactone
GHB	gamma hydroxybutyrate
GPA	Global Program for AIDS
HBV	hepatitis B

HCV	hepatitis C
HIV	human immunodeficiency virus
HLA	human leucocyte antigens
HPV	human papillomavirus
HSV	herpes simplex virus
HTLV	human T-lymphotropic virus
IBD	inflammatory bowel disease
INSTI	integrases
ITV	Independent Television
LAV	lymphadenopathy associated virus
LGB	lesbian, gay and bisexual
LGBT	lesbian, gay, bisexual and transgender
LGV	lymphogranuloma venereum
MSM	men who have sex with men
NHS	National Health Service
NNRTI	non-nucleoside reverse transcriptase inhibitor
NRTI	nucleoside reverse transcriptase inhibitor
PCP	pneumocystis pneumonia
PEP	post-exposure prophylaxis
PI	protease inhibitors
PJP	pneumocystis jiroveci pneumonia
PML	progressive multifocal leucoencephalopathy
PrEP	pre-exposure prophylaxis
RNA	ribonucleic acid
RT	reverse transcriptase
SIV	simian immunodeficiency virus
STI	sexually transmitted infection
TasP	treatment as prevention
TB	tuberculosis
U=U	undetectable equals untransmittable
UK	United Kingdom
UN	United Nations
UNAIDS	The Joint United Nations Programme on HIV/AIDS
US	United States

References

Abdool Karim, Q., Abdool Karim, S. S., Frohlich, J. A., Grobler, A. C., Baxter, C., Mansoor, L. E., … CAPRISA 004 Trial Group. (2010). Effectiveness and safety of tenofovir gel, an antiretroviral microbicide, for the prevention of HIV infection in women. *Science, 329*(5996), 1168–1174.

Abizadeh, A. (2001). Ethnicity, race, and a possible humanity. *World Order, 33*(1), 23–34.

Acheson, E. D. (1986). AIDS: A challenge for public health. *Public Health, 327*(8482), P662–P666.

Ahmedani, B. K., Peterson, E. L., Hu, Y., Rossom, R. C., Lynch, F., Lu, C. Y., … Simon, G. E. (2017). Major physical health conditions and risk of suicide. *American Journal of Preventive Medicine, 53*(3), 308–315.

Ajzen, I. (1991). The theory of planned behavior. *Organizational Behavior and Human Decision Processes, 50*(2), 179–211.

Al-Ajlouni, Y. A., Park, S. H., Schneider, J. A., Goedel, W. C., Rhodes Hambrick, H., Hickson, D. A., … Duncan, D. T. (2018). Partner meeting venue typology and sexual risk behaviors among French men who have sex with men. *International Journal of STD & AIDS, 29*(13), 1282–1288.

Auvert, B., Taljaard, D., Lagarde, E., Sobngwi-Tambekou, J., Sitta, R., & Puren, A. (2005). Randomized, controlled intervention trial of male circumcision for reduction of HIV infection risk: The ANRS 1265 Trial. *PLoS Medicine, 2*(11), e298. https://doi.org/10.1371/journal.pmed.0020298

Ayala, G., Bingham, T., Kim, J., Wheeler, D. P., & Millett, G. A. (2012). Modeling the impact of social discrimination and financial hardship on the sexual risk of HIV among Latino and Black men who have sex with men. *American Journal of Public Health, 102*(Suppl 2), S242–S249. https://doi.org/10.2105/AJPH.2011.300641

Babowitch, J. D., Mitzel, L. D., Vanable, P. A., & Sweeney, S. M. (2018). Depressive symptoms and condomless sex among men who have sex with men living with HIV: A curvilinear association. *Archives of Sexual Behavior, 47*(7), 2035–2040.

Baggaley, R. F., White, R. G., & Boily, M. C. (2008). Systematic review of orogenital HIV-1 transmission probabilities. *International Journal of Epidemiology, 37*(6), 1255–1265.

Bailey, R. C., Moses, S., Parker, C. B., Agot, K., Maclean, I., & Krieger, J. N. ... Ndinya-Achola, J. O. (2007). Male circumcision for HIV prevention in young men in Kisumu, Kenya: A randomised controlled trial. *Lancet, 369*(9562), 643–656.

Bancroft, J., Janssen, E., Strong, D., Carnes, L. C., Vukadinovic, Z., & Long, J. S. (2003). The relationship between mood and sexuality in heterosexual men. *Archives of Sexual Behavior, 32*, 217–230.

Bandura, A. (1997). *Self-efficacy: The exercise of control.* New York: W. H. Freeman.

Bardi, A., Jaspal, R., Polek, E., & Schwartz, S. (2014). Values and IPT: Theoretical integration and empirical interactions. In R. Jaspal & G. M. Breakwell (Eds.), *Identity process theory: Identity, social action and social change* (pp. 175–200). Cambridge: Cambridge University Press.

Baron, S., Poast, J., & Cloyd, M. W. (1999). Why is HIV rarely transmitted by oral secretions? Saliva can disrupt orally shed, infected leukocytes. *Archives of Internal Medicine, 159*(3), 303–310.

Barre-Sinoussi, F., Chermann, J. C., Rey, F., Nugeyre, M. T., Chamaret, S., Gruest, J., ... Montagnier, L. (1983). Isolation of a T-lymphotropic retrovirus from a patient at risk for acquired immune deficiency syndrome (AIDS). *Science, 220*(4599), 868–871.

Baumeister, R. F., & Leary, M. R. (1995). The need to belong: Desire for interpersonal attachments as a fundamental human motivation. *Psychological Bulletin, 117*(3), 497–529.

Bayley, J., Williams, A., & Singh, S. (2017). Dramatic reductions in new HIV diagnoses for MSM in England are not uniform for all ethnicities in a large London clinic. *Sexually Transmitted Infections, 93*(S1), A43. https://doi.org/10.1136/sextrans-2017-053232.125

Belshaw, R., Pereira, V., Katzourakis, A., Talbot, G., Pačes, J., Burt, A., & Tristem, M. (2004). Long-term reinfection of the human genome by endogenous retroviruses. *Proceedings of the National Academy of Sciences, 101*(14), 4894–4899.

Beltrami, E. M., Luo, C.-C., de la Torre, N., & Cardo, D. M. (2002). Transmission of drug-resistant HIV after an occupational exposure despite postexposure prophylaxis with a combination drug regimen. *Infection Control and Hospital Epidemiology, 23*(6), 345–348.

Benn, P., Fisher, M., Kulasegaram, R., & BASHH, & PEPSE Guidelines Writing Group Clinical Effectiveness Group. (2011). UK guideline for the use of post-exposure prophylaxis for HIV following sexual exposure (2011). *International Journal of STD & AIDS, 22*(12), 695–708.

Berg, R. C., Tikkanen, R., & Ross, M. W. (2013). Barebacking among men who have sex with men recruited through a Swedish website: Associations with sexual activities at last sexual encounter. *Eurosurveillance, 18*(13), pii=20438. https://doi.org/10.2807/ese.18.13.20438-en

Bérubé, A. (1996). The history of gay bathhouses. *Journal of Homosexuality, 44*(3), 33–53.

Bhatia, R., Hartman, C., Kallen, M. A., Graham, J., & Giordano, T. P. (2011). Persons newly diagnosed with HIV infection are at high risk for depression and poor linkage to care: Results from the Steps Study. *AIDS and Behavior, 15*(6), 1161–1170.

Biancotto, A., Iglehart, S. J., Vanpouille, C., Condack, C. E., Lisco, A., Ruecker, E., … Grivel, J.-C. (2008). HIV-1 induced activation of CD4+ T cells creates new targets for HIV-1 infection in human lymphoid tissue ex vivo. *Blood, 111*(2), 699–704.

Binson, D., Pollack, L. M., Blair, J., & Woods, W. J. (2010). HIV transmission risk at a gay bathhouse. *Journal of Sex Research, 47*(6), 580–588.

Binson, D., Woods, W. J., Pollack, L., Paul, J., Stall, R., & Catania, J. A. (2001). Differential HIV risk in bathhouses and public cruising areas. *American Journal of Public Health, 91*(9), 1482–1486.

Blackwell, C., & Birnholtz, J. (2015). Seeing and being seen: Co-situation and impression formation using Grindr, a location-aware gay dating app. *New Media & Society, 17*(7), 1117–1136.

Blashill, A. J., Gordon, J. R., & Safren, S. A. (2012). Appearance concerns and psychological distress among HIV-infected individuals with injection drug use histories: prospective analyses. *AIDS Patient Care and STDs, 26*(9), 557–561. https://doi.org/10.1089/apc.2012.0122

Blashill, A. J., Gordon, J. R., & Safren, S. A. (2014). Depression longitudinally mediates the association of appearance concerns to ART non-adherence in HIV-infected individuals with a history of injection drug use. *Journal of Behavioral Medicine, 37*(1), 166–172.

Blashill, A. J., & Vander Wal, J. S. (2010). Gender role conflict as a mediator between social sensitivity and depression in a sample of gay men. *International Journal of Men's Health, 9*(1), 26–39.

Bogart, L. M., Landrine, H., Galvan, F. H., Wagner, G. J., & Klein, D. J. (2013). Perceived discrimination and physical health among HIV-positive Black and Latino men who have sex with men. *AIDS and Behavior, 17*(4), 1431–1441.

Bogart, L. M., Wagner, G. J., Galvan, F. H., Landrine, H., Klein, D. J., & Sticklor, L. A. (2011). Perceived discrimination and mental health symptoms among Black men with HIV. *Cultural Diversity & Ethnic Minority Psychology, 17*(3), 295–302.

Bond, K. T., Frye, V., Taylor, R., Williams, K., Bonner, S., Lucy, D., … Straight Talk Study Team. (2015). Knowing is not enough: A qualitative report on HIV testing among heterosexual African-American men. *AIDS Care, 27*(2), 182–188.

Bonn, D. (2003). Chimp SIV could come from monkeys. *The Lancet Infectious Diseases, 3*(8), 457.

Bourne, A., Reid, D., Hickson, F., Torres Rueda, S., & Weatherburn, P. (2014). *The Chemsex study: Drug use in sexual settings among gay & bisexual men in Lambeth, Southwark & Lewisham.* London: Sigma Research, London School of Hygiene & Tropical Medicine. Retrieved June 2, 2020, from https://www.lambeth.gov.uk/sites/default/files/ssh-chemsex-study-final-main-report.pdf.

Bragança, M., & Palha, A. (2011). Depression and neurocognitive performance in Portuguese patients infected with HIV. *AIDS and Behavior, 15*(8), 1879–1887.

Brandt, C., Zvolensky, M. J., Woods, S. P., Gonzalez, A., Safren, S. A., & O'Cleirigh, C. M. (2017). Anxiety symptoms and disorders among adults living with HIV and AIDS: A critical review and integrative synthesis of the empirical literature. *Clinical Psychology Review, 51*, 164–184.

Brandt, C. P., Gonzalez, A., Grover, K. W., & Zvolensky, M. J. (2013). The relation between emotional dysregulation and anxiety and depressive symptoms, pain-related anxiety, and HIV-symptom distress among adults with HIV/AIDS. *Journal of Psychopathology and Behavioral Assessment, 35*(2), 197–204.

Braunstein, J. W. (2004). An investigation of irrational beliefs and death anxiety as a function of HIV status. *Journal of Rational-Emotive & Cognitive-Behavior Therapy, 22*(1), 21–38.

Breakwell, G. M. (1986). *Coping with threatened identities*. London: Methuen.

Breakwell, G. M. (2007). *The psychology of risk*. Cambridge: Cambridge University Press.

Breakwell, G. M. (2014). Identity and social representations. In R. Jaspal & G. M. Breakwell (Eds.), *Identity process theory: Identity, social action and social change* (pp. 118–134). Cambridge: Cambridge University Press.

Breakwell, G. M., Wright, D., & Barnett, J. (2020). *Research methods in psychology* (5th ed.). London: SAGE.

Breet, E., Kagee, A., & Seedat, S. (2014). HIV-related stigma and symptoms of post-traumatic stress disorder and depression in HIV-infected individuals: Does social support play a mediating or moderating role? *AIDS Care, 26*(8), 947–951.

Brooks, R. A., Nieto, O., Landrian, A., & Donohoe, T. J. (2019). Persistent stigmatizing and negative perceptions of pre-exposure prophylaxis (PrEP) users: Implications for PrEP adoption among Latino men who have sex with men. *AIDS Care, 31*(4), 427–435.

Broun, S. N. (1998). Understanding "post-AIDS survivor syndrome": A record of personal experiences. *AIDS Patient Care and STDs, 12*(6), 481–488.

Bruner, K. M., Murray, A. J., Pollack, R. A., Soliman, M. G., Laskey, S. B., Capoferri, A. A., … Siliciano, R. F. (2016). Defective proviruses rapidly accumulate during acute HIV-1 infection. *Nature Medicine, 22*(9), 1043–1049.

Bruner, K. M., Wang, Z., Simonetti, F. R., Bender, A. M., Kwon, K. J., Sengupta, S., … Siliciano, R. F. (2019). A quantitative approach for measuring the reservoir of latent HIV-1 proviruses. *Nature, 566*(7742), 120–125.

Buchbinder, S. P., Mehrotra, D. V., Duerr, A., Fitzgerald, D. W., Mogg, R., Li, D., … Step Study Protocol Team. (2008). Efficacy assessment of a cell-mediated immunity HIV-1 vaccine (the Step Study): A double-blind, randomised, placebo-controlled, test-of-concept trial. *Lancet, 372*(9653), 1881–1893.

Cahn, P., Madero, J. S., Arribas, J. R., Antinori, A., Ortiz, R., Clarke, A. E., … Ustianowski, A. (2019). Dolutegravir plus lamivudine versus dolutegravir plus tenofovir disoproxil fumarate and emtricitabine in antiretroviral-naive adults with HIV-1 infection (GEMINI-1 and GEMINI-2): Week 48 results from two multicentre, double-blind, randomised, non-inferiority, phase 3 trials. *The Lancet, 393*(10167), 143–155.

Cameron, D. W., Simonsen, J. N., D'Costa, L. J., Ronald, A. R., Maitha, G. M., Gakinya, M. N., … Brunham, R. C. (1989). Female to male transmission of human immunodeficiency virus type 1: Risk factors for sero-conversion in men. *Lancet, 2*(8660), 403–407.

Cannon, M. J., Schmid, D. S., & Hyde, T. B. (2010). Review of cytomegalovirus seroprevalence and demographic characteristics associated with infection. *Reviews in Medical Virology, 20*(4), 202–213.

Cao, K., Hollenbach, J., Shi, X., Shi, W., Chopek, M., & Fernández-Viña, M. A. (2001). Analysis of the frequencies of HLA-A, B, and C alleles and haplotypes in the five major ethnic groups of the United States reveals high levels of diversity in these loci and contrasting distribution patterns in these populations. *Human Immunology, 62*(9), 1009–1030.

Carballo-Diéguez, A., Balán, I. C., Brown, W., Giguere, R., Dolezal, C., Leu, C.-S., … Cranston, R. D. (2017). High levels of adherence to a rectal microbicide gel and to oral Pre-Exposure Prophylaxis (PrEP) achieved in MTN-017 among men who have sex with men (MSM) and transgender women. *PloS One, 12*(7), e0181607. https://doi.org/10.1371/journal.pone.0181607

Cardo, D. M., Culver, D. H., Ciesielski, C. A., Srivastava, P. U., Marcus, R., Abiteboul, D., … Bell, D. M. (1997). A case-control study of HIV seroconversion in health care workers after percutaneous exposure. Centers for Disease Control and Prevention Needlestick Surveillance Group. *The New England Journal of Medicine, 337*(21), 1485–1490.

Carlson, D. (1997). Gayness, multicultural education and community. In M. S. Seller & L. Weis (Eds.), *Beyond black and white* (pp. 233–256). Albany, NY: State University of New York Press.

Carrico, A. W. (2010). Elevated suicide rate among HIV-positive persons despite benefits of antiretroviral therapy: Implications for a stress and coping model of suicide. *The American Journal of Psychiatry, 167*(2), 117–119. https://doi.org/10.1176/appi.ajp.2009.09111565

Carrico, A. W., Neilands, T. B., & Johnson, M. O. (2010). Suicidal ideation is associated with HIV transmission risk in men who have sex with men. *Journal of Acquired Immune Deficiency Syndromes, 54*(4), e3–e4. https://doi.org/10.1097/QAI.0b013e3181da1270

Carrieri, M. P., Marcellin, F., Fressard, L., Préau, M., Sagaon-Teyssier, L., Suzan-Monti, M., … ANRS-VESPA2 Study Group. (2017). Suicide risk in a representative sample of people receiving HIV care: Time to target most-at-risk populations (ANRS VESPA2 French national survey). *PloS One, 12*(2), e0171645. https://doi.org/10.1371/journal.pone.0171645

Castro-Nallar, E., Crandall, K. A., & Pérez-Losada, M. (2012). Genetic diversity and molecular epidemiology of HIV transmission. *Future Virology, 7*(3), 239–252.

Catalan, J., Harding, R., Sibley, E., Clucas, C., Croome, N., & Sherr, L. (2011). HIV infection and mental health: Suicidal behaviour—systematic review. *Psychology, Health & Medicine, 16*(5), 588–611.

Celum, C., Wald, A., Hughes, J., Sanchez, J., Reid, S., Delany-Moretlwe, S., ... HPTN 039 Protocol Team. (2008). Effect of aciclovir on HIV-1 acquisition in herpes simplex virus 2 seropositive women and men who have sex with men: A randomised, double-blind, placebo-controlled trial. *Lancet, 371*(9630), 2109–2119.

Celum, C., Wald, A., Lingappa, J. R., Magaret, A. S., Wang, R. S., Mugo, N., ... Partners in Prevention HSV/HIV Transmission Study Team. (2010). Acyclovir and transmission of HIV-1 from persons infected with HIV-1 and HSV-2. *The New England Journal of Medicine, 362*(5), 427–439.

Chaney, M. P., & Burns-Wortham, C. M. (2015). Examining coming out, loneliness, and self-esteem as predictors of sexual compulsivity in gay and bisexual men. *Sexual Addiction & Compulsivity, 22*(1), 71–88.

Chaudoir, S. R., Norton, W. E., Earnshaw, V. A., Moneyham, L., Mugavero, M. J., & Hiers, K. M. (2012). Coping with HIV stigma: Do proactive coping and spiritual peace buffer the effect of stigma on depression? *AIDS and Behavior, 16*, 2382–2391.

Cheingsong-Popov, R., Weiss, R. A., Dalgleish, A., Tedder, R. S., Shanson, D. C., Jeffries, D. J., ... Mitton, S. (1984). Prevalence of antibody to human T-lymphotropic virus type III in AIDS and AIDS-risk patients in Britain. *Lancet, 2*(8401), 477–480.

Chen, W.-T. (2013). Side effects of antiretroviral therapy (ART) are associated with depression in Chinese individuals with HIV: A mixed methods study. *Journal of Midwifery & Women's Health, 58*, 585–585.

Choi, K. H., Han, C. S., Paul, J., & Ayala, G. (2011). Strategies for managing racism and homophobia among U.S. ethnic and racial minority men who have sex with men. *AIDS Education and Prevention: Official Publication of the International Society for AIDS Education, 23*(2), 145–158.

Clifton, S., Mercer, C. H., Sonnenberg, P., Tanton, C., Field, N., Gravningen, K., ... Johnson, A. M. (2018). STI risk perception in the British population and how it relates to sexual behaviour and STI healthcare use: Findings from a cross-sectional survey (Natsal-3). *EClinicalMedicine, 2–3*, 29–36.

Clucas, C., Sibley, E., Harding, R., Liu, L., Catalan, J., & Sherr, L. (2011). A systematic review of interventions for anxiety in people with HIV. *Psychology, Health & Medicine, 16*(5), 528–547.

Cohen, M. S., Chen, Y. Q., McCauley, M., Gamble, T., Hosseinipour, M. C., Kumarasamy, N., ... Fleming, T. R. (2011). Prevention of HIV-1 infection with early antiretroviral therapy. *New England Journal of Medicine, 365*(6), 493–505.

Cohen, M. S., Council, O. D., & Chen, J. S. (2019). Sexually transmitted infections and HIV in the era of antiretroviral treatment and prevention: The biologic basis for epidemiologic synergy. *Journal of the International AIDS Society, 22*(Suppl 6), e25355. https://doi.org/10.1002/jia2.25355

Coleman, E., Horvath, K. J., Miner, M., Ross, M. W., Oakes, M., Rosser, B. R., & Men's INTernet Sex (MINTS-II) Team. (2010). Compulsive sexual behavior and risk for unsafe sex among internet using men who have sex with men. *Archives of Sexual Behavior, 39*(5), 1045–1053.

Concorde Coordinating Committee. (1994). Concorde: MRC/ANRS randomised double-blind controlled trial of immediate and deferred zidovudine in symptom-free HIV infection. *Lancet (London, England), 343*(8902), 871–881.

Connor, E. M., Sperling, R. S., Gelber, R., Kiselev, P., Scott, G., O'Sullivan, M. J., ... Balsley, J. (1994). Reduction of maternal-infant transmission of human immunodeficiency virus type 1 with zidovudine treatment. *New England Journal of Medicine, 331*(18), 1173–1180.

Cook, M., Mills, R., Trumbach, R., & Cocks, H. G. (2007). *A gay history of Britain: Love and sex between men since the middle ages.* Oxford: Greenwood World Publishing.

Coyle, A., & Rafalin, D. (2000). Jewish gay men's accounts of negotiating cultural, religious and sexual identity: A qualitative study. *Journal of Psychology and Human Sexuality, 12,* 21–48.

Cresswell, F., Waters, L., Briggs, E., Fox, J., Harbottle, J., Hawkins, D., ... Fisher, M. (2016). UK guideline for the use of HIV post-exposure prophylaxis following sexual exposure, 2015. *International Journal of STD and AIDS, 27*(9), 713–738.

de Silva, S., Miller, R. F., & Walsh, J. (2006). Lack of awareness of HIV post-exposure prophylaxis among HIV-infected and uninfected men attending an inner London clinic. *International Journal of STD & AIDS, 17*(9), 629–630.

Debattista, J. (2015). Health promotion within a sex on premises venue: Notes from the field. *International Journal of STD and AIDS, 26*(14), 1017–1021.

Desai, M., Gafos, M., Dolling, D., McCormack, S., Nardone, A., & PROUD study (2016). Healthcare providers' knowledge of, attitudes to and practice of pre-exposure prophylaxis for HIV infection. *HIV Medicine, 17*(2), 133–142. https://doi.org/10.1111/hiv.12285

DiClemente, R. J., Zorn, J., & Temoshok, L. (1986). Adolescents and AIDS: A survey of knowledge, attitudes and beliefs about AIDS in San Francisco. *American Journal of Public Health, 76*(12), 1443–1445.

Dillon, S. M., Lee, E. J., Kotter, C. V., Austin, G. L., Dong, Z., Hecht, D. K., … Wilson, C. C. (2014). An altered intestinal mucosal microbiome in HIV-1 infection is associated with mucosal and systemic immune activation and endotoxemia. *Mucosal Immunology, 7*(4), 983–994.

Dillon, S. M., Frank, D. N., & Wilson, C. C. (2016). The Gut microbiome and HIV-1 pathogenesis: A two way street. *AIDS, 30*(18), 2737–2751.

Dolling, D. I., Desai, M., McOwan, A., Gilson, R., Clarke, A., Fisher, M., … PROUD Study Group. (2016). An analysis of baseline data from the PROUD study: An open-label randomised trial of pre-exposure prophylaxis. *Trials, 17*, 163. https://doi.org/10.1186/s13063-016-1286-4

Donnell, D., Mimiaga, M. J., Mayer, K., Chesney, M., Koblin, B., & Coates, T. (2010). Use of non-occupational post-exposure prophylaxis does not lead to an increase in high risk sex behaviors in men who have sex with men participating in the EXPLORE trial. *AIDS and Behavior, 14*(5), 1182–1189.

Dubov, A., Galbo, P., Altice, F. L., & Fraenkel, L. (2018). Stigma and shame experiences by MSM who take PrEP for HIV prevention: A qualitative study. *American Journal of Men's Health, 12*(6), 1843–1854.

Elopre, L., McDavid, C., Brown, A., Shurbaji, S., Mugavero, M. J., & Turan, J. M. (2018). Perceptions of HIV pre-exposure prophylaxis among young, Black Men who have sex with men. *AIDS Patient Care and STDs, 32*(12), 511–518.

Escaut, L., Liotier, J. Y., Albengres, E., Cheminot, N., & Vittecoq, D. (1999). Abacavir rechallenge has to be avoided in case of hypersensitivity reaction. *AIDS, 13*(11), 1419–1420.

Evangeli, M., Pady, K., & Wroe, A. L. (2016). Which psychological factors are related to HIV testing? A quantitative systematic review of global studies. *AIDS and Behavior, 20*(4), 880–918.

Exner, T. M., Meyer-Bahlburg, H. F., & Ehrhardt, A. A. (1992). Sexual self control as a mediator of high risk sexual behavior in a New York City cohort of HIV+ and HIV- gay men. *Journal of Sex Research, 29*(3), 389–406.

Ferlatte, O., Salway, T., Oliffe, J. L., & Trussler, T. (2017). Stigma and suicide among gay and bisexual men living with HIV. *AIDS Care, 29*(11), 1346–1350.

Ferrando, S. J. (2009). Psychopharmacologic treatment of patients with HIV/AIDS. *Current Psychiatry Reports, 11*(3), 235–242.

Fidler, S., Stöhr, W., Pace, M., Dorrell, L., Lever, A., Pett, S., … Murray, T. (2020). Antiretroviral therapy alone versus antiretroviral therapy with a kick and kill approach, on measures of the HIV reservoir in participants with recent HIV infection (the RIVER trial): A phase 2, randomised trial. *The Lancet, 395*(10227), 888–898.

Fife, B. L., & Wright, E. R. (2000). The dimensionality of stigma: A comparison of its impact on the self of persons with HIV/AIDS and cancer. *Journal of Health and Social Behavior, 41*(1), 50–67.

Figueroa, C., Johnson, C., Verster, A., & Baggaley, R. (2015). Attitudes and acceptability on HIV self-testing among key populations: A literature review. *AIDS and Behavior, 19*(11), 1949–1965.

Finneran, C., Chard, A., Sineath, C., Sullivan, P., & Stephenson, R. (2012). Intimate partner violence and social pressure among gay men in six countries. *Western Journal of Emergency Medicine, 13*, 260–271.

Fischl, M. A., Richman, D. D., Grieco, M. H., Gottlieb, M. S., Volberding, P. A., Laskin, O. L., … Schooley, R. T. (1987). The efficacy of azidothymidine (AZT) in the treatment of patients with AIDS and AIDS-related complex. A double-blind, placebo-controlled trial. *The New England Journal of Medicine, 317*(4), 185–191.

Fish, J., Papaloukas, P., Jaspal, R., & Williamson, I. (2016). Equality in sexual health promotion: A systematic review of effective interventions for black and minority ethnic men who have sex with men. *BMC Public Health, 16*, 810.

Flowers, P., Smith, J. A., Sheeran, P., & Beail, N. (1997). Health and romance: Understanding unprotected sex in relationships between gay men. *British Journal of Health Psychology, 2*, 73–86.

Ford, N., Irvine, C., Shubber, Z., Baggaley, R., Beanland, R., Vitoria, M., … Calmy, A. (2014). Adherence to HIV postexposure prophylaxis: A systematic review and meta-analysis. *AIDS (London, England), 28*(18), 2721–2727.

Ford, N., Shubber, Z., Pozniak, A., Vitoria, M., Doherty, M., Kirby, C., & Calmy, A. (2015). Comparative safety and neuropsychiatric adverse events associated with efavirenz use in first-line antiretroviral therapy: A systematic review and meta-analysis of randomized trials. *Journal of Acquired Immune Deficiency Syndromes, 69*(4), 422–429.

Frankis, J., Flowers, P., McDaid, L., & Bourne, A. (2018). Low levels of chemsex among men who have sex with men, but high levels of risk among men who engage in chemsex: Analysis of a cross-sectional online survey across four countries. *Sexual Health, 15*(2), 144–150.

Frankis, J., Young, I., Flowers, P., & McDaid, L. (2014). Understanding the acceptability of pre-exposure prophylaxis (PrEP) for HIV prevention amongst gay and bisexual men in Scotland: A mixed methods study. Retrieved from https://researchonline.gcu.ac.uk/en/publications/understanding-the-acceptability-of-pre-exposure-prophylaxis-prep-

Frankis, J., Young, I., Flowers, P., & McDaid, L. (2016). Who will use pre-exposure prophylaxis (PrEP) and why?: Understanding PrEP awareness and acceptability amongst men who have sex with men in the UK—A mixed methods study. *PLoS One, 11*(4). https://doi.org/10.1371/journal.pone.0151385

Frankis, J. S., & Flowers, P. (2006). Cruising for sex: Sexual risk behaviours and HIV testing of men who cruise, inside and out with public sex environments (PSE). *AIDS Care, 18*(1), 54–59.

Freeman, E. E., Weiss, H. A., Glynn, J. R., Cross, P. L., Whitworth, J. A., & Hayes, R. J. (2006). Herpes simplex virus 2 infection increases HIV acquisition in men and women: Systematic review and meta-analysis of longitudinal studies. *AIDS, 20*(1), 73–83.

Gallegos, M., Bradly, D., Jakate, S., & Keshavarzian, A. (2012). Lymphogranuloma venereum proctosigmoiditis is a mimicker of inflammatory bowel disease. *World Journal of Gastroenterology, 18*(25), 3317–3321.

Gallo, R. C., Sarin, P. S., Gelmann, E. P., Robert-Guroff, M., Richardson, E., Kalyanaraman, V. S., ... Popovic, M. (1983). Isolation of human T-cell leukemia virus in acquired immune deficiency syndrome (AIDS). *Science, 220*(4599), 865–867.

Galvin, S. R., & Cohen, M. S. (2004). The role of sexually transmitted diseases in HIV transmission. *Nature Reviews Microbiology, 2*(1), 33–42.

Gama, A., Abecasis, A., Pingarilho, M., Mendão, L., Martins, M. O., Barros, H., & Dias, S. (2017). Cruising venues as a context for HIV risky behavior among men who have sex with men. *Archives of Sexual Behavior, 46*(4), 1061–1068.

Garey, L., Bakhshaie, J., Sharp, C., Neighbors, C., Zvolensky, M. J., & Gonzalez, A. (2015). Anxiety, depression, and HIV symptoms among persons living with HIV/AIDS: The role of hazardous drinking. *AIDS Care, 27*(1), 80–85.

Garry, R. F., Witte, M. H., Gottlieb, A. A., Elvin-Lewis, M., Gottlieb, M. S., Witte, C. L., ... Drake, W. L. (1988). Documentation of an AIDS virus infection in the United States in 1968. *JAMA, 260*(14), 2085–2087.

Gayner, B., Esplen, M. J., DeRoche, P., Wong, J., Bishop, S., Kavanagh, L., & Butler, K. (2012). A randomized controlled trial of mindfulness-based stress reduction to manage affective symptoms and improve quality of life in gay men living with HIV. *Journal of Behavioral Medicine, 35*(3), 272–285.

George, L. (1998). Self and identity in later life: Protecting and enhancing the self. *Journal of Aging and Identity, 3*, 133–152.

Gerrard, M., Gibbons, F. X., & McCoy, S. B. (1993). Emotional inhibition of effective contraception. *Anxiety, Stress & Coping: An International Journal, 6*(2), 73–88.

Gerschenson, M., & Brinkman, K. (2004). Mitochondrial dysfunction in AIDS and its treatment. *Mitochondrion, 4*(5), 763–777.

Gesink, D., Wang, S., Guimond, T., Kimura, L., Connell, J., Salway, T., ... Grace, D. (2018). Conceptualizing geosexual archetypes: Mapping the sexual travels and egocentric sexual networks of gay and bisexual men in Toronto, Canada. *Sexually Transmitted Diseases, 45*(6), 368–373.

Geskus, R. B., Prins, M., Hubert, J.-B., Miedema, F., Berkhout, B., Rouzioux, C., ... Meyer, L. (2007). The HIV RNA setpoint theory revisited. *Retrovirology, 4*(1), 65. https://doi.org/10.1186/1742-4690-4-65

Gibb, B. E., Chelminski, I., & Zimmerman, M. (2007). Childhood emotional, physical, and sexual abuse, and diagnoses of depressive and anxiety disorders in adult psychiatric outpatients. *Depression and Anxiety, 24*(4), 256–263.

Goedel, W. C., & Duncan, D. T. (2015). Geosocial-networking app usage patterns of gay, bisexual and other men who have sex with men: Survey among users of Grindr, a mobile dating app. *JMIR Public Health and Surveillance, 1*(1), e4. https://doi.org/10.2196/publichealth.4353

Goedert, J. J., Biggar, R. J., Winn, D. M., Mann, D. L., Byar, D. P., Strong, D. M., ... Blattner, W. A. (1985). Decreased helper T lymphocytes in homosexual men. I. Sexual contact in high-incidence areas for the acquired immunodeficiency syndrome. *American Journal of Epidemiology, 121*(5), 629–636.

Goldenberg, T., Finneran, C., Sullivan, S. P., Andes, K. L., & Stephenson, R. (2016). "I consider being gay a very high risk factor": How perceptions of a partner's sexual identity influence perceptions of HIV risk among gay and bisexual men. *Sexuality Research and Social Policy, 14*(1), 32–41.

Gonzalez, J. S., Batchelder, A. W., Psaros, C., & Safren, S. A. (2011). Depression and HIV/AIDS treatment nonadherence: A review and meta-analysis. *Journal of Acquired Immune Deficiency Syndromes, 58*(2), 181–187. https://doi.org/10.1097/QAI.0b013e31822d490a

Goodwin, R., Realo, A., Kwiatkowska, A., Kozlova, A., Luu, L. A. N., & Nizharadze, G. (2002). Values and sexual behaviour in central and eastern Europe. *Journal of Health Psychology, 7*(1), 45–56.

Gounden, V., van Niekerk, C., Snyman, T., & George, J. A. (2010). Presence of the CYP2B6 516G> T polymorphism, increased plasma Efavirenz concentrations and early neuropsychiatric side effects in South African HIV-infected patients. *AIDS Research and Therapy, 7*, 32. https://doi.org/10.1186/1742-6405-7-32

Grant, R. M., Lama, J. R., Anderson, P. L., McMahan, V., Liu, A. Y., Vargas, L., ... Glidden, D. V. (2010). Preexposure chemoprophylaxis for HIV prevention in men who have sex with men. *New England Journal of Medicine,* *363*(27), 2587–2599.

Gray, R. H., Kigozi, G., Serwadda, D., Makumbi, F., Watya, S., Nalugoda, F., … Wawer, M. J. (2007). Male circumcision for HIV prevention in men in Rakai, Uganda: A randomised trial. *Lancet, 369*(9562), 657–666.

Gregson, S., Adamson, S., Papaya, S., Mundondo, J., Nyamukapa, C. A., Mason, P. R., … Anderson, R. M. (2007). Impact and process evaluation of integrated community and clinic-based HIV-1 control: A cluster-randomised trial in Eastern Zimbabwe. *PLoS Medicine, 4*(3). https://doi.org/10.1371/journal.pmed.0040102

Grosskurth, H., Mosha, F., Todd, J., Mwijarubi, E., Klokke, A., Senkoro, K., … Ka-Gina, G. (1995). Impact of improved treatment of sexually transmitted diseases on HIV infection in rural Tanzania: Randomised controlled trial. *Lancet, 346*(8974), 530–536.

Grov, C., Breslow, A. S., Newcomb, M. E., Rosenberger, J. G., & Bauermeister, J. A. (2014). Gay and bisexual men's use of the Internet: Research from the 1990s through 2013. *Journal of Sex Research, 51*(4), 390–409.

Grov, C., Golub, S. A., Parsons, J. T., Brennan, M., & Karpiak, S. E. (2010). Loneliness and HIV-related stigma explain depression among older HIV-positive adults. *AIDS Care, 22*(5), 630–639. https://doi.org/10.1080/09540120903280901

Grov, C., Parsons, J. T., & Bimbi, D. S. (2010). Sexual compulsivity and sexual risk in gay and bisexual men. *Archives of Sexual Behavior, 39*(4), 940–949. https://doi.org/10.1007/s10508-009-9483-9

Halkitis, P. N., & Wilton, L. (2005). The meanings of sex for HIV-positive gay and bisexual men: Emotions, physicality, and affirmations of self. In P. N. Halkitis, C. A. Gómez, & R. J. Wolitski (Eds.), *HIV+ sex: The psychological and interpersonal dynamics of HIV-seropositive gay and bisexual men's relationships* (pp. 21–37). American Psychological Association.

Han, C. S. (2008). A qualitative exploration of the relationship between racism and unsafe sex among Asian Pacific Islander gay men. *Archives of Sexual Behavior, 37*(5), 827–837.

Han, C. S., Ayala, G., Paul, J. P., Boylan, R., Gregorich, S. E., & Choi, K. H. (2015). Stress and coping with racism and their role in sexual risk for HIV among African American, Asian/Pacific Islander, and Latino men who have sex with men. *Archives of Sexual Behavior, 44*(2), 411–420.

Hart, T. A., & Heimberg, R. G. (2005). Social anxiety as a risk factor for unprotected intercourse among gay and bisexual male youth. *AIDS and Behavior, 9*(4), 505–512.

Haubrich, D. J., Myers, T., Calzavara, L., Ryder, K., & Medved, W. (2004). Gay and bisexual men's experiences of bathhouse culture and sex: 'looking for love in all the wrong places'. *Culture, Health & Sexuality, 6*(1), 19–29.

Heijnders, M., & Van Der Meij, S. (2006). The fight against stigma: An overview of stigma-reduction strategies and interventions. *Psychology, Health & Medicine, 11*(3), 353–363.

Hennelly, S. (2010). Public space, public morality: The media construction of sex in public places. *Liverpool Law Review, 31*(1), 69–91.

Herek, G. M. J., Gillis, R., & Cogan, J. C. (2009). Internalized stigma among sexual minority adults: Insights from a social psychological perspective. *Journal of Counseling Psychology, 56*, 32–43.

Heywood, W., & Lyons, A. (2016). HIV and elevated mental health problems: Diagnostic, treatment, and risk patterns for symptoms of depression, anxiety, and stress in a national community-based cohort of gay men living with HIV. *AIDS and Behavior, 20*(8), 1632–1645.

Hintze, J., Templer, D., Cappelletty, G. G., & Frederick, W. (1993). Death depression and death anxiety in HIV-infected males. *Death Studies, 17*(4), 333–341.

Hirsch, V. M., Edmondson, P., Murphey-Corb, M., Arbeille, B., Johnson, P. R., & Mullins, J. I. (1989). SIV adaption to human cells. *Nature, 341*(6243), 573–574.

Holt, M. (2011). Gay men and ambivalence about 'gay community': From gay community attachment to personal communities. *Culture, Health & Sexuality, 13*(8), 857–871.

Horwood, J., Ingle, S. M., Burton, D., Woodman-Bailey, A., Horner, P., & Jeal, N. (2016). Sexual health risks, service use, and views of rapid point-of-care testing among men who have sex with men attending saunas: A cross-sectional survey. *International Journal of STD and AIDS, 27*(4), 273–280.

Hoyle, R. H., Fejfar, M. C., & Miller, J. D. (2000). Personality and sexual risk taking: A quantitative review. *Journal of Personality, 68*(6), 1203–1231.

Huebner, D. M., Binson, D., Pollack, L. M., & Woods, W. J. (2012). Implementing bathhouse-based voluntary counselling and testing has no adverse effect on bathhouse patronage among men who have sex with men. *International Journal of STD and AIDS, 23*(3), 182–184.

Huet, T., Cheynier, R., Meyerhans, A., Roelants, G., & Wain-Hobson, S. (1990). Genetic organization of a chimpanzee lentivirus related to HIV-1. *Nature, 345*(6273), 356–359.

Hughes, A. R., Mosteller, M., Bansal, A. T., Davies, K., Haneline, S. A., Lai, E. H., ... on behalf of the CNA30027 and CNA30032 study teams. (2004). Association of genetic variations in HLA-B region with hypersensitivity to abacavir in some, but not all, populations. *Pharmacogenomics, 5*(2), 203–211.

Illing, P. T., Purcell, A. W., & McCluskey, J. (2017). The role of HLA genes in pharmacogenomics: Unravelling HLA associated adverse drug reactions. *Immunogenetics, 69*(8–9), 617–630.

INSIGHT START Study Group, Lundgren, J. D., Babiker, A. G., Gordin, F., Emery, S., ... Neaton, J. D. (2015). Initiation of antiretroviral therapy in early asymptomatic HIV infection. *The New England Journal of Medicine, 373*(9), 795–807.

Ironson, G., O'Cleirigh, C., Fletcher, M. A., Laurenceau, J. P., Balbin, E., Klimas, N., ... Solomon, G. (2005). Psychosocial factors predict CD4 and viral load change in men and women with human immunodeficiency virus in the era of highly active antiretroviral treatment. *Psychosomatic Medicine, 67*(6), 1013–1021.

Jaspal, R. (2012a). "I never faced up to being gay": Sexual, religious and ethnic identities among British South Asian gay men. *Culture, Health and Sexuality: An International Journal for Research, Intervention and Care, 14*(7), 767–780.

Jaspal, R. (2012b). Coping with religious and cultural homophobia: Emotion and narratives of identity threat from British Muslim gay men. In P. Nynäs & A. K. T. Yip (Eds.), *Religion, gender and sexuality in everyday life* (pp. 71–90). Farnham: Ashgate.

Jaspal, R. (2014a). Arranged marriage, identity and psychological wellbeing among British Asian gay men. *Journal of GLBT Family Studies, 10*(5), 425–448.

Jaspal, R. (2014b). Sexuality, migration and identity among gay Iranian migrants to the UK. In Y. Taylor & R. Snowdon (Eds.), *Queering religion, religious queers* (pp. 44–60). London: Routledge.

Jaspal, R. (2015). The experience of relationship dissolution among British Asian gay men: Identity threat and protection. *Sexuality Research & Social Policy, 12*(1), 34–46.

Jaspal, R. (2017a). Coping with ethnic prejudice on the gay scene: British South Asian gay men. *Journal of LGBT Youth, 14*(2), 172–190.

Jaspal, R. (2017b). Gay men's construction and management of identity on Grindr. *Sexuality & Culture, 21*(1), 187–204.

Jaspal, R. (2018a). *Enhancing sexual health, self-identity and wellbeing among men who have sex with men: A guide for practitioners.* London: Jessica Kingsley Publishers.

Jaspal, R. (2018b). Perceptions of HIV testing venues among men who have sex with men in London and the Midlands, United Kingdom. *Journal of Gay & Lesbian Social Services, 30*(4), 336–355.

Jaspal, R., & Breakwell, G. M. (Eds.). (2014). *Identity process theory: Identity, social action and social change.* Cambridge: Cambridge University Press.

Jaspal, R., & Cinnirella, M. (2010). Coping with potentially incompatible identities: Accounts of religious, ethnic and sexual identities from British Pakistani men who identify as Muslim and gay. *British Journal of Social Psychology, 49*(4), 849–870.

Jaspal, R., & Cinnirella, M. (2012a). Identity processes, threat and interpersonal relations: Accounts from British Muslim gay men. *Journal of Homosexuality, 59*(2), 215–240.

Jaspal, R., & Cinnirella, M. (2012b). The construction of ethnic identity: Insights from identity process theory. *Ethnicities, 12*(5), 503–530.

Jaspal, R., & Cinnirella, M. (2013). The construction of British national identity among British South Asians. *National Identities, 15*(2), 157–175.

Jaspal, R., & Cinnirella, M. (2014). Hyper-affiliation to the religious ingroup among British Pakistani Muslim gay men. *Journal of Community and Applied Social Psychology, 24*(4), 265–277.

Jaspal, R., & Daramilas, C. (2016). Perceptions of pre-exposure prophylaxis (PrEP) among HIV-negative and HIV-positive men who have sex with men. *Cogent Medicine, 3,* 1256850. https://doi.org/10.1080/2331205X.2016.1256850

Jaspal, R., Fish, J., Williamson, I., & Papaloukas, P. (2016). *Public Health England black and minority ethnic men who have sex with men project evaluation report.* London: Public Health England.

Jaspal, R., Lopes, B., Jamal, Z., Paccoud, I., & Sekhon, P. (2017). Sexual abuse and HIV risk behaviour among black and minority ethnic men who have sex with men in the UK. *Mental Health, Religion & Culture, 20*(8), 841–853.

Jaspal, R., Lopes, B., Bayley, J., & Papaloukas, P. (2019). A structural equation model to predict pre-exposure prophylaxis acceptability in men who have sex with men in Leicester, UK. *HIV Medicine, 20*(1), 11–18.

Jaspal, R., Lopes, B., Jamal, Z., Yap, C., Paccoud, I., & Sekhon, P. (2019). HIV knowledge, sexual health and behaviour among black and minority ethnic men who have sex with men in the UK: A cross-sectional study. *Sexual Health, 16*(1), 25–31.

Jaspal, R., Lopes, B., & Rehman, Z. (2019). A structural equation model for predicting depressive symptomatology in Black, Asian and Minority Ethnic lesbian, gay and bisexual people in the UK. *Psychology and Sexuality.* https://doi.org/10.1080/19419899.2019.1690560

Jaspal, R., & Lopes, B. (2020). Psychological wellbeing facilitates accurate HIV risk appraisal in gay and bisexual men. *Sexual Health, 17*(3), 288–295.

Jaspal, R., Lopes, B., & Breakwell, G. M. (2020). British national identity and life satisfaction in ethnic minority groups in the United Kingdom. *National Identities.* https://doi.org/10.1080/14608944.2020.1822793.

Jaspal, R., & Nerlich, B. (2016). A 'morning-after' pill for HIV? Social representations of post-exposure prophylaxis for HIV in the British print media. *Health, Risk & Society, 18*(5–6), 225–246.

Jaspal, R., & Nerlich, B. (2017). Polarised reporting about HIV prevention: Social representations of pre-exposure prophylaxis (PrEP) in the UK press. *Health: An Interdisciplinary Journal for the Social Study of Health, Illness and Medicine, 21*(5), 478–497.

Jaspal, R., & Nerlich, B. (2020). HIV stigma in UK press reporting of a case of intentional HIV transmission. *Health: An Interdisciplinary Journal for the Social Study of Health, Illness & Medicine.* https://doi.org/10.1177/1363459320949901

Jaspal, R., & Nerlich, B. (2020). Social representations, identity threat and coping amid COVID-19. *Psychological Trauma: Theory, Research, Practice and Policy, 2*(S1), S249–S251.

Jaspal, R., & Papaloukas, P. (2020). Identity, social connectedness and sexual health in the gay sauna. *Sexuality Research & Social Policy.* https://doi.org/10.1007/s13178-020-00442-0

Jaspal, R., & Siraj, A. (2011). Perceptions of 'coming out' among British Muslim gay men. *Psychology and Sexuality, 2*(3), 183–197.

Jaspal, R., & Williamson, I. (2017). Identity management strategies among HIV-positive Colombian gay men in London. *Culture, Health and Sexuality: An International Journal for Research, Intervention and Care, 19*(2), 1374–1388.

Jayappa, K. D., Ao, Z., & Yao, X. (2012). The HIV-1 passage from cytoplasm to nucleus: The process involving a complex exchange between the components of HIV-1 and cellular machinery to access nucleus and successful integration. *International Journal of Biochemistry and Molecular Biology, 3*(1), 70–85.

Jeffries, W. L., Marks, G., Lauby, J., Murrill, C. S., & Millett, G. A. (2013). Homophobia is associated with sexual behavior that increases risk of acquiring and transmitting HIV infection among black men who have sex with men. *AIDS and Behavior, 17*(4), 1442–1453.

Joffe, H. (1995). Social representations of AIDS: Towards encompassing issues of power. *Papers on Social Representations, 4*(1), 29–40.

Joffe, H. (2007). Identity, self-control, and risk. In G. Moloney & I. Walker (Eds.), *Social representations and identity* (pp. 197–213). London: Palgrave Macmillan.

Johnson, C., Baggaley, R., Forsythe, S., van Rooyen, H., Ford, N., Napierala Mavedzenge, S., ... Taegtmeyer, M. (2014). Realizing the potential for HIV self-testing. *AIDS and Behavior, 18*(Suppl 4), S391–S395. https://doi.org/10.1007/s10461-014-0832-x

Joiner, T. E. (2005). *Why people die by suicide.* Cambridge, MA: Harvard University Press.

Jose, S., Quinn, K., Dunn, D., Cox, A., Sabin, C., & Fidler, S. (2016). Virological failure and development of new resistance mutations according to CD4 count at combination antiretroviral therapy initiation. *HIV Medicine, 17*(5), 368–372.

Kalichman, S. C., Heckman, T., Kochman, A., Sikkema, K., & Bergholte, J. (2000). Depression and thoughts of suicide among middle-aged and older persons living with HIV-AIDS. *Psychiatric Services* (Washington, D.C.), *51*(7), 903–907.

Kamali, A., Quigley, M., Nakiyingi, J., Kinsman, J., Kengeya-Kayondo, J., Gopal, R., ... Whitworth, J. (2003). Syndromic management of sexually-transmitted infections and behaviour change interventions on transmission of HIV-1 in rural Uganda: A community randomised trial. *The Lancet, 361*(9358), 645–652.

Karasavvas, N., Billings, E., Rao, M., Williams, C., Zolla-Pazner, S., Bailer, R. T., ... de Souza, M. S. (2012). The Thai Phase III HIV Type 1 Vaccine Trial (RV144) regimen induces antibodies that target conserved regions within the V2 loop of gp120. *AIDS Research and Human Retroviruses, 28*(11), 1444–1457.

Kavanagh, D. J., & Bower, G. H. (1985). Mood and self-efficacy: Impact of joy and sadness on perceived capabilities. *Cognitive Therapy and Research, 9*(5), 507–525.

Keele, B. F., Jones, J. H., Terio, K. A., Estes, J. D., Rudicell, R. S., Wilson, M. L., ... Hahn, B. H. (2009). Increased mortality and AIDS-like immuno-pathology in wild chimpanzees infected with SIVcpz. *Nature, 460*(7254), 515–519.

Kelley, H. H. (1967). Attribution theory in social psychology. In D. Levine (Ed.), *Nebraska Symposium on motivation* (Vol. 15, pp. 192–238). Lincoln: University of Nebraska Press.

Kemppainen, J. K., Eller, L. S., Bunch, E., Hamilton, M. J., Dole, P., Holzemer, W., ... Tsai, Y. F. (2006). Strategies for self-management of HIV-related anxiety. *AIDS Care, 18*(6), 597–607.

Kendrick, S. R., Kroc, K. A., Withum, D., Rydman, R. J., Branson, B. M., & Weinstein, R. A. (2005). Outcomes of offering rapid point-of-care HIV testing in a sexually transmitted disease clinic. *JAIDS Journal of Acquired Immune Deficiency Syndromes, 38*(2), 142–146.

Ko, N. Y., Lee, H. C., Hung, C. C., Chang, J. L., Lee, N. Y., Chang, C. M., ... Ko, W. C. (2009). Effects of structural intervention on increasing condom availability and reducing risky sexual behaviours in gay bathhouse attendees. *AIDS Care, 21*(12), 1499–1507.

Körner, H., Ellard, J. M., Hendry, O., Kippax, S. C., Grulich, A. E., & Hodge, S. R. (2003). Taking post-exposure prophylaxis: Managing risk, reclaiming control. National Centre in HIV Social Research, Sydney.

Körner, H., Hendry, O., & Kjppax, S. (2005). Negotiating risk and social relations in the context of post-exposure prophylaxis for HIV: Narratives of gay men. *Health, Risk & Society, 7*(4), 349–360. https://doi.org/10.1080/13698570500390218

Kraaij, V., van der Veek, S. M., Garnefski, N., Schroevers, M., Witlox, R., & Maes, S. (2008). Coping, goal adjustment, and psychological well-being in HIV-infected men who have sex with men. *AIDS Patient Care and STDs, 22*(5), 395–402.

Kugle, S. S. H. (2010). *Homosexuality in Islam: Critical reflection on gay, lesbian, and transgender muslims.* Oxford: Oneworld Publications.

Kurka, T., Soni, S., & Richardson, D. (2015). Sexual health services for men who have sex with men (MSM): Are they acceptable? *Sexually Transmitted Infections, 91*, A51. https://doi.org/10.1136/sextrans-2015-052126.150

Lampe, F. C., Harding, R., Smith, C. J., Phillips, A. N., Johnson, M., & Sherr, L. (2010). Physical and psychological symptoms and risk of virologic rebound among patients with virologic suppression on antiretroviral therapy. *Journal of Acquired Immune Deficiency Syndromes (1999), 54*(5), 500–505.

Landovitz, R. J., Tseng, C. H., Weissman, M., Haymer, M., Mendenhall, B., Rogers, K., ... Shoptaw, S. (2013). Epidemiology, sexual risk behavior, and HIV prevention practices of men who have sex with men using Grindr in Los Angeles, California. *Journal of Urban Health: Bulletin of the New York Academy of Medicine, 90*(4), 729–739.

Lasala, M. C. (2000). Gay male couples: The importance of coming out and being out to parents. *Journal of Homosexuality, 39*(2), 47–71.

Lee, M., Hegazi, A., Barbour, A., Bavithra, N., Green, S., Simms, R., & Pakianathan, M. (2015). O11 Chemsex and the city: Sexualised substance use in gay bisexual and other men who have sex with men. *Sexually Transmitted Infections, 91,* A4. Retrieved from https://sti.bmj.com/content/91/Suppl_1/A4.2.info

Leichliter, J. S., Haderxhanaj, L. T., Chesson, H. W., & Aral, S. O. (2013). Temporal trends in sexual behavior among men who have sex with men in the United States, 2002 to 2006–10. *Journal of Acquired Immune Deficiency Syndromes (1999), 63*(2), 254–258.

Levi, J., Raymond, A., Pozniak, A., Vernazza, P., Kohler, P., & Hill, A. (2016). Can the UNAIDS 90-90-90 target be achieved? A systematic analysis of national HIV treatment cascades. *BMJ Global Health, 1*(2), e000010. https://doi.org/10.1136/bmjgh-2015-000010

Li, J., Gilmour, S., Zhang, H., Koyanagi, A., & Shibuya, K. (2012). The epidemiological impact and cost-effectiveness of HIV testing, antiretroviral treatment and harm reduction programs. *AIDS, 26*(16), 2069–2078.

Lima, V. D., Geller, J., Bangsberg, D. R., Patterson, T. L., Daniel, M., Kerr, T., … Hogg, R. S. (2007). The effect of adherence on the association between depressive symptoms and mortality among HIV-infected individuals first initiating HAART. *AIDS, 21*(9), 1175–1183.

Liu, L., Pang, R., Sun, W., Wu, M., Qu, P., Lu, C., & Wang, L. (2013). Functional social support, psychological capital, and depressive and anxiety symptoms among people living with HIV/AIDS employed full-time. *BMC Psychiatry, 13,* 324. https://doi.org/10.1186/1471-244X-13-324

Loewenberg, S. (2008). Selma Dritz. *The Lancet, 372*(9646), 1296.

Lopes, B., & Jaspal, R. (2020). Understanding the mental health burden of COVID-19 in the United Kingdom. *Psychological Trauma: Theory, Research, Practice and Policy, 12*(5), 465–467.

Lorenc, T., Marrero-Guillamón, I., Llewellyn, A., Aggleton, P., Cooper, C., Lehmann, A., & Lindsay, C. (2011). HIV testing among men who have sex with men (MSM): Systematic review of qualitative evidence. *Health Education Research, 26*(5), 834–846.

Lyons, A., Pitts, M., & Grierson, J. (2012). Exploring the psychological impact of HIV: Health comparisons of older Australian HIV-positive and HIV-negative gay men. *AIDS and Behavior, 16*(8), 2340–2349.

Maatouk, I., & Jaspal, R. (2019). HIV in men who have sex with men in Lebanon: Clinical & psychosocial aspects. *BMJ Journal of Sexual & Reproductive Health, 45*(3), 175–176.

Maatouk, I., & Jaspal, R. (2020a). Barriers to HIV treatment as prevention (TasP) in men who have sex with men in the Eastern Mediterranean Region. *Journal of Public Health.* https://doi.org/10.1093/pubmed/fdz186

Maatouk, I., & Jaspal, R. (2020b). Religion, male bisexuality and sexual health in Lebanon. In A. K. T. Yip & A. Toft (Eds.), *Bisexuality, spirituality and identity: Critical perspectives* (pp. 137–155). London: Routledge.

MacKellar, D. A., Valleroy, L. A., Secura, G. M., Behel, S., Bingham, T., Celentano, D. D., … Young Men's Survey Study Group. (2005). Unrecognized HIV infection, risk behaviors, and perceptions of risk among young men who have sex with men: Opportunities for advancing HIV prevention in the third decade of HIV/AIDS. *Journal of Acquired Immune Deficiency Syndromes (1999), 38*(5), 603–614.

Mallal, S., Nolan, D., Witt, C., Masel, G., Martin, A. M., Moore, C., … Christiansen, F. T. (2002). Association between presence of HLA-B*5701, HLA-DR7, and HLA-DQ3 and hypersensitivity to HIV-1 reverse-transcriptase inhibitor abacavir. *Lancet, 359*(9308), 727–732.

Manetta, A. M., & Cox, L. E. (2014). Suicidal behavior and HIV/AIDS: A partial test of Joiner's Theory of why people die by suicide. *Social Work in Mental Health, 12*(1), 20–35. https://doi.org/10.1080/1533298 5.2013.832717

Marcus, U., Gassowski, M., & Drewes, J. (2016). HIV risk perception and testing behaviours among men having sex with men (MSM) reporting potential transmission risks in the previous 12 months from a large online sample of MSM living in Germany. *BMC Public Health, 16*(1), 1111. https://doi.org/10.1186/s12889-016-3759-5

Mazick, A., Howitz, M., Rex, S., Jensen, I. P., Weis, N., Katzenstein, T. L., … Molbak, K. (2005). Hepatitis A outbreak among MSM linked to casual sex and gay saunas in Copenhagen, Denmark. *Eurosurveillance, 10*(4–6), 111–114.

McCormack, S., Dunn, D. T., Desai, M., Dolling, D. I., Gafos, M., Gilson, R., … Gill, O. N. (2016). Pre-exposure prophylaxis to prevent the acquisition of HIV-1 infection (PROUD): Effectiveness results from the pilot phase of a pragmatic open-label randomised trial. *The Lancet, 387*(10013), 53–60.

McKeown, E., Doerner, R., Nelson, S., Low, N., Robinson, A., Anderson, J., … Elford, J. (2012). The experiences of ethnic minority MSM using NHS sexual health clinics in Britain. *Sexually Transmitted Infections, 88*(8), 595–600.

Melendez-Torres, G. J., Hickson, F., Reid, D., Weatherburn, P., & Bonell, C. (2016). Drug use moderates associations between location of sex and unprotected anal intercourse in men who have sex with men: Nested cross-sectional study of dyadic encounters with new partners. *Sexually Transmitted Infections, 92*(1), 39–43.

Memon, A., Taylor, K., Mohebati, L. M., Sundin, J., Cooper, M., Scanlon, T., & de Visser, R. (2016). Perceived barriers to accessing mental health services among black and minority ethnic (BME) communities: A qualitative study in Southeast England. *BMJ Open, 6*(11), e012337. https://doi.org/10.1136/bmjopen-2016-012337

Mercer, C. H., Prah, P., Field, N., Tanton, C., Macdowall, W., Clifton, S., ... Sonnenberg, P. (2016). The health and well-being of men who have sex with men (MSM) in Britain: Evidence from the third National Survey of Sexual Attitudes and Lifestyles (Natsal-3). *BMC Public Health, 16*(1), 525. https://doi.org/10.1186/s12889-016-3149-z

Messiaen, P., Wensing, A. M. J., Fun, A., Nijhuis, M., Brusselaers, N., & Vandekerckhove, L. (2013). Clinical use of HIV integrase inhibitors: A systematic review and meta-analysis. *PLoS ONE, 8*(1). https://doi.org/10.1371/journal.pone.0052562

Michaels, M. S., Parent, M. C., & Torrey, C. L. (2016). A minority stress model for suicidal ideation in gay men. *Suicide and Life-Threatening Behavior, 46*(1), 23–34.

Miller, A. K., Lee, B. L., & Henderson, C. E. (2012). Death anxiety in persons with HIV/AIDS: A systematic review and meta-analysis. *Death Studies, 36*(7), 640–663.

Millett, G. A., Flores, S. A., Marks, G., Reed, J. B., & Herbst, J. H. (2008). Circumcision status and risk of HIV and sexually transmitted infections among men who have sex with men: A meta-analysis. *JAMA, 300*(14), 1674–1684.

Millett, G. A., Peterson, J. L., Flores, S. A., Hart, T. A., Jeffries, W. L., Wilson, P. A., ... Remis, R. S. (2012). Comparisons of disparities and risks of HIV infection in black and other men who have sex with men in Canada, UK, and USA: A meta-analysis. *Lancet, 380*(9839), 341–348.

Mizuno, Y., Borkowf, C. B., Ayala, G., Carballo-Diéguez, A., & Millett, G. A. (2015). Correlates of sexual risk for HIV among US-born and foreign-born Latino men who have sex with men (MSM): An analysis from the Brothers y Hermanos study. *Journal of Immigrant and Minority Health, 17*(1), 47–55.

Mohammed, H., Blomquist, P., Ogaz, D., Duffell, S., Furegato, M., Checchi, M., … Hughes, G. (2018). 100 years of STIs in the UK: A review of national surveillance data. *Sexually Transmitted Infections, 94*(8), 553–558.

Mohammed, H., Furegato, M., & Hughes, G. (2016). P068 Inequalities in sexually transmitted infection risk among black and minority ethnic men who have sex with men in England. *Sexually Transmitted Infections, 92*, A42.

Molina, J.-M., Capitant, C., Spire, B., Pialoux, G., Cotte, L., Charreau, I., … Delfraissy, J.-F. (2015). On-demand preexposure prophylaxis in men at high risk for HIV-1 infection. *New England Journal of Medicine, 373*(23), 2237–2246.

Morin, S. F., Vernon, K., Harcourt, J. J., Steward, W. T., Volk, J., Riess, T. H., … Coates, T. J. (2003). Why HIV infections have increased among men who have sex with men and what to do about it: Findings from California focus groups. *AIDS and Behavior, 7*(4), 353–362.

Morris, Z. S., Wooding, S., & Grant, J. (2011). The answer is 17 years, what is the question: Understanding time lags in translational research. *Journal of the Royal Society of Medicine, 104*(12), 510–520.

Moscovici, S. (1988). Notes towards a description of social representations. *European Journal of Social Psychology, 18*, 211–250.

Moseng, B. U., & Bjørnshagen, V. (2017). Are there any differences between different testing sites? A cross-sectional study of a Norwegian low-threshold HIV testing service for men who have sex with men. *BMJ Open, 7*(10), e017598. https://doi.org/10.1136/bmjopen-2017-017598

Murphy, P. J., Garrido-Hernansaiz, H., Mulcahy, F., & Hevey, D. (2018). HIV-related stigma and optimism as predictors of anxiety and depression among HIV-positive men who have sex with men in the United Kingdom and Ireland. *AIDS Care, 30*(9), 1173–1179.

Murtagh, N., Gatersleben, B., & Uzzell, D. (2014). Identity threat and resistance to change: Evidence and implications from transport-related behavior. In R. Jaspal & G. M. Breakwell (Eds.), *Identity process theory: Identity, social action and social change* (pp. 335–356). Cambridge: Cambridge University Press.

Nahmias, A. J., Weiss, J., Yao, X., Lee, F., Kodsi, R., Schanfield, M., … Motulsky, A. (1986). Evidence for human infection with an HTLV III/LAV-like virus in Central Africa, 1959. *Lancet, 1*(8492), 1279–1280.

Ni, J., Wang, D., & Wang, S. (2018). The CCR5-Delta32 genetic polymorphism and HIV-1 infection susceptibility: A meta-analysis. *Open Medicine, 13*, 467–474.

Norton, R. (2007). *Mother clap's molly house: The gay subculture in England, 1700–1830*. London: Chalford Press.

O'Cleirigh, C., Newcomb, M. E., Mayer, K. H., Skeer, M., Traeger, L., & Safren, S. A. (2013). Moderate levels of depression predict sexual transmission risk in HIV-infected MSM: A longitudinal analysis of data from six sites involved in a "prevention for positives" study. *AIDS and Behavior, 17*(5), 1764–1769.

O'Connor, J., Smith, C., Lampe, F. C., Johnson, M. A., Chadwick, D. R., Nelson, M., ... Delpech, V. (2017). Durability of viral suppression with first-line antiretroviral therapy in patients with HIV in the UK: An observational cohort study. *The Lancet HIV, 4*(7), e295–e302. https://doi.org/10.1016/S2352-3018(17)30053-X

O'Halloran, C., Sun, S., Nash, S. Brown, A., Croxford S, Connor, N., ... Gill, O. N. (2020). *HIV in the United Kingdom: Towards zero 2030*. London: Public Health England. Retrieved March 20, 2020, from https://assets.publishing.service.gov.uk/government/uploads/system/uploads/attachment_data/file/858559/HIV_in_the_UK_2019_towards_zero_HIV_transmissions_by_2030.pdf

O'Leary, A., Purcell, D., Remien, R. H., & Gomez, C. (2003). Childhood sexual abuse and sexual transmission risk behaviour among HIV-positive men who have sex with men. *AIDS Care, 15*(1), 17–26.

Oettle, A. G. (1962). Geographical and racial differences in the frequency of Kaposi's sarcoma as evidence of environmental or genetic causes. *Acta—Unio Internationalis Contra Cancrum, 18*, 330–363.

Ong, K. J., van Hoek, A. J., Harris, R. J., Figueroa, J., Waters, L., Chau, C., ... Delpech, V. (2019). HIV care cost in England: A cross-sectional analysis of antiretroviral treatment and the impact of generic introduction. *HIV Medicine, 20*(6), 377–391.

Pachankis, J. E., Rendina, H. J., Restar, A., Ventuneac, A., Grov, C., & Parsons, J. T. (2015). A minority stress—emotion regulation model of sexual compulsivity among highly sexually active gay and bisexual men. *Health Psychology: Official Journal of the Division of Health Psychology, American Psychological Association, 34*(8), 829–840.

Pakianathan, M., Whittaker, W., Lee, M. J., Avery, J., Green, S., Nathan, B., & Hegazi, A. (2018). Chemsex and new HIV diagnosis in gay, bisexual and other men who have sex with men attending sexual health clinics. *HIV Medicine*. https://doi.org/10.1111/hiv.12629.

Parsons, J. T., Grov, C., & Golub, S. A. (2012). Sexual compulsivity, co-occurring psychosocial health problems, and HIV risk among gay and bisexual men: Further evidence of a syndemic. *American Journal of Public Health, 102*(1), 156–162.

Passos, S. M., Souza, L. D., & Spessato, B. C. (2014). High prevalence of suicide risk in people living with HIV: Who is at higher risk? *AIDS Care, 26*(11), 1379–1382.

Paz-Bailey, G., Mendoza, M. C. B., Finlayson, T., Wejnert, C., Le, B., Rose, C., … NHBS Study Group. (2016). Trends in condom use among MSM in the United States: The role of antiretroviral therapy and seroadaptive strategies. *AIDS, 30*(12), 1985–1990.

Pence, B. W., O'Donnell, J. K., & Gaynes, B. N. (2012). Falling through the cracks: The gaps between depression prevalence, diagnosis, treatment, and response in HIV care. *AIDS (London, England), 26*(5), 656–658.

Phillips, G., Birkett, M., Hammond, S., & Mustanski, B. (2016). Partner preference among men who have sex with men: Potential contribution to spread of HIV within minority populations. *LGBT Health, 3*(3), 225–232.

Pilkington, V., Hill, A., Hughes, S., Nwokolo, N., & Pozniak, A. (2018). How safe is TDF/FTC as PrEP? A systematic review and meta-analysis of the risk of adverse events in 13 randomised trials of PrEP. *Journal of Virus Eradication, 4*(4), 215–224.

Pinkerton, S. D., & Abramson, P. R. (1992). Is risky sex rational? *Journal of Sex Research, 29*(4), 561–568.

Pollack, L. M., Woods, W. J., Blair, J., & Binson, D. (2014). Presence of an HIV testing program lowers the prevalence of unprotected insertive anal intercourse inside a gay bathhouse among HIV-negative and HIV-unknown patrons. *Journal of HIV/AIDS & Social Services, 13*(3), 306–323.

Pollard, A., Nadarzynski, T., & Llewellyn, C. (2017). O13 'I was struggling to feel intimate, the drugs just helped'. Chemsex and HIV-risk among men who have sex with men (MSM) in the UK: Syndemics of stigma, minority-stress, maladaptive coping and risk environments. *Sexually Transmitted Infections, 93*, A5.

Préau, M., Bouhnik, A. D., Peretti-Watel, P., Obadia, Y., Spire, B., & ANRS-EN12-VESPA Group. (2008). Suicide attempts among people living with HIV in France. *AIDS Care, 20*(8), 917–924.

Price, J. H., Desmond, S., & Kukulka, G. (1985). High school students' perceptions and misperceptions of AIDS. *Journal of School Health, 55*(3), 107–109.

Prior, J. (2009). Experiences beyond the threshold: Sydney's gay bathhouses. *Australian Cultural History, 27*(1), 61–77.

Prost, A., Sseruma, W. S., Fakoya, I., Arthur, G., Taegtmeyer, M., Njeri, A., … Imrie, J. (2007). HIV voluntary counselling and testing for African communities in London: Learning from experiences in Kenya. *Sexually Transmitted Infections, 83*(7), 547–551.

Public Health England. (2016). *HIV in the UK: 2016 report*. London: Public Health England. Retrieved June 2, 2020, from https://assets.publishing.service.gov.uk/government/uploads/system/uploads/attachment_data/file/602942/HIV_in_the_UK_report.pdf.

Public Health England. (2018). *Prevalence of HIV infection in the UK in 2018*. Health Protection Report, 13(39). Retrieved May 5, 2020, from https://assets.publishing.service.gov.uk/government/uploads/system/uploads/attachment_data/file/843766/hpr3919_hiv18.pdf.

Pufall, E., Kall, M., Shahmanesh, M., Nardone, A., Gilson, R., Delpech, V., … the Positive Voices Study Group. (2016). Chemsex and high-risk sexual behaviours in HIV-positive men who have sex with men. In *Poster presented at the Conference on Retroviruses and Opportunistic Infections Conference, Hynes Convention Center, Boston, Massachusetts*, March 4–7, 2018. Retrieved August 13, 2017, from http://www.croiconference.org/sessions/%C2%93chemsex%C2%94-and-high-risk-sexual-behaviours-hiv-positive-men-who-have-sex-men.

Pufall, E. L., Kall, M., Shahmanesh, M., Nardone, A., Gilson, R., Delpech, V., … Positive Voices study Group. (2018). Sexualized drug use ('chemsex') and high-risk sexual behaviours in HIV-positive men who have sex with men. *HIV Medicine, 19*(4), 261–270.

Quinn, T. C., Wawer, M. J., Sewankambo, N., Serwadda, D., Li, C., Wabwire-Mangen, F., … Gray, R. H. (2000). Viral load and heterosexual transmission of human immunodeficiency virus Type 1. *New England Journal of Medicine, 342*(13), 921–929.

Raifman, J., Dean, L. T., Montgomery, M. C., Almonte, A., Arrington-Sanders, R., Stein, M., … Chan, P. A. (2019). Racial and ethnic disparities in HIV pre-exposure prophylaxis awareness among men who have sex with men. *AIDS and Behavior, 23*(10), 2706–2709.

Raymond, H. F., & McFarland, W. (2009). Racial mixing and HIV risk among men who have sex with men. *AIDS and Behavior, 13*(4), 630–637.

Reece, M., & Dodge, B. (2003). Exploring the physical, mental and social well-being of gay and bisexual men who cruise for sex on a college campus. *Journal of Homosexuality, 46*(1–2), 111–136.

Rehman, Z., Lopes, B., & Jaspal, R. (2020). Predicting self-harm in an ethnically diverse sample of lesbian, gay and bisexual people in the United Kingdom. *International Journal of Social Psychiatry, 66*(4), 349–360.

Rice, C. E., Maierhofer, C., Fields, K. S., Ervin, M., Lanza, S. T., & Turner, A. N. (2016). Beyond anal sex: Sexual practices of men who have sex with men and associations with HIV and other sexually transmitted infections. *The Journal of Sexual Medicine, 13*(3), 374–382.

Richens, J. (2005). Can the promotion of post-exposure prophylaxis following sexual exposure to HIV (PEPSE) cause harm? *Sexually Transmitted Infections, 81*(3), 190–191.

Rivera-Rivera, Y., Vázquez-Santiago, F. J., Albino, E., Sánchez, M. D., & Rivera-Amill, V. (2016). Impact of depression and inflammation on the progression of HIV disease. *Journal of Clinical & Cellular Immunology, 7*(3), 423. https://doi.org/10.4172/2155-9899.1000423

Robinson, P., Turk, D., Jilka, S., & Cella, M. (2019). Measuring attitudes towards mental health using social media: Investigating stigma and trivialisation. *Social Psychiatry and Psychiatric Epidemiology, 54*(1), 51–58.

Rockstroh, J. K., DeJesus, E., Lennox, J. L., Yazdanpanah, Y., Saag, M. S., Wan, H., ... STARTMRK Investigators. (2013). Durable efficacy and safety of raltegravir versus efavirenz when combined with tenofovir/emtricitabine in treatment-naive HIV-1-infected patients: Final 5-year results from STARTMRK. *Journal of Acquired Immune Deficiency Syndromes, 63*(1), 77–85.

Rodger, A. J., Cambiano, V., Bruun, T., Vernazza, P., Collins, S., Degen, O., ... PARTNER Study Group. (2019). Risk of HIV transmission through condomless sex in serodifferent gay couples with the HIV-positive partner taking suppressive antiretroviral therapy (PARTNER): Final results of a multicentre, prospective, observational study. *Lancet, 393*(10189), 2428–2438.

Rodger, A. J., Cambiano, V., Bruun, T., Vernazza, P., Collins, S., van Lunzen, J., ... PARTNER Study Group. (2016). Sexual activity without condoms and risk of HIV transmission in serodifferent couples when the HIV-positive partner is using suppressive antiretroviral therapy. *JAMA, 316*(2), 171–181.

Rodkjaer, L., Laursen, T., Balle, N., & Sodemann, M. (2010). Depression in patients with HIV is under-diagnosed: A cross-sectional study in Denmark. *HIV Medicine, 11*(1), 46–53.

Roland, M. E., Neilands, T. B., Krone, M. R., Katz, M. H., Franses, K., Grant, R. M., … Martin, J. N. (2005). Seroconversion following nonoccupational postexposure prophylaxis against HIV. *Clinical Infectious Diseases: An Official Publication of the Infectious Diseases Society of America, 41*(10), 1507–1513.

Root-Bernstein, R. S., & Hobbs, S. H. (1993). Does HIV 'Piggyback' on CD4-like surface proteins of sperm, viruses, and bacteria? Implications for co-transmission, cellular tropism and the induction of autoimmunity in AIDS. *Journal of Theoretical Biology, 160*(2), 249–264.

Rosario, M., Hunter, J., Maguen, S., Gwadz, M., & Smith, R. (2001). The coming-out process and its adaptational and health-related associations among gay, lesbian, and bisexual youths: Stipulation and exploration of a model. *American Journal of Community Psychology, 29*(1), 133–160.

Rosengren, A. L., Huang, E., Daniels, J., Young, S. D., Marlin, R. W., & Klausner, J. D. (2016). Feasibility of using GrindrTM to distribute HIV self-test kits to men who have sex with men in Los Angeles, California. *Sexual Health, 13*, 389–392.

Rosser, B. R., Horvath, K. J., Hatfield, L. A., Peterson, J. L., Jacoby, S., & Stately, A. (2008). Predictors of HIV disclosure to secondary partners and sexual risk behavior among a high-risk sample of HIV-positive MSM: Results from six epicenters in the US. *AIDS Care, 20*(8), 925–930.

Røttingen, J. A., Cameron, D. W., & Garnett, G. P. (2001). A systematic review of the epidemiologic interactions between classic sexually transmitted diseases and HIV: How much really is known? *Sexually Transmitted Diseases, 28*(10), 579–597.

Roy, A. (2003). Characteristics of HIV patients who attempt suicide. *Acta Psychiatrica Scandinavica, 107*(1), 41–44.

Rudicell, R. S., Holland Jones, J., Wroblewski, E. E., Learn, G. H., Li, Y., Robertson, J. D., … Wilson, M. L. (2010). Impact of Simian immunodeficiency virus infection on chimpanzee population dynamics. *PLoS Pathogens, 6*(9). https://doi.org/10.1371/journal.ppat.1001116

Ruffieux, Y., Lemsalu, L., Aebi-Popp, K., Calmy, A., Cavassini, M., Fux, C. A., … Swiss HIV Cohort Study and the Swiss National Cohort. (2019). Mortality from suicide among people living with HIV and the general Swiss population: 1988–2017. *Journal of the International AIDS Society, 22*(8), e25339. https://doi.org/10.1002/jia2.25339

Ruiter, R. A., Kessels, L. T., Peters, G. J., & Kok, G. (2014). Sixty years of fear appeal research: Current state of the evidence. *International Journal of Psychology: Journal International de psychologie, 49*(2), 63–70.

Ruiter, R. A. C., Abraham, C., & Kok, G. (2001). Scary warnings and rational precautions: A review of the psychology of fear appeals. *Psychology & Health, 16*(6), 613–630.

Ryom, L., Lundgren, J. D., De Wit, S., Kovari, H., Reiss, P., Law, M., ... D:A:D Study Group. (2016). Use of antiretroviral therapy and risk of end-stage liver disease and hepatocellular carcinoma in HIV-positive persons. *AIDS, 30*(11), 1731–1743.

Sáez-Cirión, A., Bacchus, C., Hocqueloux, L., Avettand-Fenoel, V., Girault, I., Lecuroux, C., ... Rouzioux, C. (2013). Post-treatment HIV-1 controllers with a long-term virological remission after the interruption of early initiated antiretroviral therapy ANRS VISCONTI study. *PLoS Pathogens, 9*(3). https://doi.org/10.1371/journal.ppat.1003211

Safren, S. A., Gershuny, B. S., & Hendriksen, E. (2003). Symptoms of post-traumatic stress and death anxiety in persons with HIV and medication adherence difficulties. *AIDS Patient Care and STDs, 17*(12), 657–664. https://doi.org/10.1089/108729103771928717

Sahassanon, P., Pisitsungkagarn, K., & Taephant, N. (2019). The effect of cognitive-behavioral group therapy using art as a medium on depressive symptoms and HIV antiretroviral medication adherence. *International Journal for the Advancement of Counselling, 41*, 530–543.

Salfas, B., Rendina, H. J., & Parsons, J. T. (2019). What is the role of the community? Examining minority stress processes among gay and bisexual men. *Stigma and Health, 4*(3), 300–309.

Sandfort, T. G., Bakker, F., Schellevis, F. G., & Vanwesenbeeck, I. (2006). Sexual orientation and mental and physical health status: Findings from a Dutch population survey. *American Journal of Public Health, 96*(6), 1119–1125.

Sauter, D., Schindler, M., Specht, A., Landford, W. N., Münch, J., Kim, K.-A., ... Kirchhoff, F. (2009). Tetherin-driven adaptation of Vpu and Nef function and the evolution of pandemic and nonpandemic HIV-1 strains. *Cell Host & Microbe, 6*(5), 409–421.

Sax, P. E., Tierney, C., Collier, A. C., Fischl, M. A., Mollan, K., Peeples, L., ... AIDS Clinical Trials Group Study A5202 Team. (2009). Abacavir-lamivudine versus tenofovir-emtricitabine for initial HIV-1 therapy. *The New England Journal of Medicine, 361*(23), 2230–2240.

Sayer, C., Fisher, M., Nixon, E., Nambiar, K., Richardson, D., Perry, N., & Llewellyn, C. (2009). Will I? Won't I? Why do men who have sex with men present for post-exposure prophylaxis for sexual exposures? *Sexually Transmitted Infections, 85*(3), 206–211.

Schlebusch, L., & Govender, R. D. (2015). Elevated risk of suicidal ideation in HIV-positive persons. *Depression Research and Treatment*, 609172. https://doi.org/10.1155/2015/609172

Schmitt, D. P. (2004). The Big Five related to risky sexual behaviour across 10 world regions: Differential personality associations of sexual promiscuity and relationship infidelity. *European Journal of Personality*, *18*, 301–319.

Schuster, R., Bornovalova, M., & Hunt, E. (2012). The influence of depression on the progression of HIV: Direct and indirect effects. *Behavior Modification*, *36*(2), 123–145.

Schwartz, J., & Grimm, J. (2019). Stigma communication surrounding PrEP: The experiences of a sample of men who have sex with men. *Health Communication*, *34*(1), 84–90.

Semple, S. J., Strathdee, S. A., Zians, J., McQuaid, J., & Patterson, T. L. (2011). Psychosocial and behavioral correlates of anxiety symptoms in a sample of HIV-positive, methamphetamine-using men who have sex with men. *AIDS Care*, *23*(5), 628–637.

Serrero, M., Peyrin-Biroulet, L., & Grimaud, J.-C. (2017). IBD and HIV: 'Dangerous liaisons'. *Hepato-Gastro & Oncologie Digestive*, *24*(1), 34–41.

Sewell, J., Miltz, A., Lampe, F. C., Cambiano, V., Speakman, A., Phillips, A. N., … Attitudes to and Understanding of Risk of Acquisition of HIV (AURAH) Study Group. (2017). Poly drug use, chemsex drug use, and associations with sexual risk behaviour in HIV-negative men who have sex with men attending sexual health clinics. *The International Journal on Drug Policy*, *43*, 33–43.

Sewell, M. C., Goggin, K. J., Rabkin, J. G., Ferrando, S. J., McElhiney, M. C., & Evans, S. (2000). Anxiety syndromes and symptoms among men with AIDS: A longitudinal controlled study. *Psychosomatics*, *41*(4), 294–300.

Shacham, E., Morgan, J. C., Önen, N. F., Taniguchi, T., & Overton, E. T. (2012). Screening anxiety in the HIV clinic. *AIDS and Behavior*, *16*(8), 2407–2413.

Sharma, A., Howard, A. A., Klein, R. S., Schoenbaum, E. E., Buono, D., & Webber, M. P. (2007). Body image in older men with or at-risk for HIV infection. *AIDS Care*, *19*(2), 235–241.

Shernoff, M. (2006). *Without condoms: Unprotected sex, gay men & barebacking*. New York, NY: Routledge.

Sherr, L., Clucas, C., Harding, R., Sibley, E., & Catalan, J. (2011). HIV and depression—a systematic review of interventions. *Psychology, Health & Medicine*, *16*(5), 493–527.

Sherr, L., Lampe, F., Fisher, M., Arthur, G., Anderson, J., Zetler, S., ... Harding, R. (2008). Suicidal ideation in UK HIV clinic attenders. *AIDS, 22*(13), 1651–1658.

Shilo, G., & Savaya, R. (2012). Mental health of lesbian, gay, and bisexual youth and young adults: Differential effects of age, gender, religiosity, and sexual orientation. *Journal of Research on Adolescence, 22*(2), 310–325.

Simpson, D. M., & Tagliati, M. (1995). Nucleoside analogue-associated periph-eral neuropathy in human immunodeficiency virus infection. *Journal of Acquired Immune Deficiency Syndromes and Human Retrovirology: Official Publication of the International Retrovirology Association, 9*(2), 153–161.

Soni, S., Bond, K., Fox, E., Grieve, A. P., & Sethi, G. (2008). Black and minor-ity ethnic men who have sex with men: A London genitourinary medicine clinic experience. *International Journal of STD & AIDS, 19*(9), 617–619.

Spence, J. M. (2003). Should emergency departments offer postexposure pro-phylaxis for non-occupational exposure to HIV? *CJEM, 5*(01), 38–45.

Spieldenner, A. (2016). PrEP whores and HIV prevention: The queer commu-nication of HIV pre-exposure prophylaxis (PrEP). *Journal of Homosexuality, 63*, 1685–1697.

Spies, G., Asmal, L., & Seedat, S. (2013). Cognitive-behavioural interventions for mood and anxiety disorders in HIV: A systematic review. *Journal of Affective Disorders, 150*(2), 171–180.

St. Lawrence, J. S., Kelly, J. A., Dickson-Gomez, J., Owczarzak, J., Amirkhanian, Y. A., & Sitzler, C. (2015). Attitudes toward HIV voluntary counseling and testing (VCT) among African American men who have sex with men: Concerns underlying reluctance to test. *AIDS Education and Prevention, 27*(3), 195–211.

Stegmann, K., Scott, C., Jones, R., & Rayment, M. (2019). P97 Mind the gap: New diagnoses of HIV in a London clinic (2016–2018). In *Poster presented at the 25th Annual Conference of the British HIV Association (BHIVA)*, Bournemouth, UK, 2–5 April 2019. Retrieved from https://onlinelibrary.wiley.com/doi/full/10.1111/hiv.12739

Stein, D. S., Korvick, J. A., & Vermund, S. H. (1992). CD4+ lymphocyte cell enumeration for prediction of clinical course of human immunodeficiency virus disease: A review. *The Journal of Infectious Diseases, 165*(2), 352–363.

Stonewall. (2012). *One minority at a time: Being black and gay*. London: Stonewall. Retrieved June 2, 2020, from https://www.stonewall.org.uk/sys-tem/files/One_Minority_At_A_Time__2012_.pdf.

Stonewall. (2017). *LGBT in Britain: Hate crime and discrimination*. London: Stonewall. Retrieved June 3, 2020, from https://www.stonewall.org.uk/sys-tem/files/lgbt_in_britain_hate_crime.pdf.

Strategies for Management of Antiretroviral Therapy (SMART) Study Group, El-Sadr, W. M., Lundgren, J. D., Neaton, J. D., Gordin, F., Abrams, D., ... Rappoport, C. (2006). CD4+ count-guided interruption of antiretroviral treatment. *The New England Journal of Medicine, 355*(22), 2283–2296.

Strömdahl, S., Hoijer, J., & Eriksen, J. (2019). Uptake of peer-led venue-based HIV testing sites in Sweden aimed at men who have sex with men (MSM) and trans persons: A cross-sectional survey. *Sexually Transmitted Infections, 95*(8), 575–579.

Stutterheim, S. E., Sicking, L., Brands, R., Baas, I., Roberts, H., van Brakel, W. H., ... Bos, A. E. R. (2014). Patient and provider perspectives on HIV and HIV-related stigma in Dutch health care settings. *AIDS Patient Care and STDs, 28*(12), 652–665.

Summers, J., Zisook, S., Atkinson, J. H., Sciolla, A., Whitehall, W., Brown, S., ... Grant, I. (1995). Psychiatric morbidity associated with acquired immune deficiency syndrome-related grief resolution. *The Journal of Nervous and Mental Disease, 183*(6), 384–389.

Tajfel, H., & Turner, J. C. (1986). The social identity theory of intergroup behaviour. In S. Worchel & W. G. Austin (Eds.), *Psychology of intergroup relations* (pp. 7–24). Chicago, IL: Nelson-Hall.

Tan, R. K. J., Lim, J. M., & Chan, J. K. W. (2020). "Not a walking piece of meat with disease": Meanings of becoming undetectable among HIV-positive gay, bisexual and other men who have sex with men in the U = U era. *AIDS Care, 32*(3), 325–329.

Temoshok, L., Sweet, D. M., & Zich, J. (1987). A three city comparison of the public's knowledge and attitudes about AIDS. *Psychology & Health, 1*(1), 43–60.

Thomas, F., Mience, M. C., Masson, J., & Bernoussi, A. (2014). Unprotected sex and internalized homophobia. *The Journal of Men's Studies, 22*(2), 155–162.

Thornton, A. C. (2015). Viral hepatitis and HIV co-infection in the UK collaborative HIV cohort (UK CHIC) study [Doctoral, UCL (University College London)]. In Doctoral thesis, UCL (University College London). UCL. Retrieved from https://discovery.ucl.ac.uk/id/eprint/1473437/

Thornton, A. C., Delpech, V., Kall, M. M., & Nardone, A. (2012). HIV testing in community settings in resource-rich countries: A systematic review of the evidence. *HIV Medicine, 13*(7), 416–426.

Tostevin, A., White, E., Dunn, D., Croxford, S., Delpech, V., Williams, I., ... UK HIV Drug Resistance Database. (2017). Recent trends and patterns in HIV-1 transmitted drug resistance in the United Kingdom. *HIV Medicine, 18*(3), 204–213.

Tovar-y-Romo, L. B., Bumpus, N. N., Pomerantz, D., Avery, L. B., Sacktor, N., McArthur, J. C., & Haughey, N. J. (2012). Dendritic spine injury induced by the 8-hydroxy metabolite of efavirenz. *The Journal of Pharmacology and Experimental Therapeutics, 343*(3), 696–703.

Traeger, M. W., Schroeder, S. E., Wright, E. J., Hellard, M. E., Cornelisse, V. J., Doyle, J. S., & Stoové, M. A. (2018). Effects of pre-exposure prophylaxis for the prevention of human immunodeficiency virus infection on sexual risk behavior in men who have sex with men: A systematic review and meta-analysis. *Clinical Infectious Diseases: An Official Publication of the Infectious Diseases Society of America, 67*(5), 676–686.

Treisman, G., Fishman, M., Schwartz, J., Hutton, H., & Lyketsos, C. (1998). Mood disorders in HIV infection. *Depression and Anxiety, 7*(4), 178–187.

Treisman, G. J., & Soudry, O. (2016). Neuropsychiatric effects of HIV antiviral medications. *Drug Safety, 39*(10), 945–957.

Tsai, C. C., Follis, K. E., Sabo, A., Beck, T. W., Grant, R. F., & Bischofberger, N. ... Black, R. (1995). Prevention of SIV infection in macaques by (R)-9-(2-phosphonylmethoxypropyl)adenine. *Science, 270*(5239), 1197–1199.

UK Census. (2011). UK population by ethnicity. Retrieved May 10, 2020, from https://www.ethnicity-facts-figures.service.gov.uk/uk-population-by-ethnicity.

UNAIDS. (2019). Global HIV & AIDS statistics—2019 fact sheet. Retrieved May 27, 2020, from https://www.unaids.org/en/resources/fact-sheet.

United Kingdom Collaborative HIV Cohort Study Group. (2012). Uptake and outcome of combination antiretroviral therapy in men who have sex with men according to ethnic group: The UK CHIC Study. *Journal of Acquired Immune Deficiency Syndromes, 59*(5), 523–529.

Uthman, O. A., Magidson, J. F., Safren, S. A., & Nachega, J. B. (2014). Depression and adherence to antiretroviral therapy in low-, middle- and high-income countries: A systematic review and meta-analysis. *Current HIV/AIDS Reports, 11*(3), 291–307.

Vaccher, S. J., Kaldor, J. M., Callander, D., Zablotska, I. B., & Haire, B. G. (2018). Qualitative insights into adherence to HIV pre-exposure prophylaxis (PrEP) among Australian gay and bisexual men. *AIDS Patient Care and STDs, 32*(12), 519–528.

Van Damme, L., Ramjee, G., Alary, M., Vuylsteke, B., Chandeying, V., Rees, H., ... COL-1492 Study Group. (2002). Effectiveness of COL-1492, a nonoxynol-9 vaginal gel, on HIV-1 transmission in female sex workers: A randomised controlled trial. *Lancet, 360*(9338), 971–977.

van Wyk, J., Ajana, F., Bisshop, F., De Wit, S., Osiyemi, O., Portilla, J., ... Smith, K. Y. (2020). Efficacy and safety of switching to dolutegravir/lamivudine fixed-dose two-drug regimen versus continuing a tenofovir alafenamide-based three- or four-drug regimen for maintenance of virologic suppression in adults with HIV-1: Phase 3, randomized, non-inferiority TANGO Study. *Clinical Infectious Diseases: An Official Publication of the Infectious Diseases Society of America.* https://doi.org/10.1093/cid/ciz1243

Varni, S. E., Miller, C. T., McCuin, T., & Solomon, S. E. (2012). Disengagement and engagement coping with HIV/AIDS stigma and psychological well-being of people with HIV/AIDS. *Journal of Social and Clinical Psychology, 31*(2), 123–150.

Velter, A., Bouyssou-Michel, A., Arnaud, A., & Semaille, C. (2009). Do men who have sex with men use serosorting with casual partners in France? Results of a nationwide survey (ANRS-EN17-Presse Gay 2004). *Eurosurveillance, 14*(47), pii=19416. https://doi.org/10.2807/ese.14.47.19416-en

Verma, R. (2014). Decline in CD4 counts in HIV patients. *Medical Journal, Armed Forces India, 70*(3), 301. https://doi.org/10.1016/j.mjafi.2014.06.012

Vignoles, V. L., Regalia, C., Manzi, C., Golledge, J., & Scabini, E. (2006). Beyond self-esteem: Influence of multiple motives on identity construction. *Journal of Personality and Social Psychology, 90*(2), 308–333.

Vincke, J., Bolton, R., & De Vleeschouwer, P. (2001). The cognitive structure of the domain of safe and unsafe gay sexual behaviour in Belgium. *AIDS Care, 13*(1), 57–70.

Wald, A., & Link, K. (2002). Risk of human immunodeficiency virus infection in herpes simplex virus type 2-seropositive persons: A meta-analysis. *The Journal of Infectious Diseases, 185*(1), 45–52.

Walensky, R. P., Goldberg, J. H., & Daily, J. P. (1999). Anaphylaxis after rechallenge with abacavir. *AIDS, 13*(8), 999–1000.

Wang, X., Nutland, W., Brady, M., Green, I., Boffito, M., & McClure, M. (2019). Quantification of tenofovir disoproxil fumarate and emtricitabine in generic pre-exposure prophylaxis tablets obtained from the internet. *International Journal of STD & AIDS, 30*(8), 765–768.

Wawer, M. J., Gray, R. H., Sewankambo, N. K., Serwadda, D., Li, X., Laeyendecker, O., ... Quinn, T. C. (2005). Rates of HIV-1 transmission per coital act, by stage of HIV-1 infection, in Rakai, Uganda. *The Journal of Infectious Diseases, 191*(9), 1403–1409.

Wawer, M. J., Sewankambo, N. K., Serwadda, D., Quinn, T. C., Paxton, L. A., Kiwanuka, N., ... Gray, R. H. (1999). Control of sexually transmitted diseases for AIDS prevention in Uganda: A randomised community trial. Rakai Project Study Group. *Lancet (London, England), 353*(9152), 525–535.

Weatherburn, P., Hickson, F., Reid, D., Torres-Rueda, S., & Bourne, A. (2017). Motivations and values associated with combining sex and illicit drugs ('chemsex') among gay men in South London: Findings from a qualitative study. *Sexually Transmitted Infections, 93*(3), 203–206.

Weatherburn, P., Hickson, F., Reid, D. S., Schink, S. B., Marcus, U., Schmidt, A. J., & European Centre for Disease Prevention and Control, Sigma Research (London School of Hygiene and Tropical Medicine), & Robert Koch-Institut. (2019). EMIS-2017: The European men-who-have-sex-with-men Internet survey: Key findings from 50 countries. Retrieved from http://publications.europa.eu/publication/manifestation_identifier/PUB_TQ0319440ENN

Wiegand, A., Spindler, J., Hong, F. F., Shao, W., Cyktor, J. C., Cillo, A. R., … Kearney, M. F. (2017). Single-cell analysis of HIV-1 transcriptional activity reveals expression of proviruses in expanded clones during ART. *Proceedings of the National Academy of Sciences of the United States of America, 114*(18), E3659–E3668. https://doi.org/10.1073/pnas.1617961114

Williamson, I., Papaloukas, P., Jaspal, R., & Lond, B. (2019). 'There's this glorious pill': Gay and bisexual men in the English midlands navigate risk responsibility and pre-exposure prophylaxis. *Critical Public Health, 29*(5), 560–571.

Winetrobe, H., Rice, E., Bauermeister, J., Petering, R., & Holloway, I. W. (2014). Associations of unprotected anal intercourse with Grindr-met partners among Grindr-using young men who have sex with men in Los Angeles. *AIDS Care, 26*(10), 1303–1308.

Witzel, T. C., Rodger, A. J., Burns, F. M., Rhodes, T., & Weatherburn, P. (2016). HIV self-testing among men who have sex with men (MSM) in the UK: A qualitative study of barriers and facilitators, intervention preferences and perceived impacts. *PLoS One, 11*(9), e0162713. https://doi.org/10.1371/journal.pone.0162713

Wiysonge, C. S., Kongnyuy, E. J., Shey, M., Muula, A. S., Navti, O. B., Akl, E. A., & Lo, Y.-R. (2011). Male circumcision for prevention of homosexual acquisition of HIV in men. *The Cochrane Database of Systematic Reviews, 6*, CD007496. https://doi.org/10.1002/14651858.CD007496.pub2

Wolbers, M., Babiker, A., Sabin, C., Young, J., Dorrucci, M., Chêne, G., … on behalf of the CASCADE Collaboration. (2010). Pretreatment CD4 cell slope and progression to AIDS or death in HIV-infected patients initiating antiretroviral therapy—The CASCADE collaboration: A collaboration of 23 cohort studies. *PLOS Medicine, 7*(2), e1000239. https://doi.org/10.1371/journal. pmed.1000239

Woods, W. J., Lippman, S. A., Agnew, E., Carroll, S., & Binson, D. (2016). Bathhouse distribution of HIV self-testing kits reaches diverse, high-risk population. *AIDS Care, 28*(Suppl 1), 111–113.

World Health Organization. (2001). *Strengthening mental health promotion (Fact sheet No. 220)*. Geneva: World Health Organization.

Worobey, M., Watts, T. D., McKay, R. A., Suchard, M. A., Granade, T., Teuwen, D. E., … Jaffe, H. W. (2016). 1970s and 'Patient 0' HIV-1 genomes illuminate early HIV/AIDS history in North America. *Nature, 539*(7627), 98–101.

Yi, M. S., Mrus, J. M., Wade, T. J., Ho, M. L., Hornung, R. W., Cotton, S., … Tsevat, J. (2006). Religion, spirituality, and depressive symptoms in patients with HIV/AIDS. *Journal of General Internal Medicine, 21*(Suppl 5), S21– S27. https://doi.org/10.1111/j.1525-1497.2006.00643.x

Young, S. D., Nussbaum, A. D., & Monin, B. (2007). Potential moral stigma and reactions to sexually transmitted diseases: Evidence for a disjunction fallacy. *Personality and Social Psychology Bulletin, 33*(6), 789–799.

Yuan, T., Fitzpatrick, T., Ko, N.-Y., Cai, Y., Chen, Y., Zhao, J., … Zou, H. (2019). Circumcision to prevent HIV and other sexually transmitted infections in men who have sex with men: A systematic review and meta-analysis of global data. *The Lancet Global Health, 7*(4), e436–e447. https:// doi.org/10.1016/S2214-109X(18)30567-9

Zagefka, H. (2009). The concept of ethnicity in socio-psychological research: Definitional issues. *International Journal of Intercultural Relations, 33*, 228–241.

Zarwell, M., Ransome, Y., Barak, N., Gruber, D., & Robinson, W. T. (2019). PrEP indicators, social capital and social group memberships among gay, bisexual and other men who have sex with men. *Culture, Health & Sexuality, 21*(12), 1349–1366.

Zicari, S., Sessa, L., Cotugno, N., Ruggiero, A., Morrocchi, E., Concato, C., … Palma, P. (2019). Immune activation, inflammation, and non-AIDS co-morbidities in HIV-infected patients under long-term ART. *Viruses, 11*(3). https://doi.org/10.3390/v11030200

Zuckerman, M. (1994). *Behavioral expressions and biosocial bases of sensation seeking*. Cambridge: Cambridge University Press.

Index